The Persisting Osler—V

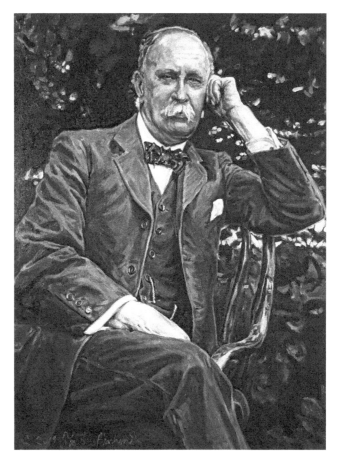

Sir William Osler, by Tarleton Blackwell. 1999. Oil on canvas, 48 × 36 in. Collection of Charles S. Bryan.

This portrait is based on a photograph of Osler taken at the Johns Hopkins Hospital in 1913 during his last return trip to North America.

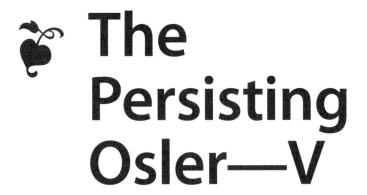

The Persisting Osler—V

Selected Transactions of the American Osler Society 2011–2020

Edited by

Charles S. Bryan, M.D.
J. Mario Molina, M.D.
Marvin J. Stone, M.D.

Science History Publications/USA
Sagamore Beach
2021

First published in the United States of America by
Science History Publications/USA
a division of
Watson Publishing International LLC
Post Office Box 1240, Sagamore Beach, MA 02562-1240

ISBN 978-0-88135-300-6

Publisher's Cataloging-in-Publication Data
Names: Bryan, Charles S., editor. | Molina, J. Mario, editor. | Stone, Marvin J., editor. |
    American Osler Society. Meeting.
Title: The persisting Osler. V, Selected transactions of the American Osler Society 2011-
    2020 / edited by Charles S. Bryan, M.D., J. Mario Molina, M.D., Marvin J. Stone,
    M.D.
Other Titles: Selected transactions of the American Osler Society 2011-2020
Description: Sagamore Beach, MA : Science History Publications/USA, 2021. | Includes
    bibliographical references and index.
Identifiers: ISBN 9780881353006
Subjects: LCSH: Osler, William, Sir, 1849-1919. | American Osler Society--Anniversaries.
    | Physicians--Canada--Biography--Congresses. | LCGFT: Biographies.
Classification: LCC R464.O8 P4725 2021 | DDC 610.92 B--dc23

Manufactured the U.S.A.

To Jeremiah A. Barondess, M.D.,
who conceived The Persisting Osler,
and to all who pursue the Oslerian ideals
of technical competence, humane caring,
and clinical wisdom in the service of the sick

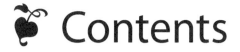 # Contents

SECTION III   Family, Friends, and Colleagues   139

SECTION IV   Influences and the Osler Diaspora   225

SECTION V   Osler's Afterlife—Moving Forward   279

Index   321

🍎 Contributors

Ian B. Anderson, CD, M.D., CM, FRCSC, is a twice-retired trauma surgeon, first as a colonel in the Canadian Armed Forces Medical Services and later from practice at Foothills Medical Centre and the University of Calgary, Calgary, Alberta.

Charles S. Bryan, M.D., MACP, FRCP(Edin.), FRCP(London), is Heyward Gibbes Distinguished Professor of Internal Medicine Emeritus at the University of South Carolina, Columbia.

John D. Bullock, M.D., MPH, MSc, is a research epidemiologist, ophthalmologist, and microbiologist, and forensic scientist, and is the CEO of the Ophthalmic History Research Institute, Inc.

Dee Canale, M.D., is a retired neurosurgeon and associate professor of surgery, emeritus, at the University of Tennessee College of Medicine, Memphis.

Richard Colgan, M.D., is professor in the Department of Family and Community Medicine at the University of Maryland School of Medicine, Baltimore.

William N. Evans, M.D., is professor of clinical pediatrics at the University of Nevada Las Vegas School of Medicine and director of the Children's Heart Center—Nevada.

Meg Fairfax Fielding, B.A., is director of the History of Maryland Medicine, Med-Chi, The Maryland State Medical Society, Baltimore.

Marilyn A. Gendek R.N., M.A., M.N., Dip. Fam. Hist., FACN, is an advisor in nurse education, professional development, and regulation.

John M. Harris, Jr., M.D., MBA, is a retired internist and former executive director of continuing medical education at the University of Arizona College of Medicine, Tucson.

Mark Hoffer, M.D., is emeritus professor and emeritus chief of orthopaedic surgery, University of California (Irvine).

Ernest B. Hook, M.D., FACMG, is professor emeritus at the School of Public Health, University of California, Berkeley.

H. Michael Jones, M.D., is an attending pathologist at the University of North Carolina School of Medicine, Chapel Hill, after a long career in the private practice of pathology.

Susan Kelen, Ph.D., C Psych, is a consulting psychologist in Ottawa, Ontario.

Dennis M. Kratz, Ph.D., is the Ignacy and Celina Rockover Professor of Humanities at The University of Texas at Dallas.

Vivien E. Lane RN., B.A.(Hons)., Ph.D., FACN, is a freelance nurse clinical practitioner in Sydney, Australia.

C. Ronald MacKenzie, M.D., is professor of clinical medicine and medical ethics, Weill Cornell College of Medicine, and also the C. Ronald MacKenzie Chair in Ethics and Medicine, Hospital for Special Surgery, New York, New York.

Michael H. Malloy, M.D., M.S., is professor of pediatrics (neonatology) and the John P. McGovern Chair in Oslerian Education at the University of Texas Medical Branch, Galveston.

J. Mario Molina, M.D., is adjunct professor at the School of Global and Community Health, Claremont Graduate University, Claremont, California.

Michael E. Moran, M.D., is professor of urology at Prisma Health and the University of South Carolina School of Medicine, Columbia, South Carolina.

T. Jock Murray, M.D., OC, ONS, FRCPC, FAAN, FRCP(London), MACP, FCAHS, LLD (Hon.), DSc (Hon.), MCFP (Hon.), DSc (Hon.), LLD (Hon.), D. Litt (Hon), DFA (Hon.), LLD (Hon.), is professor emeritus of medicine and neurology, professor of medical humanities, dean emeritus, and founding director of the Dalhousie Multiple Sclerosis Unit, and founder of the Dalhousie Society for the History of Medicine, Dalhousie University, Halifax, Nova Scotia

Clyde Partin, M.D., is the Gary W. Rollins Professor of Medicine & Master Clinician at Emory University School of Medicine, Atlanta, Georgia.

Sutchin R. Patel, M.D., FACS, is adjunct clinical assistant professor of urology at the University of Wisconsin School of Medicine and Public Health, Madison, Wisconsin.

Milton Roxanas MB., BS., FRANZCP, is retired associate professor of psychiatry, University of Sydney, Sydney Adventist Hospital, Wahroonga, Australia.

Marvin J. Stone, M.D., MACP, FRCP(London), is chief emeritus of hematology and oncology, Baylor University Medical Center/Dallas, professor of medicine, Texas A&M College of Medicine, and clinical professor of humanities, University of Texas, Dallas.

Herbert M. Swick, M.D., is a retired pediatric neurologist; director emeritus of the Institute of Medicine and Humanities and retired professor at the University of Montana, both in Missoula; and emeritus clinical professor at the University of Washington School of Medicine, Seattle.

Henry Travers, M.D., FACP, is clinical professor of pathology, Sanford School of Medicine of the University of South Dakota, Sioux Falls.

John W.K. Ward, M.B., Ch. B, (St. Andrews), FRCP(Edin.), FRCGP, DObst. RCOG, DFFP, is a retired general practitioner in Oxfordshire, England.

Ruth Ward, M.A. (St. Andrews), Dip. Ed. (Dundee), is a retired teacher of modern languages and a past president of the Oxford Guild of Tour Guides.

James R. Wright, Jr., M.D., Ph.D., is professor of pathology and laboratory medicine and professor of paediatrics at the University of Calgary, Alberta, Canada.

🍎 Preface

The Persisting Osler—V commemorates the fiftieth anniversary of the American Osler Society (AOS) and the centenary of the death of its namesake, Sir William Osler (1849–1919). Because of its anniversary significance, we chose to limit papers to those pertaining to Osler, his circle, his influence, and his ideas and opinions. Over the past half-century, the AOS has evolved to be more broadly concerned with medical history, medical biography, and the humanities as these relate to medicine than was the case at its inception. We predict that any future volumes of this series will contain a more diverse range of subject matter, since it has become increasingly difficult to say anything new or fresh about Osler. Few if any physicians have been studied so extensively with the obvious exception of St. Luke.[1]

The AOS was formed in 1970 to address concerns that science and technology were eroding the humanistic dimensions of medicine. A trial run that year took the form of a symposium on "Humanism in Medicine" held in Galveston, Texas, and published as a monograph.[2] A small group of individuals—notably, John P. McGovern (1921–2007), Alfred R. Henderson (1920–2019), Wilburt C. Davison (1892–1972), Thomas M. Durant (1905–1977), Charles G. Roland (1933–2009), H. Grant Taylor (1903–1995), William B. Bean (1909–1989), and George T. Harrell (1908–1999)—laid the groundwork "to continually place before the profession [of medicine] a reminder of the high principles of life and humanism in practice of Osler" and "to introduce these things to those entering the profession."[3,4] Most of the founding members knew people who had known Osler and they saw him as an avatar for humanism in medicine.[5]

Only two papers were presented at the first formal meeting of the AOS on 1 April 1971, but the number of papers steadily increased as the meetings became longer and more elaborate. During the early 1980s Jeremiah A. Barondess (b. 1924), impressed by the quality of papers given during the organization's first decade, proposed a compendium of selected papers and worked with McGovern and Roland to bring out the first volume of *The Persisting Osler* (1985). The founding editors perceived the volume as "an expression of a broader continuing interest in William Osler," published to "stimulate thought and further exploration of those timeless issues that captured Sir William's energies, and that remain vital to the modern physician."[6,7]

The first volume of *The Persisting Osler* contained 31 articles, the second (1994) 28 articles, the third (2002) 24 articles, and the fourth (2011) 33 articles. The present volume's 33 articles, drawn from 456 presentations at AOS meetings between 2011 and 2019 (not including the canceled 2020 meeting), brings the total to 148 articles, a small but meaningful fraction of the secondary literature pertaining to Osler. To date there have been at least 15 biographies and quasi-biographies of Osler and more than 2,000 articles about him in peer-reviewed medical journals. In 2020 the AOS, with a subvention from the Molina Family Foundation, brought out an encyclopedia to summarize and consolidate most of this information.[8]

Why does Osler command such attention? The editors of the inaugural volume of *The Persisting Osler* asked and answered this question as follows:

> What characteristics of the man and his career were so powerful that now, 65 years after his death and nearly 80 years after his departure from this continent, his example still strike responsive chords in so many? Certainly he epitomized, both personally and in his writings, the traditional elements in the supporting and helpful role of the physician. He exemplified clinical excellence and the charisma of the gifted teacher. He emphasized the importance of collegial relationships among physicians and the vital necessity of a life of continued learning in medicine and in the broader reaches of humanism. Perhaps most importantly, he helped his contemporaries and his professional progeny to see themselves as part of a distinguished lineage that includes not only the great physicians who have gone before, but also the philosophers, the poets, the essayists, and in fact all who had concerned themselves with the human condition.[6]

Osler straddled "The Old Humanities and the New Science," to use the title of his last published address, reassuring his generation that humanism and the humanities remained relevant in the face of the new science-based medicine steeped in technology.

With the arguable exception of Hippocrates. a shadowy figure of whom we know little with certainty, Osler influenced his generation and those that followed more than any physician in history. The eminent Richard C. Cabot (1868–1939) of Boston wrote two days after Osler's death: "I doubt if any single man has ever so deeply influenced any other profession."[9] Nearly a century after his death, in 2016, Osler was voted "the most influential physician in history" in an Internet-based poll of North American physicians.[10] In the preface to *Humanism in Medicine* (1973), the compilation of papers given at the trial run for the AOS at the 1970 Galveston meeting, Grant Taylor quoted from an earlier paper by Davison:

> No one has taken Osler's place. We must demonstrate to this generation not only what he was and meant to us, but what he did for them and for medicine, and can continue to do if the medical youth will try to emulate him as we attempted to do. He embodied, applied, and transmitted all that is finest and best in a physician.[11,12]

The balkanization of medicine into specialties and subspecialties that began even before Osler's era and continues to accelerate makes it unlikely a single individual will again symbolize the ideals of medicine the way Osler did.

The penumbra of Osler's personality—his vitality, kindness, helpfulness ("Do the kind thing and do it first"), and charisma, to name just a few attributes that made him so beloved by contemporaries—is now confined to the written word. His legacy will predictably bear scrutiny and criticism from generations far removed from those who knew him and who, as Wilburt Davison put it, "regarded him as perfect."[13,14] In 2018 two Australian physicians cherry-picked negative observations about Osler and fired a shot across the bow: "It is now time to set the record straight, for the sake of historical truth, the values of science, and the integrity of medicine itself."[15]

These and other recent critics[16] give rise in certain quarters to the idea that the AOS is largely about hero-worship and hagiography. We disagree.[17] Founding members of the AOS such as Harrell and Roland pointed out chinks in Osler's armor and other AOS members have continued to do so down to the present. The recently published encyclopedia, which contains 1,145 articles by 138 scholars on four continents, was edited with an eye toward pointing out anything about Osler that might be seen as questionable from a twenty-first-century perspective. Thirty such criticisms were listed in approximate order of egregiousness, ranging from his sometimes-insensitive practical jokes to his being "excessively sweet" or "too good to be true." He was thoroughly human. And we should recognize that Osler, like most thoughtful people, evolved and for the better. The Osler of his later Oxford period was not the prankster who in Montreal, Philadelphia, and Baltimore signed practical jokes under the *nom de plume* Egerton Yorrick Davis.

Roland and others asserted that Osler was not a cardboard saint, and few if any of today's AOS members view him as a flawless role model for the twenty-first century. How could he be? Our times are so different from his, as are the conditions of medical practice. Osler did not have to contend with third-party payers, bureaucracies, the Internet, electronic medical records, cell phones and pagers—in Baltimore he resisted having a telephone in his house—nor did he use such terms as "bioethics," "professionalism," "bioinformatics," and "healthcare providers." What matters are the ideals and principles for which he stood, his eloquent restating in word and deed of the Hippocratic maxim of *philanthropia* and *philotechnia*, love of humanity combined with love of the science and art of medicine.

In 1999 the French medical historian Danielle Gourevitch (b. 1941) predicted the twenty-first century will witness the triumph of medicine, but also the wide replacement of physicians by technicians. She called Osler "the last *maître à penser* of a noble-minded general medicine."[18] Osler was many things to many people, but his lasting gift to physicians—let us now substitute "the global community of healthcare workers"—was the sense of belonging to a portion of humanity committed to the scientific method and the proposition that in humanized science rests the fondest hopes not only for individuals but also for preserving higher life forms on a fragile planet.[19] Hence, *The Persisting Osler*.

We departed from previous volumes in this series in several ways. We constituted an editorial board to review and rank manuscripts, and we thank Michael Jones, Michael Malloy, Rob Stone, and Henry Travers for serving in that capacity. We allowed authors to update information presented at AOS meetings. Finally, we allowed authors to combine papers in a few instances. All three editors reviewed each manuscript prior to its final approval.

On behalf of the AOS, the authors represented herein, and others concerned with the interface between medicine, the humanities, and humanism (understood as the promotion of human flourishing), we are pleased to add this volume to the Oslerian corpus.

Charles S. Bryan
J. Mario Molina
Marvin J. Stone

References

1. Madison DL. Review of *Osler: Inspirations from a Great Physician*, by Charles S. Bryan. *New England Journal of Medicine* 1997; 337(18): 1324–1325.
2. McGovern JP, Burns CR. *Humanism in Medicine*. Springfield, Illinois: Charles C. Thomas, Publisher; 1973.
3. Roland CG. The formative years of the American Osler Society. In Barondess JA, Roland CG, eds., The formative years of the American Osler Society. In Barondess JA, Roland CG, eds. *The Persisting Osler—III*. Malabar, Florida: Krieger Publishing Company; 2002: 189–201.
4. Bryan CS, Partin C Jr. American Osler Society. In Bryan CS, ed. *Sir William Osler: An Encyclopedia*. Novato, California: Norman Publishing/ HistoryofScience.com; 2020: 26–28.
5. Roland CG. The palpable Osler: a study in survival. *Perspectives in Biology and Medicine* 1984; 27(2): 299–313.
6. Barondess JA, McGovern JP, Roland CG, eds. Preface. In Barondess JA, McGovern JP, Roland CG. *The Persisting Osler. Selected Transactions of the First Ten Years of the American Osler Society*. Baltimore: University Park Press; 1985: xiii–xiv.
7. Barondess JA. *Persisting Osler, The*. In: Bryan CS, ed. *Sir William Osler: An Encyclopedia*. Novato, California: Norman Publishing/HistoryofScience. com; 2020: 628.
8. Bryan CS, ed. *Sir William Osler: An Encyclopedia*. Novato, California: Norman Publishing/HistoryofScience.com; 2020.
9. Cabot RC. Osler's influence on the medical profession. *The Evening Post* [New York]. 31 December 1919.
10. Rourke S, Ellis G. The most influential physicians in history, part 4. The top ten. https://www.medscape.com/features/slideshow/influential-physicians -part-4, accessed 22 February 2021.
11. Davison WC. Sir William Osler—memories. *Virginia Medical Monthly* 1950; 77(6): 271–272.
12. Taylor G. In McGovern JP, Burns CR. *Humanism in Medicine*. Springfield, Illinois: Charles C. Thomas, Publisher; 1973: ix–x.
13. Bryan CS, Toodayan N. Osler studies enter second century. *Journal of Medical Biography* 2019; 27(4): 186–188.
14. Davison WC. The basis of Sir William Osler's influence on medicine. *Annals of Allergy* 1969; 27(8): 366–372.
15. Fiddes P, Komesaroff PA. An emperor unclothed: the virtuous Osler. *Hektoen International* 2018(Winter). https://hekint.org/2018/03/20/ emperor-unclothed-virtuous-osler/, accessed 22 February 2021.
16. Persaud N, Butts H, Berger P. William Osler: saint in a "White man's dominion." *Canadian Medical Association Journal* 2020; 192(45): E1414–1416. https://doi.org/10.1503/cmaj.201567, accessed 22 February 2020.
17. Bryan CS. Sir William Osler, eugenics, racism, and the *Komagata Maru* incident. *Baylor University Medical Center Proceedings* 2021; 34(1): 194–198.
18. Gourevitch D. The history of medical teaching. *Lancet* 1999; 354 Supplement: SIV33.
19. Bryan CS, Podolsky SH. Sir William Osler (1849–1919)—The uses of history and the singular beneficence of medicine. *New England Journal of Medicine* 2019; 381(23): 2194–2195.

SECTION I

Professional Activities

Osler's Attendance at International Medical Congresses: From Reporter to Section President

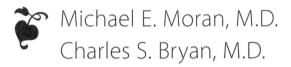
Michael E. Moran, M.D.
Charles S. Bryan, M.D.

Sir William Osler was many things to many people during his lifetime, but his most enduring legacy to physicians was the sense of belonging to a great world-wide profession.[1] He taught, for example, that the "great Republic of Medicine knows and has no national boundaries"[2]; that medicine "is the only world-wide profession"[3]; and that "the profession in truth is a sort of guild or brotherhood, any member of which can take up his calling in any part of the world."[4] Osler's sense of the catholicity of the medical profession derived in no small measure from his attendance at International Medical Congresses between 1881 and 1913. Our purpose is to review these congresses and Osler's participation.

The International Medical Congresses

In 1865 Dr. Henri Gintrac (1820–1878), dean of the Bordeaux School of Medicine, proposed at the third annual French medical convention that a unique meeting with delegates from various nations be held in conjunction with the *Exposition Universelle* (World's Exposition) scheduled for Paris two years later. Organized by

Presented at the forty-sixth annual meeting of the American Osler Society, Minneapolis, Minnesota, on 2 May 2016.

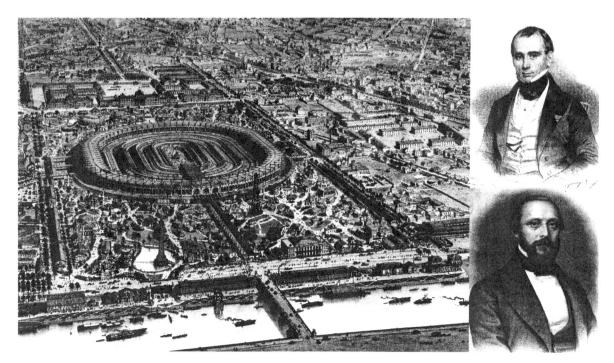

Figure 1.   Birds-eye view of the *Exposition Universelle* of 1867, showing the large central pavilion and nearly 100 smaller buildings on the Champ de Mars, the great military parade ground of Paris. At right: Jean-Baptiste de Bouillaud, president of the congress (*above*). and Rudolf Virchow, one of six foreign vice-presidents (*below*). *Credits:* Library of Congress; Wikimedia Commons (Bouillaud); National Library of Medicine (Pasteur).

decree of Napoleon III (1800–1873), promoted by the likes of Victor Hugo and Alexandre Dumas, lasting seven months (1 April–3 November 1867), featuring 50,226 exhibitors spread out over 171 acres (Figure 1), and now known as the Second World's Fair, the *Exposition Universelle* has been called the most frivolous event of the nineteenth century. The concomitant meeting organized by Gintrac and his colleagues lasted only 12 days (16–28 August 1867) and was a mixed success. Now known as the First International Medical Congress, it presaged a 46-year tradition during which medicine as a worldwide profession—at least in Western countries—was on display as it had never been before, and perhaps has not been since, specialties and subspecialties notwithstanding.

The First International Congress was held at the School of Medicine in Paris and conducted entirely in French.[5] Jean-Baptiste Bouillaud (1796–1881) (Figure 1), professor at the Charité in Paris, president of the Académie de Médecine, and consultant to the Emperor, was elected president of the meeting. Bouillaud is best known today for studies involving cerebral localization, the relationship between rheumatism and heart disease, and the differentiation between normal and abnormal cardiac rhythms. The six foreign (international) vice-presidents included Rudolf Virchow (1821–1902) of Berlin, who needs no introduction to members of the American Osler Society (Figure 1).

Bouillaud opened by stating: "The present occasion is the carrying out of a desire long since entertained by many of the eminent physicians and surgeons in France." He quoted an old French proverb to the effect that international barriers were breaking down, "the Pyrenees have ceased to exist . . . all barriers to the advance of civilization have now ceased to exist, save only the line which divides the domains of civilization from barbarism." Bouillaud continued: "We celebrate to-day a great fête . . . [indeed] the history of medicine can cite no greater."

Bouillaud was an optimist. Of the participants—estimated between 1,200 and 1,500—only 333 Frenchmen attended as "founder members." Tickets were issued to 300 medical students, but most of the 922 physician-attendees came from other European countries. Only three of the active participants came from the British Isles, but a reporter for the *British Medical Journal* wrote critically:

> In Paris there were all the elements of success except the knowledge how to use them. . . . There was a pedantic bureau, with questions cut and dried, to which the discussion must be limited. Questions of medical interest, of medical legislation, were beyond the programme, and were stifled. . . . There was no official reception of the members, or even of the delegates; there was not even a reading-room or common meeting room of any sort during the day. A large number of delegates from America [there were 60 attendees from the US] were utterly ignored. There was an entire absence of hospitality, or even of public courtesies, of any kind. . . . The Congress degenerated into a schoolboy reading of papers. . . . The Congress was a great fact and a great success, by reason of the great number of distinguished men who attended it from all quarters. But it is a success which was due wholly to the guests, and they were soon tired of contributing to it, seeing how awkwardly they were received. . . . Many complaints were heard in Paris. . . . Another such success would be destructive of the idea of international congresses; and we utter the warning lest it might be in any sense initiated in a city of less magnificence and attractions than Paris in the year of the Exhibition.[6]

Many of the papers concerned topics of public-health interest such as tuberculosis and its mortality in different countries, measures to control venereal diseases, and the impact of living conditions on disease occurrence. A single banquet comprised the only scheduled social event. However, the pioneering gynecologist J. Marion Sims (1813–1883), a native of South Carolina who was then living in Paris in the wake of the American Civil War, entertained with "brilliant hospitality" at his residence in the rue du Faubourg St. Honoré which, according to one reporter, "redounded greatly to the credit of America."[5,6]

Given this inauspicious start, would there be future international congresses? The Italian delegation deserves much and perhaps most of the credit for making the congress a recurring and increasingly elaborate event. On the evening of the second day, Diomede Pantaleoni (1810–1885), a surgeon, intellectual, and politician, proposed on behalf of his delegation that the Paris meeting should be the first of a series of meetings to be held in different countries. Some attendees voiced skepticism that such a congress would be successful unless held in a major city concomitant with a universal exhibition (world fair). Ferdinando Palasciano (1815–1891), who like Pantaleoni was a political figure as well as a physician, consulted with fellow Italians and, after some negotiation, Florence was chosen as the site for the Second International Medical Congress.

The organizing committee for the second congress, held in Florence during 23 September–2 October 1869, identified seven themes for formal sessions: marsh miasmas as a cause of malaria; therapeutics of cancer; treatment of gunshot wounds; hygienic conditions of hospitals; conditions predisposing to epidemics in large cities; the rights and duties of physicians; and public health measures

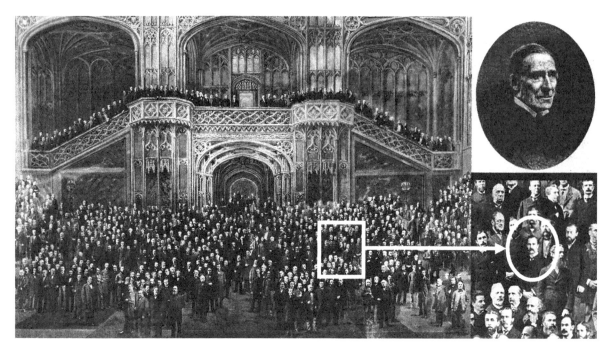

Figure 2. Attendees at the Seventh International Medical Congress, held in London, included 32-year-old William Osler (inset). *Top right:* Sir James Paget, president of the congress.
Credits: Wellcome Collection. CC BY. Chronicle/Alamy Stock Photo (Paget).

extant in various countries. The organizing committee also addressed the need for social occasions to promote collegiality and friendships. Attendees enjoyed the art treasures of Florence, a banquet, and a trip to the nearby Royal Baths of Montecatani.[7] Organizers of later congresses built on these successes, adding specialty sections and more social occasions. Attendance at these congresses was less than that of the first conference in Paris—357 at the 1869 congress in Florence; 671 at the 1873 congress in Vienna; 412 at the 1877 congress in Brussels; 365 at the 1877 congress in Geneva; and 630 at the 1879 congress in Amsterdam—but the stage was now set for the grandest congress to date, held in London during 1881 and commonly known as "Paget's Congress" after its president, the great surgeon-pathologist Sir James Paget (1814–1889) (Figure 2).[8] It was there that Osler made his debut in this forum.

Osler at the International Medical Congresses

The Seventh International Medical Congress, held in London during 2–9 August 1881 under the patronage of Queen Victoria and hosted and organized by the Irish-born surgeon Sir William Mac Cormac (1836–1901), became a huge Victorian spectacle with 3,181 attendees from many countries. This event, probably more than any other, impressed on the 32-year-old Osler the ideal of medicine as a glorious worldwide profession.[9] Attendees included Paget, Jean-Martin Charcot, Thomas Huxley, Louis Pasteur, Robert Koch, and Virchow. Seldom in the history of medicine have so many luminaries representing the best of medicine and science been present at the same place at the same time.

Osler crossed the Atlantic aboard the S.S. *Parisian* in the company of his Montreal mentor R. Palmer Howard (1823–1889), arriving in time for the opening address by Sir William Jenner (1815–1898), president of the Royal College of Physicians. Jenner, sharing the dais with the Prince of Wales and the Prince of Prussia, began:

> It would be scarcely courteous to you or congenial to my own feelings, were I not to express my idea of the sentiments and aims of those who have collected from all parts of her Majesty's dominions, and from all the great schools of the world where the science of medicine is cultivated and advanced, and through which, by means of their pupils, the science of practical medicine and the fruits it bears are diffused throughout the earth. We have been told that commerce is the golden girdle of the world. . . . But science binds men and nations together with a girdle the links of which are far stronger, and more durable, and more precious than are the links of the golden girdle of commerce. . . .
>
> If this be true of science in general, it is true in the highest and widest sense of the science of medicine. Commerce is fettered in the supposed or real interests of nations. Commerce separates as well as binds men together. Discovers in other applied sciences than medicine are stimulated by a desire for pecuniary rewards, but the discoveries in scientific and applied medicine are open to all the world. . . .

Jenner concluded: "We are here to meet each other socially; to remove in that way all prejudices, to promote kindly feeling, to renew old friendships and to lay the foundations of new friendships, and, by personal intercommunication, to knit more closely the bonds of that professional brotherhood of which we are all so justly proud."[10] Readers familiar with Osler's essays will recognize in these remarks by Jenner the germs of Osler's thoughts expressed in such addresses as "The Leaven of Science," "Chauvinism in Medicine," and "Unity, Peace and Concord."

Paget in his inaugural address amplified Jenner's call to unity and brotherhood, predicting that "in the casual conversations of this coming week there will be a larger interchange and diffusion of knowledge than in any equal time and space in the whole past history of medicine." Paget in closing exhorted attendees to "resolve to devote ourselves to the promotion of the whole science, art, and charity of medicine," as a "vow of brotherhood."[10, i: 13–21]

Addresses at plenary sessions—now available online in the four-volume, 2,552-page *Transactions* of the congress—make good reading even today. These include Huxley on "Relations of Biological Science to Medicine," Virchow "On the Value of Pathological Experimentation in Medicine," Pasteur on "Vaccination in Relation to Chicken Cholera and Splenic Fever," Richard von Volkmann (1830–1889) on "Progress of Surgery during the Last Ten Years," John Shaw Billings (1838–1913) on "Our Medical Literature," and Auguste Gabriel Maurice Raynaud (1834–1881) on "Medical Skepticism in the Past and at the Present Time" (read by Louis Henri Félix Féréol [1825–1891], since Raynaud had recently died). There were also addresses by Sir William Bowman (1816–1892), Charcot, Austin Flint (1812–1886), Sir William Gull (1816–1890), Moritz Kaposi (1837–1902), Koch, the biologist Sir Richard Owen (1804–1892), and Sir Samuel Wilks (1824–1911).

Attendees had to choose among concurrent sections. Osler concentrated on those concerned with physiology and pathology, possibly because these were the subjects he was teaching as professor of the Institutes of Medicine at McGill. At one of the pathology sessions, he presented "On Some Points in the Etiology and Pathology of Endocarditis," illustrated by seven cases in which autopsies were performed.[10, i: 341–349] He observed "micrococci" in all seven, but he questioned their causative significance:

> The relation of the micrococci to the disease has been very fully discussed by Virchow, [Karl Joseph] Eberth, [Theodor Albrecht Edwin] Klebs, and others, most of whom hold that they are the specific elements which account for the peculiar malignancy of the disease, and that they stand in the same position in this affection as the bacillus in anthrax. There are some points which should, I think, make us hesitant to accept this view without further evidence.... How far they are responsible either for the development of the endocarditis or for the subsequent character which, in the grave form, it assumes, the evidence does not, I think, warrant as yet a very positive opinion.

In retrospect, Osler was hindered by the lack of adequate blood culture techniques, observing as he did: "So far as my observation goes, the micrococci do not exist in the blood during the course of the malady."

Osler failed to grasp the significance of the presentations by Pasteur and Koch, which are now considered landmarks in the acceptance of the germ theory. Among the many distractions to Osler and other attendees were the Museum sessions, which included not only the demonstration of specimens but also the presentation of living patients by Jonathan Hutchinson (1828–1913), who stated afterwards: "The attempt to illustrate disease by the exhibition of living patients in a Museum was at once a novelty and an experiment. Our exhibition was more popular than we had expected; every morning, at the hour announced, the room filled." Osler basked in the social events, which include an opulent reception at Holly Lodge hosted by the philanthropist Angela Burdett Counts (1ˢᵗ Baroness Burdett Counts [1814–1906]) and a reception at the Crystal Palace featuring a pyrotechnic display with fire portraits of Paget, Charcot, and the German surgeon Bernhard von Langenbeck (1810–1887). Attendees received as a souvenir a circular bronze medal with Hippocrates on one side and Queen Victoria on the other (Figure 3).

The day after the congress closed, Osler submitted a detailed account to his friend George Ross, coeditor of the *Canada Medical and Surgical Journal*, describing how "the sight of above 3,000 medical men from all parts of the world, drawn together for one common purpose, and animated by one spirit was enough to quick the pulse and to arouse enthusiasm to a high pitch."[11] He apparently did not comment on the organizers' decision to limit invitations to men, which drew protests from a group of women.

Osler made a positive impression on many people including the Philadelphia surgeon Samuel Weissel Gross (1837–1889), who attended the congress only because his father, the eminent surgeon Samuel David Gross (1805–1884), was unable to attend because of a conflict. Samuel W. Gross had recently married a former Boston debutante, Grace Linzee Revere. When the elder Gross asked his son to give impressions of men he had seen at the congress, the younger Gross mentioned "a swarthy young Canadian named Osler" who gave an excellent paper, adding that perhaps someday "they might get him in Philadelphia." Three years the elder Gross was instrumental in recruiting Osler to Philadelphia. Osler

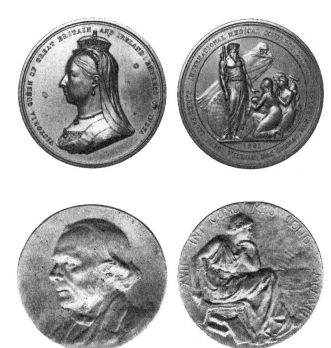

Figure 3.   *Above:* Commemorative medal created for the Seventh International Medical Congress held in London (1881) by Leonard Charles Wyon (1826–1891), based on an illustration by John Tenniel (1820–1914), showing a bust of Queen Victoria and, on the opposite side, figures kneeling before Hippocrates. *Below:* Commemorative bronze medal created for the Seventeenth International Medical Congress held in London (1913) by Cecil Hew Brown (1895–1926), showing a bust of Joseph, Lord Lister and, on the opposite side, the Goddess Hygiea. *Credits:* Wikipedia.

became a frequent guest at Sunday dinners at the home of Samuel W. Gross, and thus got to know Grace Linzee Revere Gross, whom Osler married after her husband's death from pneumonia.

Following the Seventh International Medical Congress in London were congresses in Copenhagen (1885), Washington, DC (1887), Berlin (1880), Rome (1894), Moscow (1897), Paris (1900), Madrid (1903), Lisbon (1906), Budapest. (1909), and finally London (1913), the seventeenth and last congress. The Copenhagen congress (1885) was remarkable for its public and private hospitality: banquets, excursions, provisions for women guests, and the innovation of having officers of the various sections host dinner parties for their members. So impressed was the New York laryngologist and rhinologist D. Bryson Delavan (1850–1942) that he wrote a 54-page account of "The Social History of the Eighth International Medical Congress" of sufficient interest to prompt William Bennett Bean (1909–1989), founding president of the American Osler Society, to write a review of it 76 years after its publication.[12,13] The Washington, DC, congress (1887) was a fiasco because of attempt by the American Medical Association (AMA) to overthrow the authority of John Shaw Billings, who had been named chairman of the organizing committee. Osler was among 29 Philadelphia physicians who protested the attempt by the AMA leadership to undermine Billings.[14]

Osler attended neither the eighth nor the ninth congress, but he attended the Tenth International Medical Congress, held 4–9 August 1890 in Berlin, as part of a "quinquennial brain dusting" that included extensive travels in Germany and three weeks in Paris (Figure 4). Osler and his former John Hopkins colleague William H. Welch were present on 4 August when Robert Koch announced he had found a cure for tuberculosis. The "cure" was tuberculin, an extract of cultures of the tubercle bacillus. Osler was skeptical and he and others quickly

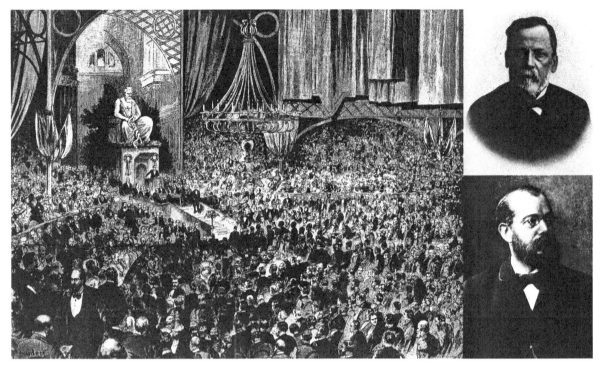

Figure 4. Artist's depiction of the opening ceremony of the Tenth International Medical Congress held in Berlin (1890). Note the gallery for women spectators on the left and the massive sculpture of Asklepios (Asclepios or Aesculapius), god of medicine. *Top right:* Louis Pasteur. *Lower right:* Robert Koch.
Credits: INTERFOTO/Alamy Stock Photo. National Library of Medicine (Pasteur and Koch).

disproved tuberculin as a treatment for tuberculosis. Koch's claim became a national scandal in Germany after he marketed tuberculin without adequate research to demonstrate efficacy and safety.

William S. Thayer (1864–1932), writing 39 years later, recalled the first time he saw Osler, which was at the 1890 congress in Berlin:

> But as clearly as if it were before my eyes, one figure stands out—the figure of a man who was not wandering about, who was not idly conversing. Alone, seemingly oblivious of those about him, with an easy, elastic, winging stride, rapidly but without haste, his open frock coat flowing in the breeze, a package of papers in his left hand, he passed by and entered the hall. He was not a large man. Rather spare and well built, he gave the impression of vigour and energy. He wore a silk hat and carried a stick. He was obviously well dressed. Among the idle groups, talking together, observing and commenting on their neighbours, he passed, a figure apart, plunged in his own thoughts. The oval, dark, almost olive face, with the long, drooping moustache, was calm and composed, and the deep, thoughtful eyes betrayed the serene, intent and active man.
>
> "Do you know who that is?" said my companion, who had followed my gaze. "That is Osler, professor of medicine at Johns Hopkins."[15]

The German scholar Karl Sudhoff (1853–1938), who perhaps more than anyone else was responsible for the professionalization of medical history as an academic discipline, recalled from a congress: "I was deeply impressed by him. I was fascinated by the generous freedom of his personality, the quiet accuracy of his judgment, his high erudition, his broad view and the nobility of his concept of man and things."[16]

Osler, who was in his own words was "not an office-seeker," nevertheless consented to serve as president of the Medical Section of the Seventeenth International Medical Congress which took place in London, 6–12 August 1913. Preparations surely taxed him, as he had recently returned from a four-week trip to North America (28 April–23 May) during which he gave the Silliman Lectures at Yale and visited Boston, New York, Philadelphia, Washington, Baltimore, Buffalo, Toronto, Montreal, and friends and relatives in small towns in Ontario. More than 7,000 attendees were expected, making the congress a daunting task for the president, Sir Thomas Barlow (1845–1945) and the principal organizer, Wilmot P. Herringham (1855–1936). Osler pitched in by recruiting Waldorf and Nancy Astor to host an afternoon reception at Cliveden and the Canadian philanthropist Lord Strathcona (Donald A. Smith [1820–1914]) to provide evening entertainment for the entire congress.[9, ii: 345] Osler also helped with the organization of a new History of Medicine Section, of which Sir Norman Moore (1847–1922) served as president and Sir Raymond Crawfurd (1865–1938) as secretary. Osler had previously arranged the groundwork to stage the grand opening of the museum assembled by Sir Henry Wellcome (1853–1936) during the congress.

The Seventeenth International Medical Congress opened with a dazzling ceremony in Royal Albert Hall in South Kensington, at the gates of Hyde Park, and continued with packed programs that included new sections, such as a Section on Urology. However, the congress lacked the scientific luster of the seventh congress in London because so many luminaries had died including Huxley, Koch, and, the previous year, Lord Lister, who was honored on the commemorative medal (Figure 3). Perhaps the most notable presenter was Paul Ehrlich (1854–1915), the German physician-scientist who four years earlier had launched the age of chemotherapy of infection with arsphenamine (Salvarsan) for syphilis. Osler presided successfully over the Medical Section, entertained throughout the meeting at a suite in the fashionable Brown's Hotel in Mayfair, and put on a dinner for 196 members of the Medical Section at the Royal Automobile Club. The congress received much attention in the lay press but, as Harvey Cushing predicted, it proved "to be the last of those unwieldly periodical gatherings of medical men from all over the world."[9, ii: 368–372]

Osler foresaw this. In a farewell address to the medical profession of the United States, delivered in Baltimore in 1905, he declared that "the International Congress . . . has proved rather an unwieldly body" and predicted that its role would be usurped by "the specialty societies which are rapidly denationalizing science." The Great War (1914–1918) erupted less than a year after the Seventeenth International Medical Congress in London, and there would never be another great congress with thousands of attendees from all walks of medicine. For 2021, for example, a single website lists 329 international medical conferences, despite the Covid-19 pandemic, but all are narrowly focused on one or another specialty or special interest.[17] Osler in that 1905 address famously proclaimed: "Linked together by the strong bonds of community of interests, the profession of medicine forms a remarkable world-unit in the progressive evolution of which there is a fuller hope for humanity than in any other direction."[3] Will it ever be possible for the profession of medicine—or, optimally, the global community of healthcare workers—to coalesce into a "remarkable world-unit" committed to humanized science and prolonged survival of higher life forms on this fragile planet we call home?[1]

References

1. Bryan CS, Podolsky SH. Sir William Osler (1849–1919)—The uses of history and the "singular beneficence" of medicine. *New England Journal of Medicine* 2019; 381(23): 2194–2195.
2. Osler W. The importance of post-graduate study. *British Medical Journal* 1900; 2(2083): 71–75.
3. Osler W. Unity, peace and concord. In Osler W. *Aequanimitas, With other Addresses to Medical Students, Nurses and Practitioners of Medicine.* Third edition, Philadelphia: P. Blakiston's Son & Co., In.; 1932: 425–443.
4. Osler W. Chauvinism in medicine. In Osler W. *Aequanimitas, With other Addresses to Medical Students, Nurses and Practitioners of Medicine.* Third edition, Philadelphia: P. Blakiston's Son & Co., In.; 1932: 263–289.
5. McMenemey WH. International Congress of Medicine 1867 and some of the personalities involved. *British Medical Journal* 1967; 3(5563): 487–489.
6. Unsigned. The International Medical Congress of Paris. *British Medical Journal* 1867; 2(351): 254–255.
7. Unsigned. The history of International Medical Congresses. *British Medical Journal* 1884; 2(1238): 561–571.
8. Unsigned. Former International Medical Congresses. *Medical Record* 1903; 63(January 24): 147–154.
9. Cushing H. *The Life of Sir William Osler.* Oxford: Clarendon Press; 1925; i: 189–192.
10. *Transactions of the International Medical Congress, seventh session, held in London, August 2d to 9th, 1881.* London: J.W. Kolckmann; 1881; volume 1: 1–2.
11. Osler W. International Medical Congress. *Canada Medical and Surgical Journal* 1881–1882; 10: 121–125.
12. Delavan DB. *The Social History of the Eighth International Medical Congress, Held in Copenhagen, August 1884.* New York: D. Appleton and Company; 1885.
13. Bean WB. *The Social History of the Eighth International Medical Congress, Held in Copenhagen, August 1884,* by D. Bryson Delavan (review). *Archives of Internal Medicine* 1963; 112(6): 989–990.
14. William Osler to Henry Pickering Bowditch 29 June 1885. Osler Letter Index, CUS417/81.19, Osler Library of the History of Medicine, McGill University.
15. Thayer WS. Reminiscences of Osler in the early Baltimore days. *California & Western Medicine* 1929; 31(September): 161–168.
16. Sudhoff K. Osler und die Geschichte der Medizin. In [Abbott ME, ed.]. Sir William Osler Memorial Number: Appreciations and Reminiscences. *Bulletin No. IX of the International Association of Medical Museums and Journal of Technical Methods.* Montreal: Privately printed; 1926: 28.
17. Medical International Conferences List | Medical Symposiums (omicsonline.org), accessed 8 February 2021.

Cliveden: The Canadian Red Cross Hospital, William Osler, and the "Taplow Affair"

Milton Roxanas, M.B., B.S.

Marilyn A. Gendek, R.N., M.A., M.N.

Vivien E. Lane, R.N., Ph.D.

Dominating the land around it and with impressive views of the River Thames, Cliveden House (with an 800-year history) is now a luxurious hotel and National Trust property. However, during the Great War (First World War [WW1], 28 July 1914 to 11 November 1918), it was a place for salvaging and rehabilitating the severely damaged bodies and minds of soldiers. It was to here that Sir William Osler (1849–1919) (Figure 1), Consultant Physician, drove from his Oxford home once a week to consult in a 'pop-up' hospital, facilitate medical research and to socialize.

An incident that climaxed in September 1916, referred to in some correspondence as the "Taplow scandal" or "Taplow affair," was a personal crisis for Osler, causing his wife to write with concern "the CAMC [Canadian Army Medical Corps] business nearly killed him with shame and annoyance," and prompting his biographer Harvey Cushing to write that Osler showed signs of depression.[1] This paper provides a brief history of the Cliveden estate, the development of the hospital facilities and soldiers' amenities. The political and sociocultural background to this crisis will be mentioned. However, the emphasis will be on Osler's ethical crisis in relation to the key local characters, namely Nancy

Presented in part at the forty-ninth annual meeting of the American Osler Society, Montreal, Quebec, on 14 May 2019. This paper was previously published in the *Journal of Medical Biography* (2019; 27[4]: 220–229) and is reprinted with permission.

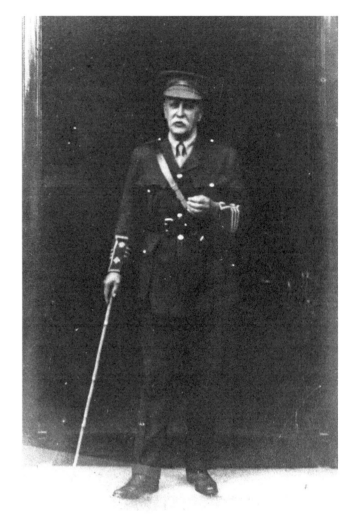

Figure 1. Sir William Osler in uniform at Cliveden.
Credit: Osler Library of the History of Medicine, McGill University.

Astor (1879–1964), Matron Edith Campbell (1871–1951), and Lieutenant-Colonel Charles Gorrell (1871–1917).

Brief History of the Cliveden Estate

The history and grandeur of Cliveden provided an extraordinary venue for injured WW1 soldiers to convalesce. The land on which Cliveden was built was originally owned by Geoffrey de Clyveden in 1237. In 1666, the estate of Cliveden was comprised of two hunting lodges in 400 acres located only 30 miles from the Palace of Westminster in London. It was bought by the Duke of Buckingham (1628–1687) in 1668 but it is said that he started building on it about 10 years later. His aim was to house his mistress, Anna Maria Talbot (1642–1702) and use it to entertain Royalty, enjoy his artistic collections, and hunt in well-stocked grounds full of horses, deer, hounds, etc.[2] The house was built in the Italianate style by the architect Captain William Winde (c. 1645–1722) and the Duke continued with extensions until the 1680s. On 5 February 1674, both Houses of Parliament passed a resolution ordering Buckingham to separate from his mistress and he consequently brought his wife, Mary, to live with him in Cliveden. The house burned down twice, and the present building was designed by Charles Barry (1795–1860) in the Italianate style, being completed in 1851. Cliveden (Figure 2) continues to attract influential people.

In 1893 William Waldorf Astor (1848–1919), a wealthy American who became a British citizen, bought Cliveden and gave it as a gift to his son Waldorf (1879–1952) when he married the Virginian divorcee Nancy Shaw (née Langhorne) in 1906.[2] In 1919 Waldorf Astor inherited the title of Viscount conferred on his father making him "Sir" and Nancy "Lady" Astor.

Queen Victoria enjoyed staying at Cliveden, as did the Duke and Duchess of Connaught in 1908,[3] and Sir Winston Churchill at a later date. More recently, millions around the world watched Meghan Markle emerge from Cliveden House to travel to Windsor Castle to marry Prince Harry in 2018.

One of Waldorf Astor's interests was the National Association for the Prevention of Consumption and he was on the same committee as Osler, hence Osler and Astor knew each other before WW1.[4] Osler also knew Nancy Astor when in 1884 he treated her as a 15-year-old at the Johns Hopkins Hospital.[5] These friendships prevailed and the onset of WW1 found them all ensconced in the war effort at Cliveden.

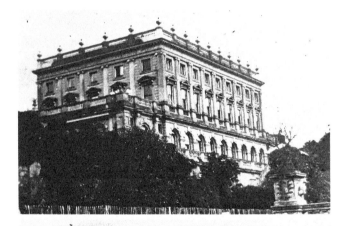

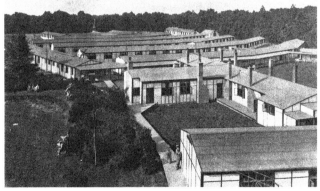

Figure 2.   *Above:* Cliveden mansion during World War I. *Below:* The Duchess of Connaught Canadian Red Cross Hospital (also known as the "Canadian Red Cross Hospital" or "Cliveden"), constructed on the Cliveden estate.
Credits: Albert James Rooks Photograph Albums, 1916–1918, the John Oxley Library, State Library of Queensland, Australia (above). Sgt. J.R. Howe, Duchess of Connaught Canadian Red Cross Hospital ("Cliveden"), Taplow Bucks, The Quails Photo Co., London. Courtesy of the Alfred Deakin Prime Ministerial Library, Deakin University, Australia (below).

The World War 1 effort and the building of the Cliveden hospital(s)

When Waldorf Astor was rejected from combat in WW1, he offered Cliveden to the British War Office four days after the war started. This offer was declined. He then approached the Canadian Government who accepted the use of Cliveden on behalf of the Canadian Red Cross. The hospital established at Cliveden was officially named the Duchess of Connaught (after the wife of the Governor-General of Canada) Canadian Red Cross Hospital (DCCRCH) from December 1914 to September 1917, after which it was reassigned as the Number 15 Canadian General Hospital. It was also affectionately known by the soldiers as "Lady Astor's hospital" or CRX (i.e., Cliveden Red Cross).

As the main house was unsuitable for a hospital, the Astors initially converted their indoor tennis court into makeshift wards. The fives court (a handball game) became a kitchen and the bowling alley was converted into a special ward for "influenza and rheumatism." The Astors paid for the conversion.[2]

The original accommodation was temporary, yet of high standard for the day. A total of 106 beds were set up into 25 bed wards under the central skylight of the covered tennis court. A gallery was added with more beds and a matron's office which had a bird's eye view of the patients. Each bed locker had a vase of flowers provided by Nancy Astor, whilst the inpatients were described as occupying their time making quilts, socks, reading, or playing games. It was said "red tape seemed in the background if it existed at all."[6] The trolleys had glass tops and tables made by the resident carpenter. The nursing sisters were accommodated in the main house and the first patients were received in April 1915.[6]

Within six months, new permanent buildings were designed by the architect Charles Frederick Skipper (1877–1936) and commissioned on 12 July 1915 (Figures 2 and 3). They consisted of five pairs of wards connected by two central corridors which contained the lavatories. On either side of each ward there was a scullery, a room for washing bedpans and a small kitchen for making tea and coffee. There was a separate isolation ward, and the hospital expanded to accommodate over 1,000 sick and injured soldiers, which necessitated a staff of over 70 nursing sisters. A total of 24,000 soldiers were treated here over the period of the war. The medical and nursing staffs were now accommodated in separate buildings and the sergeants' mess was built from the winnings of Waldorf Astor's racehorse "Winky Pop."[7] New operating theatres were built with sterilising, X-ray and dark rooms, and lavatories for the doctors. There was another building for pathology, eye, ear and dental diseases. Food was carried to the wards in heated trolleys, electricity and water were supplied by Cliveden, garbage and dressings were incinerated, and sewage disposed of in a septic tank.[8] Cliveden's gardens provided seasonal vegetables, fruit, and meat. The gardens and river boats were made available to the patients and staff as was the library.

Admitting soldiers

Osler would have understood that from admission to discharge, the overall management of the hospital was achieved by collaborative effort from multiple agencies: staff supplied by the CAMC, building by the Astors, maintenance by the British War Office and equipment by the Canadian Red Cross Society. The

Deputy Director of Medical Services, Southampton, directed patients to the hospital.[7] Patients came not only from Canada but from various countries, such as the Great Britain, the USA, Australia, Germany, with other nationalities frequently outnumbering Canadians.

Special mention was made that soldiers were received in an efficient way. It only took one hour to get soldiers from the train at Taplow station into an ambulance, take them to the reception office at the hospital, check their names against the roll from the train, wait their turn to be undressed, bathe them in hot water, give them clean clothes and put to bed.[8] The *Times* on 3 November 1916 declared DCCRCH as "one of the two best hospitals in England." Given the conditions the injured soldiers had survived in France, the setting at Cliveden must have been a surreal paradise.

Hospital staffing

Generally, middle management and clinical staff were forever in flux whereas the Astors and Osler remained constant. The initial commanding officer was Lieutenant-Colonel Ford and when he was transferred to France,[8] Lieutenant-Colonel Charles Gorrell (McGill, 1894), CAMC,[9] was appointed on 27 January 1915, together with Lieutenant-Colonels D.W. McPherson and W.L. Watts. Other CAMC appointments included 10 other medical officers, Matron Edith Campbell and E. Russell, and 20 other nurses, one dentist and 32 orderlies.[10] Canadian doctors practicing in Britain were also appointed as consultants.

Matron Campbell had an outstanding military record before and after her appointment to run the Cliveden hospital, and was eight years the senior of the high-society lady of the house, Nancy Astor. Campbell was on active duty in France with the first contingent of the Canadian Expeditionary Force before transferring to DCCRCH, was mentioned in dispatches, and awarded the Royal Red Cross 1st Class on the same day in June 1915. A recent find of three real photo postcards, taken about 1915–1916, shows Matron Campbell in the company of royalty, the Prime Minister of Canada, Sir Robert Borden (1854–1937), Waldorf Astor, Gorrell, and other visitors to DCCRCH, attesting her social standing.[11]

Osler was appointed consultant in Medicine on 2 February 1915. He did his rounds at Cliveden on Mondays and then had lunch with Nancy Astor. Osler's wife, Lady Grace Revere Osler (1854–1928) wrote to her sister on 1 December 1915: "At Cliveden if he doesn't go every Monday they are dreadfully annoyed and Nancy [Astor] telephones to know why—and says her children [referring to her patients] are weeping for him . . ." In a later letter, Grace writes: "the officers tell me they live for this Monday visit."[2, ii: 503, 530]

Cliveden staff included Osler's son Revere (Edward Revere Osler [1895–1917]) who was appointed assistant quartermaster at Cliveden in February 1915. Osler wrote on 4 March 1915 to Harvey Cushing: "Revere got his commission last week and has been ordered to join the Canadian Hospital at Cliveden where he will learn quartermaster work and look after the discipline of the convalescents. He is stationed at Taplow House. It is a big hospital and will have some 500 beds."[12] Revere left Cliveden in May 1915, had a brief visit with his parents, then joined the McGill Hospital unit in France which was set up by 7 August 1915.[13] Revere was later killed in action after he decided to enlist in the British Army when he could have served out the war with the McGill Hospital unit.

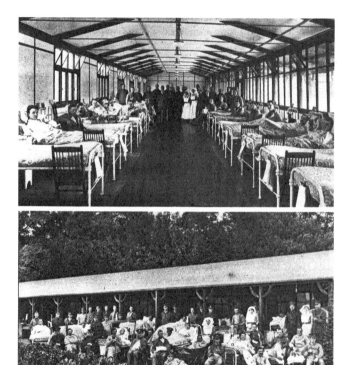

Figure 3.   *Above:* Interior of a ward at the Duchess of Connaught Canadian Red Cross Hospital at Cliveden. *Below:* Summertime outside one of the wards.
Credit: Sgt. J.R. Howe, Duchess of Connaught Canadian Red Cross Hospital ("Cliveden"), Taplow Bucks, The Quails Photo Co., London. Courtesy of the Alfred Deakin Prime Ministerial Library, Deakin University, Australia.

Activities at the Duchess of Connaught Canadian Red Cross Hospital (DCCRCH)

DCCRCH had a most enlightened and modern approach to the rehabilitation of soldiers, rewarding their war heroes with free access to all that Cliveden had to offer and encouraging them to re-socialize among people normally restricted by class and racial boundaries. Canadians were kept abreast with Canadian news and affairs.[7] In addition to physical rehabilitation, sport was encouraged which included athletics, soccer, cricket, hockey, and DCCRCH teams played against other hospitals, including the Royal Engineers, and celebrations were held when DCCRCH teams won. Entertainment was provided by visiting orchestras, ensembles, and actors, as well as cinematographic evenings. Patients were also invited into the Astors' house, for example, to their son's birthday party celebrations in August 1917, and dances were organised. Lady Annesley (1881–1959) adopted a ward at DCCRCH and frequently entertained the patients in her country cottage near Taplow.[14]

In addition, the Astors held special formal occasions in the ballroom for officers and nurses. Further diversion was provided by visits from the King and Queen of England, groups of senior American officers, the Prime Minister of Canada and other dignitaries who provided motivation to spruce up patients, staff, and buildings.[7] Vocational rehabilitation was provided for future civilian life and facilities for training were available in tailoring, woodwork, hurdle making, basket work, metal and iron work. An attempt was made to teach agricultural work but was abandoned as the duration of stay at the hospital was deemed too

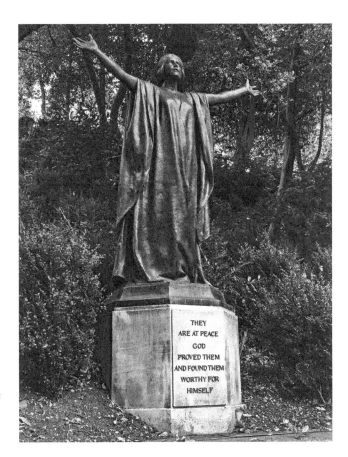

Figure 4.   Statue representing Canada with the head of Nancy Astor on the Cliveden estate, by Bertram Mackennal (1863–1931).
Credit: Vivien E. Lane and Milton G. Roxanas.

short. Items made by patients were sold and funds given to the hospital. In return, both the Canadian and American Red Cross sent presents to the soldiers.

The staff and patients started a fortnightly newspaper on 30 June 1917 and called it *The Chronicles of Cliveden* which had a circulation of 900 and cost three pence. The first issue had a welcome note from Nancy Astor, and included results of sporting fixtures, short stories, jokes, poems and advertisements from local businesses.

The patients were further stimulated by an interesting series of topics and lecturers, including one by Rudyard Kipling, who spoke in January 1916 in the recreation room.[15] Osler spoke on Ambroise Paré, presumably on his wartime experiences (bland dressings, ligatures) and showed books from his collection, whilst Colonel Major Robertson spoke on surgical anecdotes. Mr. Fletcher of Oxford spoke on "the English Army from the Norman Conquest to the Restoration." Mr. Hall presented on "The Navy in War." Other speakers included Professor J.S. Haldane, other academics from Oxford University, a Serbian priest, and others.[7]

Medical care and research publications

The variety of patients afforded an opportunity for observation, research and publication. As noted earlier, staff of a high calibre was appointed to Cliveden and innovative medical approaches were often published in reputable journals.

The hospital sent regular lists of injuries in soldiers, and autopsy reports, back to Canada. Deaths from other causes, including suicide, were also listed and there were nine deaths from tuberculosis in six months in 1918.[16] Anaesthetics used included nitrous oxide and oxygen, ether, methyl chloride and ether, chloroform and novocaine.[7]

It is difficult to know the exact influence of Osler in the day-to-day activities, but we do know that he mentored other doctors, and some made a routine of doing ward rounds with him. Dr. Walter S. Atkinson (1892–1978) showed interest in doing research on the effect of poison gases on the eyes, and on learning this, Osler arranged for a train full of soldiers who had been gassed in the preceding 48 hours to be sent to the hospital.[17] This led to publications by that author on delayed keratitis after mustard gas exposure which also influenced the Veterans Administration to accept the condition as service related. There is a humorous story about how this ophthalmologist had his longest conversation with Osler while in the toilet with Osler advising him to practice in a university town, advice which he didn't follow.[18] Further publications emanating from the hospital described three cases of "concussion aphasia" or hysterical aphasia following close contact with exploding shells. Treatment included using alcohol in one case and anaesthesia with ether in the other two. The author mentioned that Osler wrote to him about the procedure and had a patient treated with ether with good recovery.[18] Osler had a long interest in aphasic disorders and wrote several articles on them.[19,20] Ever the teacher and mentor, Osler was still encouraging others and was instrumental in pushing for the establishment of the Canadian Army Medical Service Journal edited by his friend Colonel John George Adami (1862–1926).[21]

Another report mentions the accidental poisoning of an Australian soldier with mercury who died 52 days later from renal failure and tuberculosis, with a thorough post-mortem report.[7] Patients admitted with phosgene poisoning were under the care of Lieutenant-Colonel J.C. Meakins, and a report by J.S. Haldane, J.C. Meakins and J.G. Priestley was published on reflex restriction of breathing after gas poisoning and the use of oxygen to treat it.[7,21] Another Canadian, Frank Hamilton Mewburn (1858–1929) was appointed head of the surgical division of the hospital and published a paper on "Management of lesions of peripheral nerves."[22]

The hospital had an isolation ward for those patients with infectious diseases, for example, tuberculosis and diarrhoea, the latter coming from the Dardanelles; and was periodically in quarantine from scarlet fever and measles.[7]

Special studies were conducted about nephritis/trench nephritis and deformities of the chest from gunshot wounds.[7]

Cliveden also accommodated the spiritual needs of the soldiers. A small elaborate chapel already existed but Nancy Astor then developed her sculpture garden into a consecrated memorial, known as the Cliveden War Cemetery. Osler and his wife Grace attended the consecration of the cemetery in December 1916. Nancy asked the Australian sculptor Bertram Mackennal to make a statue representing Canada to which he agreed on the proviso that she pose for the head (Figure 4). The cemetery contains 42 burial sites of soldiers and nurses from WW1, of which 29 were Canadians, two Americans and others from the UK, Australia, and New Zealand. Two further graves were added in the 1939–1945 war.[23]

As demonstrated above, the Astors, like other British aristocrats, not only attempted to enlist but also accommodated military hospitals (and other services) on their estates. The political and socio-cultural impact on the estate owners and the hospital population was significant.

Figure 5. Group photograph taken at the Duchess of Connaught Canadian Red Cross Hospital at Cliveden in 1915. *From left:* Matron Edith Campbell, RRC, Major Astor, General Carleton Jones, Willie Astor, Sir Robert Borden, Lt. Col. Gorrell. Photograph by E.R. Owen, from the Grace Waters Collection.
Credit: Community Archives of Belleville and Hastings County, Ontario.

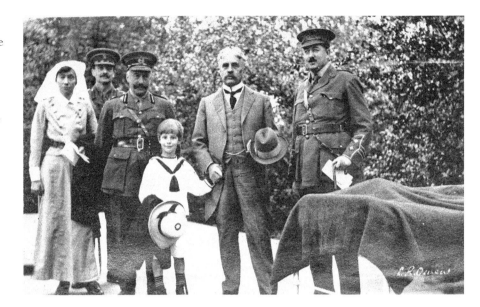

Suddenly the private space and immense resources of the British upper-class owners were shared with injured solders, nurses, doctors, and the whole military management system. The pre-existing constructions of the political and socio-cultural boundaries such as authority, national identity and gender roles were necessarily blurred, which generated tension and even conflict. Cliveden was no exception.

The controversy at DCCRCH

An anonymous telegram from DCCRCH on 28 September 1916 alerted Osler that all was not well at the hospital. It read "Matron in trouble please come at once."[24] As background, Sir Sam Hughes (1853–1921), the Canadian Minister of Militia and Defense, ordered an enquiry into the medical department of the Canadian Expeditionary Force and appointed Dr. Herbert Bruce (1868–1963), a Toronto surgeon, to conduct the enquiry. Osler's biographer Michael Bliss described Bruce as ambitious but incompetent.[5, p. 529] The enquiry was precipitated by a number of issues such as the large number of Canadian soldiers who were returned from Britain because of poor health, discrimination because of their foreign surnames (and birthplace in countries opposing Britain), and inefficient sending of reinforcements.[22] Bliss opines that Bruce and his team went around the units "collecting grievances in a fairly obvious witch-hunt aimed at bringing down [Surgeon General Carleton] Jones."[26] Hughes was unhappy with the Surgeon General Guy Carleton Jones (1864–1950) who authorised Canadian resources to be managed by the (British) War Office when Hughes hoped that the war would give an opportunity for Canada to show its independence from Britain. Hughes believed Jones's actions were regarded as subordinate to those of England. Bruce's investigations were conducted over six weeks and he visited hospitals with Hughes, and Surgeon General Carleton Jones. As a prominent member in the Canadian Conservative Party, Hughes had aspirations for a more senior position in the war effort. Bruce's report identified 23 deficiencies.[25] Hughes then leaked the report to businessmen in Toronto, recalled Carleton Jones, and replaced him with Bruce, in spite of his meagre experience in military affairs. One author wrote that the medical services after the Battle of the Somme "considered the Bruce investigation a form of madness at home that matched the madness of the battlefield...."[27] Lady Julia Drummond (1860–1942) was vehemently against the report and made this known in letters to *The Times* of London.[25]

Even before the findings were published, Osler had reservations about the composition and terms of the enquiry. Osler wrote to Hughes asking whether it was fair to appoint people subordinate to Carleton Jones to the enquiry, if he knew or was consulted about it, and whether these facts should be made public.[26] A similar letter was sent to Sir Robert Borden, Prime Minister of Canada, complaining that there were appointments from Carleton Jones's department who were "junior... (which) is contrary to all usage."[27]

Allegations of sock-selling and romance

Osler was also concerned not only at Matron Campbell's recommended dismissal but also that of Lieutenant-Colonel Gorrell.[28] Bruce's findings from Cliveden primarily focused on advising the transfer of the Matron because of an implied "liaison" with Gorrell; and the latter's dismissal because of finding him trading in Red Cross supplies with proceeds from this kept in a special cashbox in his office.[5, p. 430; 29] This accusation of 'Red Cross sock-selling' was not new. The story goes that it was the result of rumours spread in Canada when large numbers of women were harnessed into voluntary work to produce knitted comforts, food parcels and other supplementary items and received no feedback or thanks for their efforts. It was rumoured that items were sold to soldiers or remained unused in warehouses, and that Canadian Red Cross Society workers were paid large sums of money. There were even rumours that the enemy started this propaganda or spread it.[29]

Nancy Astor, military staff, and Matron Edith Campbell

A letter from Edith Campbell to Osler states that Nancy Astor wanted to get rid of Gorrell and herself as she "interfered in everything and everybody, and she can be moody and nasty when she likes, quite different person to her usual sunny self...."[30] It was reported that Nancy Astor "cleverly contrives to get into close contact with them [patients]..."[31] when she was throwing lavish parties and took guests into the grounds to show off convalescing soldiers and even tried to get access into the wards.[32] This behaviour may have interfered in the running of the wards and may have been resisted by Matron Campbell leading to animosity between the two. One author described it as a power struggle between inherited power and military power.[32] On another occasion, Nancy Astor invited a Canadian soldier to a service at the First Church of Christian Scientists in Sloane Street London. She drove him in her car but after the service, she left him at Paddington Station to find his way back to Cliveden. He was stopped by the Military Police and charged with absenteeism. Mrs. Astor then went to Marylebone Police Court to defend him.[33] She even offered a sick soldier her Cartier watch if he recovered, which he did, and she had to part with it.[2] There are many accounts indicating that Nancy Astor believed the DCCRCH to be her domain and referred to Canadian soldiers as her "children." She represented herself as a maternal figure, perhaps for political gain, which is interesting in view of the evidence that she was a somewhat neglectful mother.[32] It appears Nancy Astor paid little respect to the military culture or staff members managing the service.

A letter from the Matron-in-Chief, Major Margaret C. Macdonald (1873–1948) to Osler informs him that Campbell's "dismissal" was justified and that he (Osler) "only knows one side of the affair . . . there is much you do not know regarding the result of the enquiry."[34] There is an interesting phrase in this correspondence which says that Campbell visited Macdonald, and they discussed the subject, and Campbell "realised where she had done wrong" but without any further clarification.[37] Perhaps this relates to what Campbell wrote to Osler in that she had reported officers who were drunk and asked Gorrell to reprimand them (which he did not). She was also accused by three nurses of being "cruel and undermined their health." Campbell also mentioned that Nancy Astor enlarged her net of conspirators by enlisting the help of the Chaplain, asking him if the Matron "was in love" with Gorrell. Campbell believed that "the vulgar story was started by Mrs. Phipps, Mrs. Vidal and Mrs. Astor."[35] (Mrs. Phipps was Nancy Astor's sister and Mrs. Vidal was the Home Sister at the hospital). It could be that Osler was "blind" or overlooked the interference, attitude, and machinations of Nancy Astor to those working in the hospital because of his long and close relationship with her. She polarised people and it is not surprising that later the Nazis also hated Nancy Astor. Her name was on the Gestapo list to be captured if Germany invaded England.[2] There is little doubt that there was constant tension between the owners of Cliveden and the military/medical staff which erupted in accusations and revenge. One could speculate that Campbell, a senior decorated nurse, stood up to Nancy Astor which led to personal conflict.

Fallout from the Bruce Report

Matron Campbell was "transferred" from the DCCRCH, went on leave, and was later re-assigned to the Canadian Red Cross Special Hospital at Buxton, Derbyshire on 19 October 1916. On 11 February 1917 she returned to frontline active service with No. 1 Canadian General Hospital, Etaples, in France. She was again mentioned in dispatches and when the hospital was bombed by the enemy in 1918, Edith Campbell was awarded the Military Medal.

Gorrell was replaced in September 1916. He was admitted to Queen Alexandra Military Hospital, London, on 16 December 1916 and discharged 11 days later with the diagnosis "functional" paralysis of his legs. Several days later, he committed suicide by taking hydrocyanic or prussic acid.[9,36] Osler was so distressed with the CAMC "crisis" that he quietly resigned from his position at DCCRCH, but later retracted it at the request of Carleton Jones.

The Times reported that Colonel Bruce advised a complete reorganization of the Canadian Medical Service was required and the blame was attributed to the Director of Medical Service Surgeon General Carleton Jones. Hughes was relieved of his position after making some controversial statements based on the report to businessmen. His successor, Sir George Perley (1857–1938), set up a Special Board to enquire into the Bruce report. It advised an "unequivocal" reversal of the Bruce report. The work of the Surgeon General was praised, and he was reinstated.[37]

While Osler was quite clearly feeling wretched about the war, he continued to consult and promote scholarly efforts with his colleagues in the thick of managing wounded and damaged soldiers.[38] Letters from Lady Osler indicate his despondent mood from the beginning of hostilities. The negative disruption to the CAMC created by Sir Sam Hughes for political gain darkened his mood further. It was shortly after the "Taplow Affair" that Revere Osler had his wish and joined the British Royal Artillery. He was given a ticket to the Somme in October 1916 and by August 1917 he was dead. Osler sustained his commitment to the DCCRCH and elsewhere through the remainder of the war, but in March 1918 Harvey Cushing noted that "the poor man is a shadow of his former self . . ."[2, ii: 595]

Osler witnessed colleagues, themselves reputable military personnel, made scapegoats to appease overseas bureaucrats. Whilst this incident occurred over a century ago, we can still learn from the "Taplow Affair."

Subsequent history of the hospital

After WW1, the DCCRCH at Cliveden was dismantled and recycled. It was offered to the Public Health Committee of the Birmingham City Council who accepted the hospital and its equipment and transported it to Birmingham.[39] There are no known artefacts remaining from the original DCCRCH other than photographs. However, the covered tennis court which temporarily housed the first injured soldiers to arrive at Cliveden still exists as a large two-storey brick building which is in use by local enthusiasts for competition tennis.

In the Second World War, Waldorf Astor again offered Cliveden estate to the Canadians. The new hospital was funded by the Canadian Red Cross, and designed to be more structurally sound, modern, and larger, and was named "Canadian Red Cross Memorial Hospital."

In 1942 the Astors donated the entire Cliveden estate to the National Trust, with the proviso that the Astor family could live there as long as they wished.[40] The hospital was donated to the Government after the war and consequently became part of the National Health Service. It housed a large maternity unit (said to have delivered 60,000 babies) and a special hospital for paediatric rheumatology under Professor Bywaters and Dr. Barbara Ansell who worked there in the 1960s and made it famous. The repurposing of the hospital as a research unit in a limited medical field would have had the approval of Osler. It offered critical thought, the expansion of knowledge and clinical teaching, all of which were close to his heart.

The hospital was closed in 1985 and became a derelict site frequented by urban archaeologists. The National Trust sold part of the land for redevelopment. There is now, in place of the hospital, an over-55s residential development known as Cliveden Gages in Cliveden Village, with a commemorative stone.[41]

Within the grounds of Cliveden Gages lays the history of the establishment of a WW1 hospital and research centre, in which the "Taplow Affair" occurred causing the temporary humiliation of Canada's most distinguished army Matron, Edith Campbell, the suicide of a Lieutenant-Colonel, and aggravated Osler's miseries during the War.

References

1. Osler GR. Letter to Thomas Archibald Malloch, 19 November 1916. CUS417/122.50, William Osler Letter Index, Osler Library of the History of Medicine, McGill University; Cushing H. *The Life of Sir William Osler.* Oxford: Clarendon Press; 1925; ii: 539.
2. Livingstone N. *The Mistresses of Cliveden.* London: Arrow Books; 2015.
3. Anonymous. About Men and Women. *Islington Daily Gazette and North London Tribune*, 16 June 1908: 3.
4. Anonymous. Annotations: Tuberculosis and the National Insurance Bill. *Lancet* 1911; 178(4585): 169–170.
5. Bliss M. *William Osler: A Life in Medicine.* Oxford: Oxford University Press; 1999: 406
6. Anonymous. The Duchess of Connaught Canadian Red Cross Hospital. *British Journal of Nursing* 1915; 54: 320–321.
7. Archives and Library Canada. War Diaries—15th Canadian Field Hospital (Duchess of Connaught Red Cross Hospital).1915/07/01–1919/05/31.
8. Duchess of Connaught Canadian Red Cross Hospital. *British Medical Journal* 1915; 2(2861): 655.
9. Roland CG. Gorrell, Charles Wilson Farran. *Dictionary of Canadian Biography.* Toronto: University of Toronto, 1998.
10. Anonymous. The Duchess of Connaught Hospital. *Lancet* 1915; 185(4730): 730.
11. McDiarmid G. The story of Matron Edith Campbell's Three WW1 Real Photo Post Cards (RPPC). *The Official Journal of British North America Philatelic Society* 2013; 70: 34.
12. Osler W. Letter to Harvey Cushing, 4 March 1916. CUS417/52.106, William Osler Letter Index, Osler Library of the History of Medicine, McGill University.
13. Beckett A and Harvey EJ. No. 3 Canadian General Hospital (McGill) in the Great War: service and sacrifice. *Canadian Journal of Surgery* 2018; 61: 8–12.
14. Anonymous. Cliveden. *The Sketch*, 17 February 1917: 121.
15. Mann S. *The War Diary of Clare Gass 1915–1918.* Montreal & Kingston: McGill-Queen's University Press, 2016.
16. Anonymous. Prevention of tuberculosis. Meeting of County Care Committee. *Oxfordshire Weekly News*, 31 July 1918.
17. Atkinson WS. An Osler memorandum. *Journal of the American Medical Association* 1970; 211: 2018–2018.
18. Procter AP. Three cases of concussion aphasia: treatment by general anaesthesia. *Lancet* 1915; 186(4809): 977.
19. Osler W. Transient attacks of aphasia and paralysis in states of high blood pressure and arteriosclerosis. *Canadian Medical Association Journal* 1911; 1: 919–926.
20. Osler W. Transient aphasia and paralyses in states of high blood pressure and arteriosclerosis. *Lancet* 1911; 178(4602): 1349.
21. MacPhail SA. *The Medical Services. Official History of the Canadian Forces in the Great War 1914–1919.* Ottawa: FA Acland; 1925.
22. Mewburn FH. Observations on lesions of peripheral nerves; with special reference to pre-operative and post-operative treatment 1919. *Medical Quarterly* (Ottawa) 1: 279–294.

23. Commonwealth War Graves Commission. *Cliveden War Cemetery*. www .cwgc.org/find-a-cemetery/cemetery/36350/cliveden%20war%20 cemetery, accessed 8 December 2018.

24. Anonymous. Telegram from Sister, Canadian Hosp. Taplow to William Osler, 29 September 1916. CUS 417/2.16 William Osler Letter Index, Osler Library of the History of Medicine, McGill University.

25. Bernier J-R, McAlister VC. The Canadian Army Medical Corps affair of 1916 and Surgeon General Guy Carleton Jones. *Canadian Journal of Surgery* 2018; 61: 85–87.

26. Osler W. Letter to Sam Hughes, 24 September 1916. CUS 417/2.18, William Osler Letter Index, Osler Library of the History of Medicine, McGill University.

27. Osler W. Letter to Robert Borden, n.d. 1916. CUS 417/2.22, William Osler Letter Index, Osler Library of the History of Medicine, McGill University.

28. Osler W. Letter to Edith Campbell,12 October 1916. CUS 417/2.25, William Osler Letter Index, Osler Library of the History of Medicine, McGill University.

29. Glassford SC. *Mobilizing Mercy: A History of the Canadian Red Cross.* Montreal and Kingston, Ontario: McGill-Queen's University Press; 2017.

30. Campbell E. Letter to Sir William Osler, [n.d. 1917]. CUS 417/2.48, William Osler Letter Index, Osler Library of the History of Medicine, McGill University.

31. Stanley B. Boudoir Gossip. *Pall Mall Gazette*, 13 March 1917: 8.

32. Davies JM. *A Very Haven of Peace: The Role of the Stately Home Hospital in First World War Britain*. PhD thesis, University of Kent; 2017.

33. Anonymous. Mrs Astor and a soldier: plea for a Canadian whom she drove to Church. *Daily Gazette for Middlesborough*, 18 August 1916: 3.

34. Macdonald MC. Letter to William Osler, 17 October 1916. CUS417/2.32, William Osler Letter Index, Osler Library of the History of Medicine, McGill University.

35. Campbell E. Letter to William Osler, 30 December 1916. CUS417/2.45, William Osler Letter Index, Osler Library of the History of Medicine, McGill University.

36. Reid NC. *Canada's Great War Album*. Canada: HarperCollins; 2014.

37. Anonymous. Canadian Medical Service. *The Medical Press and Circular* 1917; 154: 24.

38. Osler GR. Letter to Mr Jonah, 10 November 1916. CUS417/56.48, William Osler Letter Index, Osler Library of the History of Medicine, McGill University.

39. Anonymous. Cliveden hospital. *Western Morning News*, 9 June 1919: 8.

40. Anonymous. Cliveden, Buckinghamshire, England. *Geni*, www.geni.com/ projects/Cliveden-Buckinghamshire- England/29066, accessed 6 January 2019.

41. Partridge C. Life is greener on the retirement side for village people. *The Observer.* 3 June 2007: 2.

"A Servant to his Brethren": Osler's Impact on Maryland MedChi and the University of Maryland School of Medicine

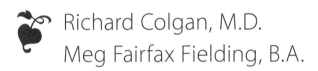

Richard Colgan, M.D.
Meg Fairfax Fielding, B.A.

Perhaps the greatest legacy William Osler has left to practicing physicians was in demonstrating, by how he has lived his life, how to care carefully with both competence and compassion.[1–3] Also well chronicled is William Osler's impact on the Johns Hopkins Hospital and School of Medicine. What is less well known however, are his relationships elsewhere in Baltimore—specifically at the University of Maryland School of Medicine and at the Medical and Chirurgical Faculty of the State of Maryland (the Maryland state medical society, commonly known then as the Faculty, and now known as the MedChi). His impact on the rest of Baltimore, and indeed on the medical profession in Maryland, were considerable as evinced by a commemorative bulletin published by the Faculty in 1920 after Osler's death.[4] Here, we review a few of Osler's specific influences.

Presented at the forty-fifth annual meeting of the American Osler Society, Baltimore, Maryland, on 28 April 2015 (Dr. Colgan), and at forty-eighth annual meeting of the American Osler Society, Pittsburgh, Pennsylvania, 14 May 2018 (Ms. Fielding). Portions of this paper were previously published in *Maryland Medicine* (2015; 16[3]: 31, 33), and are reproduced with permission.

Maryland MedChi, John Ruhräh and Marcia Crocker Noyes

John Ruhräh (1872–1935) (Figure 1), a leading pediatrician who became an accomplished amateur medical historian, remembered Osler especially for promoting medical libraries.[5] When Osler came to Baltimore, the Faculty's library was housed in the basement of the Old Maryland Historical Society Building on St. Paul Street. The library was described as not dead at that time, not moribund, but asleep. Osler succeeded in waking it and having the library moved to a remodeled dwelling on North Eutaw Street. Ruhräh quotes Osler: "A physician who does not use books and journals, who does not need a library, who does not read one or two of the best weeklies and monthlies, soon sinks to the level of the cross-counter prescriber, and not alone in practice, but in those mercenary feelings and habits which characterize a trade."

Ruhräh also credits Osler with initiating the Faculty's Book and Journal Club, writing: "With the small dues of five dollars a year a group of over one hundred men were induced to join this club, the meetings of which under Dr. Osler were a delight to all book lovers. This ability to get men out to meetings and to get them interested in things was one of his very marked traits and he succeeded because he knew so well how to deal with the human being."

Ruhräh attended the College of Physicians & Surgeons in Baltimore, but he did his clinical work at Johns Hopkins at Dr. William Osler's open clinics.

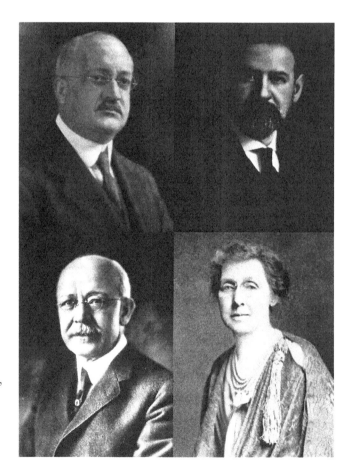

Figure 1.   Clockwise from upper left: John Ruhräh (1872–1935), Harry Friedenwald (1864–1950), Marcia Crocker Noyes (1869–1946), and Hiram Woods (1857–1931).
Credits: The MedChi, The Maryland State Medical Society (Ruhräh), National Library of Medicine (Friedenwald and Woods), and Wikipedia (Noyes).

He became a huge fan of Osler's in part because of their mutual love of books, which led to their work with the Medical Library Association (MLA). Osler served as president of the MLA and Ruhräh as Treasurer. Osler acquired books from around the world and donated many to the Faculty. His generosity knew no limit. When Osler found the library, it had a few thousand books, mostly old, and some journals. When he left, it had some 14,500 books—becoming one of the most important collections in the country.

Both belonged to the Faculty's Book & Journal Club, established by Osler. When Osler left for England, Ruhräh succeeded him as head of the Faculty's Library Committee. Ruhräh and others worked to keep Osler's memory alive. Ruhräh, who never enjoyed good health, began to write his recollections of his time with Dr. Osler, focusing on Osler's personal library with its collection of rare medical books. Shortly before his death in 1934, Ruhräh completed a short biography of Osler and submitted it to the publisher. Because of his death, it was not published and languished in a file at the Faculty for more than 80 years, when it was rediscovered and published as originally written, complete with the photographs Ruhräh originally specified.

Francis R. Packard (1870–1950) remembered Osler for urging an appreciation of the history of medicine: "The great increase in the publication of books and articles on medical history which has taken place in this country during the last twenty or thirty years, is undoubtedly largely due to his influence." Dr. Packard cites specifically *Index Medicus* and the *Catalogue of the Library of the Surgeon General* as "two great indices of medical literature in which he took such a profound and vital interest. Packard adds: "Osler was no dry as dust medical historian . . . No man ever possessed a more profound love of literature nor a more eclectic taste."

Osler was president of the Faculty during 1896–1897. His presidential address dealt with the need for physicians to get together to enjoy each other's company and to exchange ideas as a remedy to the stress of everyday practice.

Ruhräh wrote: "Osler believed in professional harmony and more that anyone who ever lived in Baltimore to secure it. What is more remarkable, he succeeded. Professional relations were less bitter during his residence there than ever before, or since." He would not listen to gossip nor speak ill of anyone. His jokes were always kindly, according to Joseph Pratt (1872–1956). "He never willingly hurt a brother's feeling, and all men were his brothers. He would never allow anyone to censure in his presence a fellow practitioner of medicine."[5]

Harry Friedenwald (1864–1950) (Figure 1), an eminent Baltimore ophthalmologist, summarized the extent to which Osler was loved by his colleagues in Baltimore and throughout Maryland: "Never has the medical profession of this city felt the loss of one of its members more keenly, never has the whole community shown greater respect and honor and love for the dead. How is it that his being here for only a short time, his almost comet like presence among us, should have impressed and influenced us so profoundly? We felt near to him, each one of us, we loved him as we have loved none other."

During his Baltimore period, and continuing after his departure from North America, Osler gave much of his time, talent, and treasury to the Medical and Chirurgical Faculty of Maryland. Under Osler's influence the Faculty became a model for other state medical societies to follow, and its library a gathering place for Maryland physicians.

The Faculty cherished his memory in 1920 with a special commemorative bulletin conveying the extent to which they had embraced the Canadian as one of their own.[4] The ophthalmologist Hiram Woods (1857–1931) (Figure 1) wrote in that issue: "I have asked myself what were Dr. Osler's basic thoughts and principles in his work for, and devotion to, the State Medical Society?" Woods then answered his own question: "How many of us have met him browsing around in the library, and soon found ourselves just talking! It was from one such talk that I took away definite impressions about the evils of narrow specialism. . . . We would sometimes find him in deep conversation with a beginner in medicine, or a man we hardly knew, and we shied off. It was perfectly clear what he was doing. . . . The comradeship was the real thing; there was nothing professorial about it."

The renowned Faculty medical librarian, Marcia Crocker Noyes (1869–1946) quoted Osler: "For the general practitioner a well-used library is one of the few correctives of the premature senility which is so apt to overtake him. Self-centered, self-taught, he leads a solitary life, and unless his everyday experience is controlled by careful reading or by the attrition of a medical society it soon ceases to be of the slightest value and becomes a mere accretion of isolated facts, without correlation."

As a young librarian in Baltimore, Marcia Noyes was personally hired by Dr. Osler in 1896 to run the Faculty's library, which was in a pitiful state. Although she lacked any medical training or indeed, even knowledge, Osler realized that Noyes had many other skills which would serve her, and the Faculty, well. Over the next nine years, Noyes and Osler accomplished much together, including founding the MLA, establishing a medical lending library, and setting the groundwork for a new Faculty headquarters and library.

Osler and Noyes sustained their friendship after Osler left Baltimore for Oxford. Noyes oversaw the opening of the Faculty's new building in 1909, expanded the library's collection to more than 65,000 volumes, organized the Book & Journal Club meetings, and remained a leading force at the MLA for several more decades.

At her funeral in 1946, held in Osler Hall at the Faculty where she had spent 50 years, it was said that Miss Noyes created a created a reality of the hopes and dreams Dr. Osler formulated while he was at Hopkins. On this foundation, she worked constantly, before and after Osler left Baltimore, as his understudy.

From Montreal, Osler's nephew, William Willoughby Francis (1879–1959), sent the following telegram: "Well done good and faithful Sister Marcia. Farewell to Osler's earliest, from his latest librarian."

Noyes and Ruhräh, who were close friends, edited the MLA's Bulletin from 1911 to 1926 and had a similar sense of humor as Dr. Osler. Fond letters between the three of them are a testament to their friendship.

After Osler departed from Baltimore, a movement took place to buy his house at 1 West Franklin Street and convert it into a memorial and library building. A considerable amount of money was raised and turned over to the Building Committee of the Faculty. It was eventually decided to use the funds for a new building at 1211 Cathedral Street. The largest meeting room in the new building was named Osler Hall. This building was dedicated in 1909, and Osler, on a return trip to the U.S., delivered one of the addresses there, entitled "Old and New."

The Faculty's 1920 special commemorative bulletin contains additional examples of how its members had Osler, and how Osler had improved medicine in Maryland. For example, Osler worked hard to strengthen the requirements for medical licensure. His efforts and those of others prompted legislation stipulating the appointment of medical examiners who would then grant licenses to practice. Osler also worked toward promoting fellowship amongst physicians. Edward N.

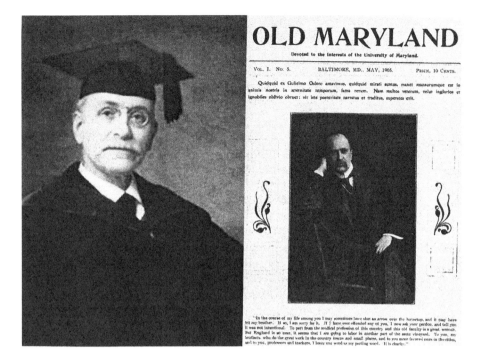

Figure 2. Eugene Fauntleroy Cordell (1943–1913); Cover of the 1905 issue of *Old Maryland*, featuring William Osler on the cover to observe his departure from Baltimore and North America.
Credits: University of Maryland School of Medicine (Cordell).

Brush (1852–1933) noted: "He so regulated his work that he always had a certain amount of time to give to his friends in social converse, or in conference over the more serious things of their everyday lives and work."

Archival records from the Faculty document how this vanguard medical society recognized Osler for his comradeship, for his promoting attendance at meetings, and for promoting medical libraries in Maryland elsewhere. Common themes in these records include Osler's wise and thoughtful advice, his cheerful disposition, and his sense of humor.

Eugene F. Cordell and the University of Maryland School of Medicine

Little is known about the relationship between William Osler and the University of Maryland School of Medicine, aside from the relationship with his friend and colleague, Eugene Fauntleroy (1943–1913) (Figure 2).

Cordell, the University of Maryland's first librarian and a prolific editor, founded a publication entitled *Old Maryland* in 1905 and continued until his death in 1914. *Old Maryland* featured many entries about Osler, including reviews of several of his works such as "After Twenty-Five Years" and cites an admonition by Osler on what to read: "The Religio Medici, one of the great English classics, should be in the hands——in the heart too—of every medical student." One of the reviews notes Osler's "charming" essay on "Science and Immortality." Another describes "Oslerism—a Review": "There is in press and will be early published a collection of medical aphorisms gathered from the bedside teaching of Dr. Osler, while Professor of medicine in Baltimore, by two of his pupils."

Osler's farewell address, "Unity, Peace and Concord." was summarized in *Old Maryland*, noting Osler's opinion that medicine is the only worldwide profession. The May 1905 issue of *Old Maryland* featured Osler on its cover. Future issues contained excerpts and enthusiastic reviews of Osler's addresses.

In 1904, Cordell founded the Library and Historical Society of the University of Maryland. Osler attended the inaugural meeting at the old medical building later known as Davidge Hall. Several hundred students and members of the Faculties of the various departments, along with guests, were present. "Much enthusiasm was exhibited." *Old Maryland* notes that Osler was "warmly welcomed" as a keynote speaker on December 20, 1904. It was reported that "Dr. Osler rose, amid the cheers of the audience . . . [and] spoke beautifully and impressively of his subject. . . . The meeting was in every way a great success and will doubtlessly be long remembered by those present, especially the students."

After his departure from Baltimore, Osler continued to receive the publication. A letter written by Osler, which he wrote from Oxford, was printed in *Old Maryland* under the headline: Dr. William Osler writes from 13 Norham Gardens, Oxford. It reads: "So glad to hear the centennial movement is prospering. How satisfactory to have a History on hand. We have just moved into this house, and I am getting my books unpacked. Many thanks for the Old Maryland, which I read with great interest."

Cordell, who may have been William Osler's principal link to the University of Maryland School of Medicine, was perhaps the first person in the U.S. to hold a professorship in medical history. Several sources, including from the University of Maryland School of Medicine, Maryland's MedChi as well as highly respected international medical journals described his impact on medicine.[6-8] He was also known in Baltimore and elsewhere as a practicing physician, medical educator, medical historiographer, and public servant.

Cordell was born in Charleston, Virginia (which became Charleston, West Virginia, after the western part of the state of Virginia, whose population was sharply divided over the issue of secession, seceded from the Confederate state of Virginia). He attended Virginia Military Institute, and between 1861 and 1865 served in the Army of the Confederate States of America. In 1866 he entered the University of Maryland Medical School, from which he graduated in 1868. He practiced medicine in Baltimore, taught medicine at his alma mater, and held many roles in MedChi.

Cordell was an early advocate for higher standards for applicants to medical school and for medical education. To that end he organized meetings of local medical schools. These efforts led to lengthening medical education from two to three years. Cordell's model for convening medical educators from various schools was replicated regionally and nationally, and thus played a part in the founding of the Association of American Medical Colleges in 1876.

In 1903, upon his retirement from practice and teaching, Cordell was named "Honorary Professor of Medical History and Librarian in the Medical School." In this capacity he created a new periodical entitled Old Maryland to celebrate his home institution and wrote a *Historical Sketch of the University of Maryland, 1807–1907* to mark its centenary.

Their mutual interest in medical libraries, the classics, medical education, and historical research naturally led to a close friendship between Cordell and Osler, and it is likely that their initial bond came through their joint commitment to promoting the library of the Medical and Chirurgical Faculty of Medicine of Maryland. Cordell was director of the library for many years and served as president of the state medical society in 1903–1904. In 1903 he brought out an

899-page history of the society, entitled *The Medical Annals of Maryland, 1799–1899*, an effort that was funded largely through Osler's support. The book was reviewed as "a model which may be followed to advantage by other medical organizations."

In a preface to his "Medical and Other Notes," Cordell wrote: "Dedicated to my friend and benefactor Dr. William Osler, *Exemplar vitae morunue* (a model of life and habits) to whom Baltimore owes a debt which words cannot express for his unselfish public spirit, his inspiring leadership and his glorious example. He has banished discord from our ranks, has created in us new and higher aspirations and has ennobled our lives."

Osler, in turn, thought so highly of Cordell that he led efforts to raise funds for a portrait of Cordell to hang in the Maryland medical school. Upon the unveiling of this portrait, Osler wrote to Cordell: You know my dear Cordell, how much I have always appreciated your devoted and unselfish labors. You have done a great work for us—and one that will be remembered by coming generations."

While still at the University of Maryland, Cordell suffered a cerebral embolism and died on August 27, 1913. Upon his death, the following acknowledgement was published in the Medical and Chirurgical Faculty of Maryland's bulletin: "No man connected with the University of Maryland has done more for its advancement, and no man connected with its work in the –past will live longer in its future life."

An unsigned obituary of Cordell in the *British Medical Journal* may well have been written by Osler. it reads in part: "Dr. Eugene Fauntleroy Cordell . . . was a man of remarkable gifts, which he used unselfishly for the benefit of his fellows. . . . Dr. Cordell had a lofty ideal of his profession regarding scientific and literary culture. His ethical standard was of the highest, and in his life, he was an example of the best type of physician."

References

1. Bliss W. *William Osler: A Life in Medicine.* New York: Oxford University Press; 1999.
2. Bryan CS. *Osler: Inspirations from a Great Physician.* New York: Oxford University Press; 1997.
3. Bryan CS. Caring carefully: Sir William Osler on the issue of competence vs compassion in medicine, *Baylor University Medical Center Proceedings* 1999; 12: 277–284.
4. Osler Memorial Bulletin of the Medical and Chirurgical Faculty of Maryland. *The Bulletin of the Medical & Chirurgical Faculty of Maryland*, 1919–1920; 12 (May 1920).
5. Pratt JH. *A Year with Osler.* Baltimore: The Johns Hopkins Press; 1949.
6. Ashby TA. Personal reminiscences of Dr. E.F. Cordell. *Bulletin of the Medical and Chirurgical Faculty of Maryland* 1914; 6: 114–116.
7. Unsigned. *The Medical Annals of Maryland, 1799–1899* (review). *Medical Library and Historical Journal* 1913; 2(1): 64–65.
8. Dr. Eugene Fauntleroy Cordell. *British Medical Journal* 1913; 2(2757): 1189.

Bloodletting in Osler's Textbook, With Emphasis on Pneumonia

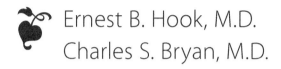 Ernest B. Hook, M.D.
Charles S. Bryan, M.D.

In the first edition of *The Principles and Practice of Medicine* (1892), William Osler endorsed unequivocally, systemic bloodletting by venesection for nine conditions, in selected cases. Michael Bliss, Osler's most recent biographer, calls bloodletting Osler's "blind spot."[1] Our purpose is to review aspects of Osler's recommendations for bloodletting, with special emphasis on pneumonia.

Background

Before the introduction of methods of blood-vessel puncture without incision, as with a hollow needle, connecting tube, and receptacle around 1907, bloodletting was done by cutting into a blood vessel as with a lancet (venesection usually, but occasionally arteriotomy); by the application of leeches; or by a process known as wet cupping, which involved making many small superficial cuts in the skin (scarification) and then applying a vacuum as with suction cups. ("Dry" cupping involved drawing serous fluid or pus away from an area without prior scarification.

Presented in part at the forty-third annual meeting of the American Osler Society, Tucson, Arizona, on 8 April 2013 (EBH); at the forty-fifth annual meeting of the American Osler Society, Baltimore, Maryland, on 27 April 2015 (EBH); and at the thirty-seventh annual meeting of the American Osler Society, Montreal Quebec, on 2 May 2007 (CSB). Portions of this paper were previously published in the *Baylor University Medical Center Proceedings* (2019; 32[3]: 372–376) (CSB) and are reproduced with permission.

Figure 1. Studies conducted between 1828 and 1835 by Pierre-Charles-Alexander-Louis (1787–1872) (left) raised questions about the efficacy of bloodletting. Addresses and essays by William Orlando Markham (1818–1891) (right) clarified the main benefit of bloodletting to be relief of heart failure. *Credit:* Wikimedia Commons (Louis); Wellcome Collection CC BY (Markham).

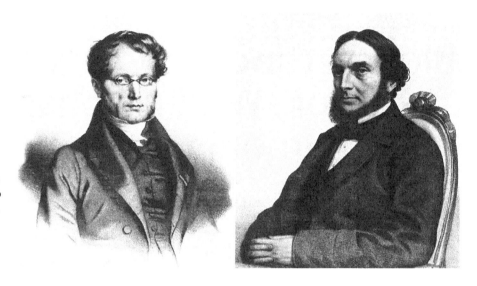

The unmodified term "cupping" always meant "wet" cupping to draw blood.)[2,3] The discussion here will concern primarily systemic bloodletting intended to alter a disease process. Osler did not use the term "systemic bloodletting" but referred instead to "venesection," "free venesection," or "free bleeding."

The rich historiography of therapeutic bloodletting lends to opposing narratives.[4,5] Bloodletting for some epitomizes the dangers of yesteryear's "heroic" style of medicine. Others, including many medical historians, suggest doctors bled because it sometimes worked and that over time bleeding became more "rational." The early decades of the nineteenth century marked what the medical historian Fielding H. Garrison called a "prow-wave of extensive and intensive bloodletting,"[6] especially in France and the US, but beginning around 1830 bleeding was gradually abandoned for most conditions.[7,8] Historians often credit Pierre-Charles-Alexandre Louis (1787–1872) (Figure 1) for stemming the tide of excessive bleeding by applying his "numerical method" (statistics) to venesection,[9] but Louis did not abandon bloodletting for what he termed deep-seated inflammatory processes. It remained for William Orlando Markham (1818–1891) (Figure 1), a Scottish-born physician practicing in London, to point out in 1864 that venesection had 'no directly beneficial influence over inflammation" and that the major benefit of bleeding was relief of what we now call heart failure—a term that did not come into wide use until the twentieth century.[10,11] Therapeutic phlebotomy for heart failure, especially for acute pulmonary edema, makes eminent sense in the absence of potent diuretics, as was the case until 1919 when mercurial diuretics were introduced.[12]

In 1964 one of us (CSB) reported an analysis of recommendations for systemic bloodletting in textbooks of medicine available to US physicians and published between 1830 and 1892 (the latter date chosen as the year Osler brought out his textbook) and has now updated these data to include 14 representative US textbooks of medicine published between 1830 and 2004 (Figure 2).[13,14] As shown in Figure 2, recommendations for venesection were abandoned in textbooks between 1830 and 1892 for acute meningitis, nephritis, and peritonitis—conditions for which today there is no good rationale. Bleeding was retained for acute pulmonary edema. Bleeding was also retained for cerebral hemorrhage—notably, subarachnoid hemorrhage accompanied by severe hypertension—as a

Figure 2.
Recommendations for systemic bloodletting for nine selected indications (chosen for consistency of nomenclature) according to 15 selected US textbooks of medicine published between 1830 and 2004. The methods for rating the strength of recommendation of bloodletting on a zero to four scale (that is, "never" to "most cases") are shown in the Appendix to a previous article.[13]

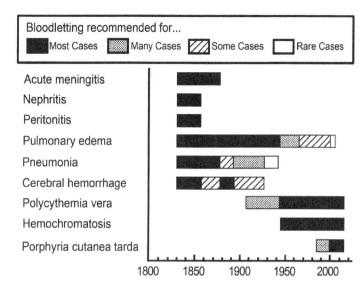

method for lowering blood pressure rapidly. Bleeding for pneumonia, discussed more fully below, was controversial.

Osler's recommendations for bloodletting in the first edition of *The Principles and Practice of Medicine* (1892)

Osler never wrote a separate article on bloodletting, and it appears that his recommendations reflect a synthesis of then-current opinion and his own experience and judgment. The first edition of his textbook endorsed venesection without qualification for nine conditions (Table 1).[15] He described symptoms and signs of heart failure in six of the disorders noted in Table 1: chronic valvular heart disease, arterio-sclerosis, cardiac hypertrophy and dilatation, thoracic aortic aneurysm with dyspnea, pulmonary edema, and emphysema with "great engorgement of the veins" [cor pulmonale]. We can appreciate today why bloodletting would relieve heart failure in these conditions.[12] In cerebral hemorrhage, Osler's rationale was "to reduce the arterial pressure," a mechanism confirmed in 1901 by Osler's friend and colleague Harvey Cushing (1869–1939).[16,17]

Osler's mention of venesection for heatstroke may puzzle some twenty-first-century readers. Note that he recommended it when "the symptoms are those of intense asphyxia, and in which death may take place in a few minutes." Pulmonary edema is a well-recognized complication of heatstroke, "occasional" or "common" according to different authors, and therefore bloodletting might help in carefully selected situations.[18–23]

Osler's discussions of bloodletting for these eight conditions remained essentially unchanged during the editions of the textbook written during his lifetime. In the eighth (1912) edition, he added polycythemia vera (erythræmia or Vaquez' disease), a disease he had helped characterize and now sometimes called Osler-Vaquez disease,[24] as an indication "when there is much fullness in the head and vertigo." Pneumonia was the only indication for bloodletting for which he altered the text significantly in sequential editions of *The Principles and Practice of Medicine* (Table 2) and will be discussed separately.

Table 1. Indications and rationale for systemic bloodletting (venesection) for nine disorders in the first edition of *The Principles and Practice of Medicine* (1892), by William Osler

Disorder	Indication and/or Rationale
Chronic valvular heart disease (p. 624)	"In cases of dilatation, from whatever cause, whether in mitral or aortic lesion or distention of the right ventricle in emphysema, when signs of venous engorgement are marked and when there is orthopnœa with cyanosis, the abstraction of from twenty to thirty ounces of blood is indicated. This is the condition in which timely venesection may save the patient's life. It is the condition in which I have had most satisfactory results from venesection. It is done much better early than late. I have on several occasions regretted its postponement, particularly in instances of acute dilatation and cyanosis in connection with emphysema . . . For illustrative cases from my wards, see paper by H.A. Lafleur *Medical News* July 1891"
Arterio-sclerosis (p. 670)	"In cases which come under observation for the first time with dyspnœa, slight lividity, and signs of cardiac insufficiency, venesection is indicated. In some instances, with very high tension, striking relief is afforded by the abstraction of twenty ounces of blood."
Cardiac hypertrophy and dilatation (p. 640)	". . . with signs of dilatation, as indicated by gallop rhythm, urgent dyspnœa, and slight lividity, venesection is in many cases the only means by which the life of the patient may be saved, and from twenty-five to thirty ounces of blood should be abstracted without delay."
Thoracic aneurism [aneurysm] (pp. 679–680)	"Pressure on veins causing engorgement, particularly of the head and arms, is sometimes promptly relieved by free venesection, and at any time during the course of a thoracic aneurism, if attacks of dyspnœa with lividity supervene, bleeding may be resorted to with great benefit. . . . Dyspnœa, if associated with cyanosis, is best relieved by bleeding."
Pulmonary edema (p. 506)	"The treatment of œdema of the lung is practically that of the condition with which it is associated. In the acute cases active catharsis, and, if there is cyanosis, free venesection should be resorted to."
Emphysema (p. 549)	"Patients who come into the hospital in a state of urgent dyspnœa and lividity, with great engorgement of the veins, particularly if they are young and vigorous, should be bled freely. On more than one occasion I have saved the lives of persons in this condition with venesection."
Cerebral hemorrhage (p. 882)	"The patient should be placed with head high, and measures immediately taken to reduce the arterial pressure. Of these the most rapid and satisfactory is venesection, which should be practiced whenever the arterial tension is much increased."
Sunstroke (heatstroke) (p. 1018)	"In the cases in which the symptoms are those of intense asphyxia, and in which death may take place in a few minutes, free bleeding should be practiced, a procedure which saved Weir Mitchell when a young man."
Pneumonia (p. 530)	See text.

*Osler mentioned venesection briefly in a few other disorders without providing a rationale; for example, in hæmophilia ("Venesection has been tried in several cases" [p. 322]) and acute meningitis ("if the subject is young and full-blooded" [p. 866]).

Brief mention should be made of Osler's comments on topical bloodletting for relief of pain in lobar pneumonia and a few other conditions. In the first and second editions of his textbook he addressed the pleuritic pain of lobar pneumonia: "The first distressing symptom is usually the pain in the side, which may be relieved by local depletion—by cupping or leeching—or, better still, by a hypodermic injection of morphia." In the third edition, however, he deleted topical bloodletting and was specific about the opiate dose: "The stitch in the side

Table 2. Recommendations for systemic bloodletting both early and later during pneumonia in seventeen editions of *The Principles and Practice of Medicine* published between 1892 and 1968*

Edition (Year)	Author(s)	Recommendations for bloodletting, both early** and later† during pneumonia
1 (1892)	Osler	Early: "... a timely venesection may save a life ... [but] to be of service, it should be done early. In a full-blooded, healthy man with high fever and bounding pulse, the abstraction of from twenty to thirty ounces of blood is in every way beneficial." Late: "... in a majority of cases bleeding is now used at a late stage, when the heart is beginning to fail, the right chambers are dilated ... Though resorted to [then] rather as a forlorn hope, it is a rational practice, and, in cases of emphysema and heart-disease, proves satisfactory under identical hydraulic indications, but unfortunately, in a majority of cases of pneumonia it proves futile."
2 (1895)	Osler	Early: The same but italicizes (i.e., emphasizes) "it should be done early." Late: No change.
3 (1898)	Osler	Early: "... to bleed at the very outset in robust, healthy individuals in whom the disease sets in with great intensity and high fever is, I believe, a good practice." Late: If heart weakness is present and due to progressive distention and overfilling of the right heart "a free venesection is sometimes helpful..."
4 (1901)	Osler	No changes from the third (1898) edition.
5 (1902)	Osler	No changes from the third (1898) edition.
6 (1905)	Osler	Early: No change. Late: There is now no comment on bloodletting later in course.
7 (1909)	Osler	No changes from the sixth (1905) edition).
8 (1912)	Osler ("with the assistance of ... McCrae")	Early: No change. Late: "Late in the course marked dilatation of the right heart is the common indication [for bleeding]. The quantity of blood removed must be decided by the effect; small amounts are often sufficient."
9 (1920)	Osler and McCrae	Early: States simply "good practice" without qualification. Late: No changes from the eighth (1912) edition.
10 (1926)	McCrae	No changes from the ninth (1920) edition.
11 (1930)	McCrae	No changes from the ninth (1920) edition.
12 (1935)	McCrae	No changes from the ninth (1920) edition.
13 (1938)	Christian	Early: No change. Late: Modified to state simply: "... small amounts are sufficient."
14 (1942)	Christian	Early: "... to bleed at the outset in robust, healthy individuals in whom the disease sets in with great intensity and high fever is, possibly still good practice." [Emphasis added.] Late: No change from the thirteenth (1938) edition.
15 (1944)	Christian	No changes from the fourteenth (1942) edition.
16 (1947)	Christian	No changes from the fourteenth (1942) edition.
17 (1968)	Harvey et al.‡ et al.	No mention of bloodletting in pneumonia.

*For bibliographical data on the textbook see Golden.[30]

**Bloodletting early in pneumonia:* Note that Osler modified the text in the third (1898) edition, but that no substantial modifications were made until the fourteenth (1942) edition when Henry Christian stated bloodletting was "possibly still" good practice.

†*Bloodletting later in pneumonia:* Observe that Osler modified the text in the third edition, but then in the sixth (1905) edition dropped discussion of bloodletting in this phase of the disorder. The ninth (1912) edition, written "with the assistance of Thomas McCrae," added "late in the course marked dilatation of the right heart is the common indication" and "[removal of] small mounts [is] often sufficient" No further changes were made during McCrae's authorship, but Henry Christian modified the text in the thirteenth (1938) edition to indicate that only "small amounts" were sufficient.

‡A multi-authored textbook edited by A. McGehee Harvey and his colleagues and written entirely by faculty members at the Johns Hopkins University School of Medicine.

at onset, which is sometimes agonizing, is best relieved by a hypodermic injection of a quarter of a grain of morphia."

Recommendations for venesection in pneumonia in the first and later editions of *The Principles and Practice of Medicine*

Accounting for the effectiveness or non-effectiveness of venesection in lobar pneumonia challenged Osler, his predecessors, his contemporaries, and his successors up until the mid-twentieth century. Alfred Lebbeus Loomis (1831–1895) opposed it in the 1885 edition of his textbook of medicine,[25] while Austin Flint (1812–1886) endorsed it in the 1894 edition of his textbook (published posthumously) and in earlier editions for cases in which there was "accumulation of blood in the cavities of the right side of the heart."[26] Here, we will review (1) Osler's recommendations for bleeding in pneumonia in the editions of his textbook published during his lifetime; (2) recommendations in editions of *The Principles and Practice of Medicine* by Thomas McCrae and Henry Christian subsequent to Osler's lifetime; and (3) papers by Osler on "The Treatment of Pneumonia" (1886) and "The Mortality of Pneumonia" (1888), which clarify his rationale for venesection in selected cases of pneumonia well before he commenced to write a textbook.

Osler distinguished between bleeding early and later in lobar pneumonia (Table 2). In the first edition of his textbook (1892), he discussed "free venesection" as follows (on page 530):

> In many cases [of lobar pneumonia] the question comes up at the onset as to the propriety of venesection. . . . During the first five decades of this century the profession bled too much, but during the last decades we have certainly bled too little. Pneumonia is one of the diseases in which a timely venesection may save life. To be of service it should be done early. In a full-blooded, healthy man with high fever and bounding pulse the abstraction of from twenty to thirty ounces of blood is in every way beneficial, relieving the pain and dyspnœa, reducing the temperature, and allaying the cerebral symptoms, so violent in some instances. Unfortunately, in a majority of the cases, bleeding is now used at a late stage in the disease, when the heart is beginning to fail, the right chambers are dilated, the face is of a dusky hue, the respirations are very rapid, and there are signs, perhaps of œdema of the uninvolved portions of the lungs. Though resorted to rather as a forlorn hope, it is a rational practice, and, in cases of emphysema and of heart-disease, proves satisfactory under identical hydraulic indications, but, unfortunately, in a majority of the cases of pneumonia it proves futile. Time and again, in such cases, have I urged free venesection, but in twelve hospital patients bled under these circumstances only one recovered.

In the second (1895) edition Osler used italics to emphasize early bleeding in selected cases of pneumonia: "Pneumonia is one of the diseases in which a timely venesection may save life. To be of service *it should be done early*."[27]

In the third (1898) edition he shortened the discussion of venesection for pneumonia writing: "We employ it nowadays much more than we did a few years ago, but more often late in the disease than early. To bleed at the very outset in robust, healthy individuals in whom the disease sets in with great intensity and high fever is, I believe a good practice. I have seen instances in which it was very beneficial in relieving the pain and dyspnœa, reducing the temperature, and allaying the cerebral symptoms."[28]

It was not until the eighth (1912) edition that it was added: "Late in the course [of lobar pneumonia] marked dilatation of the right heart is the common indication [for venesection]."[29] This edition was written "with the assistance of" Thomas McCrae (1870–1935), Osler's former resident at Hopkins, who had moved to Jefferson Medical College in Philadelphia. Osler states in the preface that McCrae revised the material on therapy. Thus, it was probably McCrae who added right-sided heart failure to the text of *The Principles and Practice of Medicine*.

One of us (EBH) tabulated recommendations for bloodletting in editions of *The Principles of Practice of Medicine* beyond Osler's lifetime (Table 2).[30] McCrae continued to endorse bloodletting for selected cases of pneumonia through the twelfth edition. When Henry A. Christian (1876–1951) assumed editorship of Osler's textbook for the thirteenth edition (1938) he made it clear that bleeding remained useful in cases with pneumonia accompanied by cyanosis and distended neck veins. Christian continued this advice through the sixteenth and last edition (1947). It was not until the seventeenth edition of *The Principles and Practice of Medicine* (1968), a multi-authored textbook edited by A. McGehee Harvey and his colleagues at the Johns Hopkins University School of Medicine, that therapeutic bloodletting was no longer recommended for lobar pneumonia. By then, potent diuretics were available to accomplish the same purpose.

Osler's 1886 and 1888 papers on pneumonia provide an informative clinical and pathological background to his comments on venesection, and show how his thinking evolved up to the time he wrote his textbook.

On 11 December 1886, Osler discussed venesection in an editorial for *The Medical News* entitled "The Treatment of Pneumonia."[31] He acknowledged Markham's conclusion that bleeding does not reduce inflammation: "So long as the disease was regarded as a local inflammation, antiphlogistic [anti-inflammatory] measures were in vogue, of which bleeding and antimony were the most important..." He discussed the 1881 discovery of the usual causative organism, now known as *Streptococcus pneumoniae*, made independently by Louis Pasteur (1822–1895) and George M. Sternberg (1838–1915). He stressed the importance of heart failure as a cause of death in pneumonia, elaborating:

> We propose to call attention to one or two practical points about which there is a wide difference of opinion among practitioners in this country. There is a tendency at present to revive venesection, and it is important to understand clearly the indications for its practice. Unquestionably, prompt and free bleeding is called for in threatened death from asphyxia *when the right heart is dilated* [emphasis added], cyanosis marked, and the pulse becoming small and rapid. The timely abstraction of sixteen to twenty ounces of blood will sometimes save life, though we must confess to some disappointment in the results, for, of five such cases observed, only one recovered. The practice of free bleeding at the onset, which is still employed by some practitioners, is not to be commended, except in rare cases.

In November 1888, the year before Osler moved to Baltimore to become professor of medicine at Johns Hopkins, he discussed venesection in pneumonia again in *The University Medical Magazine* (which later became *The University of Pennsylvania Medical Bulletin*).[32] After reviewing mortality statistics from three large hospitals—Montreal General Hospital, the Pennsylvania Hospital, and the New Orleans Charité (later Charity Hospital)—he gave some of his own observations. For example, a previously healthy 22-year-old man who died of pneumonia was found at autopsy to have "a large patch of fresh myocarditis in the septum ventriculorum" [interventricular septum]. Osler elaborated:

> I have puzzled over the cadavers of persons dead of pneumonia and asked why should this man have died? Too often the answer is the echo of the question. The cause is evident in many cases in the form of serious complications such as endocarditis and meningitis. Some years ago I was struck in the post-mortem room with the cases of young vigorous men, who had died with distended right hearts and systemic veins, though in some instances limited areas of [pulmonary] consolidation. It seemed as if the heart had failed in over-distention—asystole—and I determined, when the opportunity arose, not to let such cases die without a copious venesection. *Clinically, I think we see this condition in two different periods of the affection. There is an early cardiac embarrassment during the first few days of the disease leading to slight cyanosis; and in a later period, at the 7th—10th day, we see with increasing anxiety, the changing color, a dull suffusion, a deepening hue, then the marked cyanosis* [emphasis added]. Bleeding may be indicated at both these periods. In hospital practice we more commonly see the patients in the latter. For ten years I have practiced free bleeding to the amount of from 20 to 25 ounces in adults, and yet I have to confess disappointment in my results. I have seen but one case recover after bleeding, out of twelve or fifteen. The cases of bleeding in the late stages have been uniformly fatal. I know they [venesections] have often been performed with the patient *in extremis*, but it seems imperative to attempt to relieve an over-distended circulatory system. I know it [bleeding] does relieve the cyanosis of cardiac dilatation from other causes, but in pneumonia there are doubtless conditions other than mechanical.

From these observations it becomes clear that Osler understood the rationale for venesection in pneumonia to be relief of heart failure, predominantly right-heart failure, before he wrote *The Principles and Practice of Medicine*.

Recent observations lend further validity to Osler's recommendations for venesection in pneumonia

Several of Osler's clinical and pathological observations merit comment. His observation that there might be "œdema of the uninvolved portions of the lungs" suggests an early recognition of the acute respiratory distress syndrome (ARDS, characterized by diffuse capillary leak or permeability pulmonary edema due to lung injury or systemic inflammation).[33] His observation that bleeding often failed to relieve cyanosis in pneumonia can be attributed, at least in part, to perfusion of unventilated alveoli—hence, a high alveolar-arterial (A-a) oxygen gradient, which correlates with severity of pneumonia.[34] His emphasis on bleeding early in pneumonia resonates with the findings by Robert Austrian and Jerome Gold, since confirmed by others including one of the present authors (CSB), that much of the mortality from bacteremic pneumococcal pneumonia occurs during the first several days, irrespective of therapy.[35,36]

Osler's recognition of "hydraulic indications" for bleeding coheres with recent clinical and experimental observations pertaining to cardiac complications of pneumonia. Clinical studies, notably those by Daniel Musher and his colleagues, indicate that 19 percent to 25 percent of patients with pneumococcal pneumonia experience one or more major cardiac events, such as new or worsening heart failure, new-onset arrhythmia, or acute myocardial infarction.[37–40] A few investigators have confirmed by transthoracic echocardiography and other methods that patients with pneumonia who have elevated pulmonary artery systolic pressure and/or impairment of right-ventricular systolic function have an unfavorable prognosis.[41–44] Population-based studies suggest heart failure increases mortality from pneumonia by up to 50 percent, especially among the elderly.[45] Patients who survive hospitalization for pneumonia experience increased long-term mortality.[46,47]

Osler was intrigued by what we would now call the molecular mechanisms of pneumococcal disease. In the first edition of *The Principles and Practice of Medicine*, he devoted more than a page of discussion on (pages 513–514) to the work of two German internists, Georg Klemperer (1865–1946) and his brother Felix (1866–1932, who had recently published on a "poisonous albumen" or "pneumotoxin" produced by the pneumococcus and causing systemic effects that could be negated by an antiserum.[48] This was an early step toward serum therapy for pneumococcal pneumonia, and also toward the development of a pneumococcal vaccine.[49] Osler called these experiments "very interesting."

The effect of *Streptococcus pneumoniae* on the heart remains a lively area of research. Some conclusions from recent studies in humans, mice, and nonhuman primates include the following: (1) the pneumococcal cell wall can inhibit the contractility of heart-muscle cells (cardiomyocytes); (2) the pneumococcus can invade heart muscle (as suggested by Osler's observations at autopsy) with cytotoxic effects (causing the death of cardiomyocytes); and (3) pneumococcal infection causes scar tissue to form in the heart, leading to what cardiologists call "remodeling."[50,51] These effects result from a highly complex host-parasite interaction amenable to molecular explanations. (For example, "Pneumococcal invasion of heart tissue is dependent on the bacterial adhesion choline-binding protein A that binds to laminin receptor on vascular endothelial cells and binding of phosphorylcholine residues on pneumocccal cell wall to platelet-activating receptor."[50]) We can be certain that Osler, if alive today, would find these observations fascinating. And he would surely be grateful for drugs and other therapeutic modalities that render venesection obsolete in this setting.

Summary

Pathophysiological justification now exists for all nine of Osler's clear indications for venesection in the first edition of *The Principles and Practice of Medicine*. He endorsed venesection for treatment of heart failure in eight of these indications, and for rapid lowering of blood pressure in the remaining instance (subarachnoid hemorrhage accompanied by extreme hypertension). Pneumonia was the most problematic indication for bleeding for Osler, as it was for his predecessors and for those who succeeded him. Bleeding was still recommended for heart failure in pneumonia in the sixteenth edition (1947) of *The Principles and Practice of Medicine*, the last edition edited by Henry Christian. Recent clinical and experimental observations substantiate how venesection might be useful in selected cases of pneumonia complicated by heart failure, should one lack drugs to accomplish the same purpose. Overall, these observations lend credence to the narrative that therapeutic bleeding became more "rational" over time.

Acknowledgments

EBH thanks John T. Golden and Hector O. Ventura for providing copies of some references; J. Gordon Frierson and John A. Kastor for comments; Lily Szcyzgiel of the Osler Library of the History of Medicine, McGill University, for bibliographical advice, and Jonathan Goulian for other assistance. CSB thanks Owsei Temkin (1902–2002) for sponsoring, in 1963, a student project that prompted a career-long interest in the history of bloodletting.

References

1. Bliss M. *William Osler: A Life in Medicine.* Toronto: University of Toronto Press; 1999: 156–157.
2. Haller, JS Jr. *American Medicine in Transition,* Urbana: University of Illinois Press; 1981: 35–38.
3. Dunglison R. *Medical Lexicon: A Dictionary of Medical Science.* Philadelphia: Henry C. Lea; 1874: 281.
4. Kuriyama S. Interpreting the history of bloodletting. *Journal of the History of Medicine and Allied Sciences* 1995; 50(1): 11–46.
5. Schneeberg NG. A twenty-first century perspective on the ancient art of bloodletting. *Transactions & Studies of the College of Physician of Philadelphia* 2002; 24(December): 157–185.
6. Garrison FH. The history of bloodletting, part II. *New York Medical Journal* 1913; 97: 498–501.
7. Warner JH. *The Therapeutic Perspective: Medical Practice, Knowledge, and Identity in America, 1820–1885.* Cambridge, Massachusetts: Harvard University Press; 1986.
8. Carter KC. Change of type as an explanation for the decline of therapeutic bloodletting. *Studies in the History and Philosophy of Biological and Biomedical Sciences* 2010; 41(1): 1–11.
9. Morabia A. Pierre-Charles-Alexandre Louis and the evaluation of bloodletting. *Journal of the Royal Society of Medicine* 2006; 99(3) 158–160.
10. Markham WO. *Bleeding and Change of Type of Diseases, Being the Gulstonian Lectures for 1864.* London: John Churchill & Sons; 1866.
11. Unsigned. William Orlando Markham, M.D. Edin., F.R.C.P. Lond., F.R.C.P.I.(Hon.). *British Medical Journal* 1891; 1(1571): 323–324.
12. Ventura HO, Mehra MR. Bloodletting as a cure for dropsy: heart failure down the ages. *Journal of Cardiac Failure* 2005;11(4): 247–252.
13. Bryan LS Jr. [Bryan CS]. Blood-letting in American medicine, 1830–1892. *Bulletin of the History of Medicine* 1964; 38(6): 516–529.
14. Bryan CS. New observations support William Osler's rationale for systemic bloodletting. *Baylor University Medical Center Proceedings* 2019; 32(3): 372–376.
15. Osler W. *The Principles and Practice of Medicine.* New York: D. Appleton Company; 506, 530, 549, 624, 640, 679–680, 882, 1018.
16. Cushing H: Concerning a definite regulatory mechanism of the vasomotor centre which controls blood pressure during cerebral compression. *Bulletin of the Johns Hopkins Hospital* 1901; 12(September): 290–292.

17. Wan WH. The Cushing Response: a case for a review of its role as a physiological reflex. *Journal of Clinical Neuroscience* 2008; 15(3): 223–228.

18. Bruchim Y, Horowitz M, Aroch I. Pathophysiology of heatstroke in dogs—revisited. *Temperature* (Austin) 2017; 4(4): 356–370.

19. Zahger D, Moses A, Weiss AT. Evidence of prolonged myocardial dysfunction in heat stroke. *Chest* 1989; 95(5): 1089–1091.

20. Atar S, Rozner E, Rosenfeld T. Transient cardiac dysfunction and pulmonary edema in exertional heat stroke. *Military Medicine* 2003; 168(8): 671–673.

21. Leon LR, Helwig BG. Heat stroke: role of the systemic inflammatory response. *Journal of Applied Physiology* 2010; 109(6): 1980–1988.

22. Walter E, Venn R, Stevenson T. Exertional heat stroke: the athlete's nemesis. *Journal of the Intensive Care Society (JICS)* 2012: 13(4): 304–308.

23. Liu C-H, Wang C-C, Lin H-C, Chen I-H, Tsai M-K, Shiang J-C. Pulmonary edema complicating exertional heat stroke: a case series. *Resuscitation & Intensive Care Medicine* 2016; 1: 147–153.

24. Osler W. A clinical lecture on erythræmia (polycythæmia with cyanosis, maladie de Vaquez). *Lancet* 1908; 171(4403): 143–208.

25. Loomis AL. *A Text-book of Practical Medicine, Designed for the Use of Students and Practitioners of Medicine.* Third edition; New York: William Wood and Company; 1885: 97.

26. Flint, A. *A Treatise on the Principles and Practice of Medicine; Designed for the Use of Practitioners of Medicine.* Seventh edition revised by Henry FP. Philadelphia: Lea Brothers & Co.; 1894: 81.

27. Osler W. *The Principles and Practice of Medicine.* Second edition, New York: D. Appleton and Company; 1895: 564.

28. Osler W. *The Principles and Practice of Medicine.* Third edition, New York: D. Appleton and Company; 1898: 135.

29. Osler W. *The Principles and Practice of Medicine* Eighth edition, with the assistance of Thomas McCrae. New York: D. Appleton and Company; 1912: 99.

30. Golden RL. *A History of William Osler's* The Principles and Practice of Medicine. Osler Library Studies in the History of Medicine No. 8. Montreal: McGill University; 2004: 222–225.

31. [Osler W]. The treatment of pneumonia. *The Medical News* (Philadelphia) 1886; 49(24): 660–661.

32. Osler W. The mortality of pneumonia. *The University Medical Magazine* [University of Pennsylvania] 1888; 1(2) (November): 77–82.

33. Herrero R, Sanchez G, Lorente JA. New insights into the mechanisms of pulmonary edema in acute lung injury. *Annals of Translational Medicine* 2018; 6(2): 32. doi: 10.21037/atm.2017.12.18. Accessed 14 January 2021.

34. Moammar MQ, Azam HM, Blamoun AI, et al. Alveolar-arterial oxygen gradient, pneumonia severity index and outcomes in patients hospitalized with community acquired pneumonia. *Clinical and Experimental Pharmacology and Physiology* 2008; 35(9): 1032–1037.

35. Austrian R, Gold J. Pneumococcal pneumonia with especial reference to bacteremic pneumococcal pneumonia. *Annals of Internal Medicine* 1964; 60(5): 759–776.

36. Bryan CS, Hornung CA, Reynolds KL, Brenner ER. Endemic bacteremia in Columbia, South Carolina. *American Journal of Epidemiology* 1996; 123(1): 113–127.

37. Musher DM, Rueda AM, Kaka AS, Mapara SM. The association between pneumococcal pneumonia and acute cardiac events. *Clinical Infectious Diseases* 2007; 45(2): 158–165.

38. Corrales-Medina VF, Musher DM, Wells GA, et al. Cardiac Complications in Patients with Community-Acquired Pneumonia. Incidence, Incidence, Timing, Risk Factors, and Association with Short-Term Mortality *Circulation* 2012; 125(5): 773–781.

39. Musher DM, Abers MS, Corrals-Medina VF. Acute infection and myocardial infarction. *New England Journal of Medicine* 2019; 380(2): 171–176.

40. O'Meara ES, White M, Siscovick DS, et al. Hospitalization for pneumonia in Cardiovascular Health Study: incidence, mortality, and influence on longer-term survival. *Journal of the American Geriatrics Society* 2005; 53(7): 1108–1116.

41. Yildirim B, Biteker FS, Başaran Ö, et al. Is there a potential role for echocardiography in adult patients with CAP? *American Journal of Emergency Medicine* 2015; 33(11): 1672–1676.

42. Biteker FS, Başaran Ö, Dogan V, et al. Prognostic value of transthoracic echocardiography and biomarkers of cardiac dysfunction in community-acquired pneumonia. *Clinical Microbiology and Infection* 2016; 22: 1006e1–1006e6.

43. Streter KB, Budimir I, Golub A, et al. Changes in pulmonary artery systolic pressure correlate with radiographic severity and peripheral oxygenation in adults with community-acquired pneumonia. *Journal of Clinical Ultrasound* 2018; 46(1): 41–47.

44. See KC, Ng J, Siow WT, et al. Frequency and prognostic impact of basic critical care echocardiography abnormalities in patients with acute respiratory distress syndrome. *Ann Intensive Care* 2016; 7: 120. doi: 10.1186/s13613-017-0343-9, accessed 14 January 2021.

45. Bartlett B, Ludewick HP, Lee S, Dwivedi G. Cardiovascular complications following pneumonia: focus on pneumococcus and heart failure. *Current Opinion in Cardiology* 2019; 34(2): 233–239.

46. Kaplan V, Angus DC, Griffin MF, et al. Hospitalized community-acquired pneumonia in the elderly: age- and sex-related patterns of care and outcome in the United States. *American Journal of Respiratory and Critical Care Medicine* 2002; 165(6): 766–772.

47. Peyrani P, Arnold FW, Bordon J, et al. Incidence and mortality of adults hospitalized with community-acquired pneumonia according to clinical course. *Chest* 2020; 157(1): 34–41.

48. Klemperer G, Klemperer F. Versuche über Immunisierung und Heilung bei Pneumokokkeninfektion. *Berliner klin Wchnschrift* 1891; 28(31 August): 833–835, 869–875.

49. Grabenstein JD, Klugman KP. A century of pneumococcal vaccination research in humans. *Clinical Microbiology and Infection* 18(Supplement 5): 15–24.

50. Brown AO, Millett ERC, Quint JK, Orihuela CJ. Cardiotoxicity during invasive pneumococcal disease. *American Journal of Respiratory and Critical Care Medicine* 2015; 191(7): 739–745.

51. Reyes LF, Restrepo MI, Hinojosa CA, et al. Severe pneumococcal pneumonia causes acute cardiac toxicity and subsequent cardiac remodeling. *American Journal of Respiratory and Critical Care Medicine* 2017; 196(5): 609–620.

"Osler Warned": Was William Osler a Grave Robber While at McGill or was he a Victim (or Perpetrator) of One Final Practical Joke?

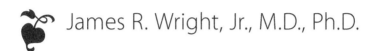 James R. Wright, Jr., M.D., Ph.D.

Bodysnatching (i.e., grave robbing or resurrectionist activities) was an illegal way to procure bodies for anatomical dissection before the existence of effective anatomy legislation. As knowledge of anatomy was fundamental to medical practice, many nineteenth-century physicians turned a blind eye to this activity as the profession benefited from it, while others, including very prominent physicians, openly admired and honored its perpetrators.[1-3]

Canada passed its first anatomy act in December 1843, a decade after the Warburton Anatomy Act in England in 1832. It was ineffective, but this did not cause major issues as there were relatively few medical students in Canada. The first medical school in Canada was the proprietary Montreal Medical Institution which was established by four physicians practicing at the Montreal General Hospital in 1823; in 1829, it evolved into the Medical Faculty of McGill College.[4] While early McGill medical students did illegally procure the dissection subjects they needed to complete their education, there appears to have been little public knowledge of this until Montreal newspaper articles began highlighting this in 1843, thus precipitating the aforementioned Canadian anatomy act. At the same

Presented in part at the forty-eighth annual meeting of the American Osler Society, Pittsburgh, Pennsylvania, on 15 May 2018. This paper was previously published in *Clinical Anatomy* (2018; 31[5]: 632–640) and is reproduced with permission.

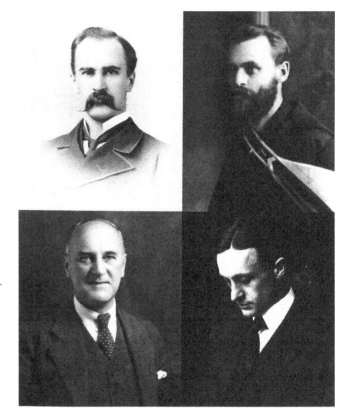

Figure 1. *Clockwise from upper left:* William Osler as a young man; Francis J. Shepherd as a young man; Harvey Cushing; and W.W. Francis—all potential suspects for authorship of the letter by "Long Seen."
Credits: Osler Library of the History of Medicine (Osler and Francis). McCord Museum, Montreal (Shepherd); and National Library of Medicine (Cushing).

time, the need for bodies increased as Quebec opened two more medical schools, L'Ecole de Médcine et Chirurgie de Montréal and the Incorporated School of Medicine of the City of Quebec, which eventually became the Faculties of Medicine at the University of Montreal and Laval University, respectively. While the need for bodysnatching in Quebec was tempered as "plenty of negroes were obtained cheap, packed in casks, and passed over the border as provisions, or flour,"[5, p. 414] the deficiencies in the anatomy act became increasingly clear. In 1867, with the passage of the British North America Act, Canada became a Dominion with a federal constitution, a federal parliament, and provincial legislatures. By 1871, there was a third medical school in Montreal, the Medical Faculty of Bishop's University, further increasing the need for cadavers. Throughout the 1870s and early 1880s, bodysnatching was rampant in Quebec. For one six-week period (12 December 1882 to 25 January 1883), one Montreal newspaper reported seven different grave robbing events, with a total of 18 resurrected bodies, prompting the Quebec Legislature to consider the issue. Eight more events and 18 more bodies were resurrected during the next 33 days. Effective anatomy legislation was passed on 31 March 1883, resulting almost immediately in the cessation of bodysnatching in Quebec.[5]

William Osler

Sir William Osler (Figure 1) is perhaps the most revered physician of all time.[6-9] He received his medical degree from McGill University in 1872 and pursued post-graduate training in Europe. Upon his return to Montreal, Osler was appointed Lecturer in the Institutes of Medicine in 1874 and taught histology. His friend and medical school classmate, Francis Shepherd (Figure 1),[8,10] was hired as Demonstrator of Anatomy in 1875. Osler also served as the first pathologist at Montreal General Hospital and at McGill University, until he moved to Philadelphia in 1884. Osler performed 786 autopsies at McGill,[11] and 162 more in at Blockley Almshouse in Philadelphia, where he was frequently in trouble with hospital administration for circumventing regulations related to obtaining family consent for performing autopsies or retaining teaching specimens obtained at autopsy.[9,12] While at the Montreal General Hospital, Osler once performed a "covert autopsy" after the next of kin had denied consent for an autopsy in order to obtain a teaching specimen (adrenals from a patient with Addison's disease) for the McGill Medical Museum; he did this in the middle of the night by greasing his forearm, dilating the sphincter and, inserting his hand into the rectum, breaking through the wall of the rectum, and bluntly dissecting using a blind arm's length approach until he located and retrieved the coveted teaching specimens.[9,13] Osler was not the only physician to use this "arm's length" covert autopsy technique; it had been developed by Howard Kelly when he was a resident in Philadelphia to circumvent autopsy consent problems and, in fact, this is how the founding professor of internal medicine (Osler) and the founding professor of gynecology (Kelly) at Johns Hopkins Medical School first met.[13] It should be noted that neither of these individuals believed what they were doing was really wrong, as the overarching ethical paradigm under which medicine was practiced in the nineteenth century (beneficence) was much different than the one embraced now (autonomy; respect for persons). In general, physicians were expected to be paternalistic and doctors made decisions for patients based upon what they believe to be in the patient's best interest. Furthermore, since "teaching specimens" were an absolute necessity to teach clinical pathological correlation, it was extremely easy to rationalize that the "good" for Society, that comes from having well-trained physicians far outweighs the need for a corpse to be buried with valuable educational materials decomposing within, especially when these could be removed by a simple sleight of hand.[13] Obviously, a similar rationale could be used by nineteenth-century physicians to justify bodysnatching.[3]

While Sir William Osler is widely admired for helping establish a scientific basis for the modern practice of medicine, for his bedside teaching style, for his writings, and for being a medical role model, there was another side of him who greatly enjoyed playing practical jokes on friends, colleagues, and students. Osler historian William B. Bean astutely noted that:

> it is a characteristic of man's nature to be full of paradoxes, even great men may have important but unorthodox features of character and personality. [He describes] Osler's imp of the perverse. An erratic spirit made him a perennial practical joker, providing a vehicle for his unquenchable ribaldry, and supplied many a nagging and not completely answered question in our efforts to evaluate the whole man.[14, p. 49]

Perhaps, nowhere was this better documented than Osler's series of off-color hoax letters published in various medical journals under the pseudonym of Dr. Egerton Yorrick Davis (EYD), ostensibly a former U.S. Army Surgeon who lived and practiced in Caughnawaga, Quebec. While Osler was in Montreal, EYD wrote fabricated papers and letters to the editor on a variety of bawdy topics including a graphic fictionalized case report of "penis captivus" (vaginismus) and

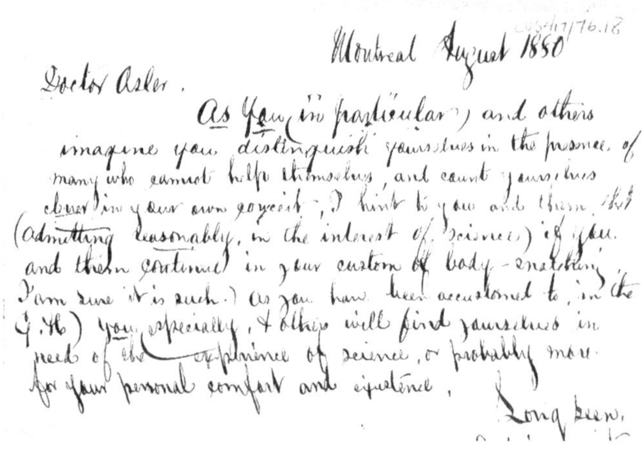

Figure 2.   The "Osler warned" letter. Handwritten letter in highly stylized copybook handwriting using black ink on lined white paper (line spacing 6/16") measuring 7 ¾" H x 8 5/16" W); it is irregularly torn across the top. The letter was previously folded in half vertically and then folded in thirds. On the opposite side of the letter, W.W. Francis has annotated the following in his handwriting: "Found at end of "1880" folder, drawer 2 of Cushing material, #8303, ED, 1940" "Entered in card cat. Under Montreal Gen Hosp with such entries OSLERAIAN and RESURRECTIONISTS."
Credit: Osler Library. Cushing Acc. 417, Box 161, 31/4/5, folder 76 1880.

a study describing bizarre aboriginal birthing methods in the Northwest Territories. When Osler moved to Philadelphia, he likely planned to dispense with EYD, and even reported that "the old rascal... was drowned in the Lachine Rapids in 1884 (The St. Lawrence River near Caughnawaga and Montreal), and the body was never recovered" (n.b., this was the year that Osler left McGill).[15, p. 532] However, before long, Osler had "resurrected" EYD, who continued to publish from Philadelphia, including a humorous paper on the conversion of extrauterine to intrauterine pregnancies via the use of electrical current. When Osler was traveling and did not want to be found, sometimes he used the pseudonym EYD to check into hotels. EYD apparently liked to travel as much as Osler as he moved to Baltimore and Oxford when Osler became professor of medicine at Johns Hopkins and Regius professor at Oxford, respectively.[14–17]

Anatomy during Osler's tenure at McGill University:

In the 1870s and early 1880s, most of the cadavers in the McGill anatomy laboratory were resurrected and his friend Francis Shepherd was "convicted of this offence on several occasions, but the judge was basically sympathetic to the problem of the medical school, and he only charged Shepherd a fifty dollar fine with no further prosecution."[18] According to Harvey Cushing's *The Life of Sir William Osler*, Osler wrote Shepherd on September 14, 1918, and asked him "to write up the story" of "the last persistence of bodysnatching in Montreal... if not for publication, send it to me to put with my Resurrectionist literature."[6, ii: 617] Shepherd did this immediately in a book entitled *Reminiscences of Student Days and Dissecting Room*; however the book was "PRINTED FOR PRIVATE CIRCULATION ONLY."[19] Osler acknowledged receipt of his copy of Shepherd's book in a letter dated January 11, 1919. Osler displayed his enjoyment of Shepherd's account by writing "I thought the denouement came with the stealing of the body of Mayor of Three Rivers (Quebec) & Bro. of the Bishop. Tis an A1 account."[20] Clearly, like most physicians of his time,[3] Osler was fascinated by the phenomenon of bodysnatching but had never been suspected of actually participating, until William Willoughby Francis (Figure 1), the first Osler Librarian at McGill University who co-edited *Bibliotheca Osleriana* (and was Osler's first cousin once-removed).[8] found the following highly accusatory (and poorly grammatical) letter addressed to Osler "among the papers returned a few years ago by his biographer, [Harvey] Cushing" (Figure 1):

> Montreal August 1880.
> Doctor Osler,
>
> As You (in particular) and others imagine you distinguish yourselves in the presence of many who cannot help themselves, and count yourselves clever in your own conceit, I hint to you and them that (admitting reasonably, in the interest of science) if you and them continue in your custom of bodysnatching, (I am sure it is such.) as you have been accustomed to, in the G.H.) You (especially, & others will find yourselves in need of the experience of science, or probably more for your personal comfort and existence,
>
> (signed) Long Seen, And In Wait[21]

Francis apparently considered the letter (Figure 2) entertaining enough that he published it along with his own letter to the editor in 1940 in the *Canadian Medical Association Journal* (*CMAJ*) under the title of "Osler Warned!"[21]

Considering that most nineteenth-century physicians either benefited from or participated in grave robbing early in their medical careers,[3] and considering that medical students sometimes procured their own dissection materials while Osler was training at McGill,[5,10,19] is it possible, or even likely, that Osler participated in bodysnatching? Let's dissect further!

There is no way to know whether Osler or Shepherd participated in resurrectionist activities as medical student classmates, but according to Shepherd, at least by the time he was the anatomy demonstrator in 1875, he "found immediately that to provide subjects for the dissecting room (he) had to accept those obtained from 'Resurrectionists.' The body-snatchers were usually medical students, chiefly French, who by the proceeds of their nefarious occupation paid their fees." Shepherd furthermore indicated that "the usual price of a subject at the time was thirty to fifty dollars!"[5, p. 417] Another Shepherd source suggests that the Irish medical students were the main culprits and includes a few humorous stories about students tobogganing with resurrected bodies while transporting them to McGill.[10] It should be noted that Osler, as a medical student, "was seriously short of money."[9, p.63] In fact, it is not entirely clear how he paid his tuition. Although one could speculate that he had some help from one of his highly accomplished older brothers, I can find no evidence to support this premise. However, it is documented that brother Edmund Osler supported his postgraduate training in Europe by advancing him $1,000. But, since the letter is dated 1880, Long Seen appears to have been accusing Osler the "baby professor" (a nickname for Professor Osler at McGill) not Osler the medical student.

Osler's troubled youth

From his youth, Osler was never one to follow the rules simply because they were the rules and he was in trouble at almost every level of education. In 1864, at the age of 15, William was expelled from Dundas Grammar School (Dundas, Ontario, Canada) for a series of pranks, which eventually adversely affected the reputation of both the school and its headmaster. The following year, William, while enrolled as a boarding student at Barrie Grammar School (Barrie,

Ontario, Canada), became the leader of "Barrie's bad boys," three boarders who feuded with the day students. Their pranks culminated in an apparent school fire precipitating a visit from the local fire department. A year later, Osler attended Trinity College in Weston, Ontario, where he was a stellar student and a school leader, and he had been selected to be the College's head prefect for the next year. Unfortunately, Osler, now almost 17 years old, and nine of his classmates were charged with assaulting the widow of a clergyman and trespassing. While it is not clear that the case had much merit and it was clear that the widow's abusive behavior precipitated the event, nine of the students were convicted and each was fined a dollar plus court costs. Osler, who was apparently the ringleader but was defended by one of his older brothers, was the only student who ended up without a criminal record. Sources differ as to whether it was Featherston Osler, later a prominent Ontario judge, or Britton Bath Osler, later considered one of the greatest criminal lawyers in Canadian history, who successfully defended William in court.[14]

Regardless, considering that bodysnatching was a necessary evil when Osler was a student at McGill, that some McGill students used this activity to pay their tuition, that Osler needed a source of tuition money, that many medical professionals of the time either turned a blind eye or participated, that Osler liked to participate in dangerous pranks, and that performing illegal arm's length covert autopsies was not beyond him, it is certainly not inconceivable that Osler could have been guilty at some time during his years in Montreal. There is simply no evidence one way or the other.

On the other hand, W.W. Francis in his letter to the editor "suspects that it (the letter) was misdirected" noting that "in 1880 Shepherd was still . . . having to deal with the body-snatchers. Surely this was meant for him and McGill, not for Osler . . ." Francis also notes that: "it has a genuine look, though it might perhaps be a reprisal concocted by a victim of Osler's pranks."[21]

I personally like Francis' latter theory. Perhaps, the accusatory letter was a reprisal directed at the antics of Osler's impish alter ego, Dr. Egerton Yorrick Davis [n.b., it is believed by some that Osler named his fun-loving second self after the court jester Yorick in William Shakespeare's *Hamlet*[15]]. If so, the irony is delicious as Yorick himself fell victim to a gravedigger, and Hamlet, on seeing a gravedigger hoisting Yorick's skull in the air, uttered his famous line: "Alas, poor Yorick! I knew him, Horatio; a fellow of infinite jest, of most excellent fancy . . ."[22]

Dissecting the letter—who was "Long Seen"?

First, it must be stressed that the provenance of the letter is not only unknown, but much about it also seems highly suspect and there are many obvious questions to address. What is the evidence that the letter was written in August 1880? The writer's given name and surnames not only appear to be fictitious, but they also have a humorous nature suggesting that the letter may be a practical joke.

The "stationary" on which the letter is written [crude white (or more likely faded yellow) lined paper appearing to have been torn irregularly from a larger page] bears no identifiers and has no return address. In his letter to the editor, Francis writes that "it is written (appropriately) on a bit of foolscap" [n.b., foolscap is defined as "a type of inexpensive writing paper, especially legal-size, lined, yellow sheets, bound in tablet form,"[23] but the term can also apply to a traditional cap or hood with bells worn by jesters.[24]

Presumably, the letter was mailed to Osler; if he thought it important enough to keep, why did he not bother to either provide a handwritten annotation on it as Osler frequently did with other documents and letters or why did he not save the envelope with its postmark, as he certainly would have known that this would be the only way to preserve its historical value and the identity of the writer?

If the letter is genuine and was really mailed to Osler in 1880, why did Osler value this letter so much that it survived his extensive travels including his moves to Philadelphia, Baltimore, and Oxford. It is not intuitive why Long Seen's letter was meaningful to Osler; perhaps, he kept it because he thought it was funny or maybe it served as a reminder that practical jokes can evoke retaliation. While it is possible that Osler retained this strange anonymous letter from 1880 until his death 39 years later simply so that it could be found after his death, this seems improbable, even though Osler was a great collector and might certainly have found it humorous to leave it amongst his papers after his death.

It seems more plausible that the letter is a fabrication, rather than a legitimate 1880 letter from Long Seen, And in Wait. If so, this leaves the questions of who wrote it, when it was written, and why? The "why" seems obvious—surely it was a practical joke. The more difficult question is whether Osler was an innocent victim or possibly even the perpetrator. Let's dissect further.

Many of the victims of bodysnatching in nineteenth-century Quebec were Francophone, but the letter was written in English not French. However, the English is atrocious and Francis points this out by injecting some humor into his accompanying letter to the editor: "the punctuation and grammar are Long-seen's, and not yours or mine!"[21] Was the letter purposefully designed to appear as if it was written by a semi-literate or non-native English speaker? Interestingly, Francis describes Long Seen's handwriting as "a would-be copybook hand," possibly suggesting that the writer's penmanship had not differentiated further since grammar school.

Was the letter really written in 1880? If not, the choice of this date is possibly instructive. Is it a coincidence that this is the year that Osler's biographer (and friend) Harvey Cushing claims EYD first appeared on the horizon. According to Cushing, it was 1880 that "there appeared on the scene a creature named Egerton Yorrick Davis, soon recognized as a pathological fabricator of ill repute, whose name became coupled with that of William Osler."[6, i: 181] However, it should be noted that not all Osler scholars date YD's emergence in 1880. Some suggest a few years later when his papers start being published. Nevertheless, Cushing said 1880.

If Long Seen's letter is not from 1880 and was fabricated in the twentieth century, its true author must have known that the letter could not be credibly dated after March 31, 1883, the date effective anatomy legislation was passed in Quebec. Furthermore, Osler was a faculty member at McGill from 1874 to 1884, at which point he moved to Philadelphia. A knowledgeable perpetrator wanting to construct a credible accusatory letter as a practical joke would have needed to take these dates into account to determine when to date the letter.

It seems very safe to assume that "Long Seen, And in Wait" is not a real name. If not, what does the letter's signatory's name mean? A Google search does not suggest a literary reference, unlike the made-up name Yorrick. Interestingly, Google consistently tries to turn the phrase into stories about long wait times for medical care, which was not a problem for paying patients in Osler's time. None of Osler's biographies mention this letter or anyone by this name. It sounds rather like the author of the letter may be suggesting that Osler should have foreseen this coming, and that the author had long waited to write it. This interpretation brings us back to the premise that the letter was not likely written and mailed to Osler in 1880, as he would have been only very early into his lifelong career of pulling practical jokes on his colleagues.

What does the text of the letter mean? The letter is comprised of only one long, complex, poorly punctuated, and incompetently grammatical sentence. It is impossible to understand it in its entirety, but it seems to speak to Osler's and other's (perhaps Shepherd's) conceit, presumably related to dissection. In this context, knowledge of anatomy gained by human dissection was actually a source of conceit for many late-nineteenth-century physicians; according to historian-sociologist Michael Sappol, physicians were all members of the "fraternity of dissectors" setting themselves apart from the public and that "medical students, teachers, and practitioners shared a set of common anatomical experiences that were vital to the making of professional medical identity . . . [including] dissecting the dead, robbing graves, transporting bodies, making and exhibiting 'anatomical preparations' obtained from dissection, and joking with bodies and body parts."[25, p. 470]

The phrase "in the presence of many who cannot help themselves" almost certainly refers to helpless cadavers. It then accuses him and others of bodysnatching for the "G.H." (Montreal General Hospital), where Osler was the pathologist. This is puzzling as Osler would have performed autopsies at the Hospital, but anatomical dissections would have been performed by Shepherd at the McGill Medical School. Francis picked up on this inconsistency in his letter to the *CMAJ*. Next, the writer seems to admit that anatomical dissection is necessary and "in the interest of science," suggesting it was written by a well-educated person or possibly a physician. Finally, it finishes with a threat. Shepherd and Osler remained friends for life and neither their extensive correspondence in the archives of the Osler Library at McGill University nor his chapter in Maude Abbott's Osler Memorial Number[26] mention the letter nor offer any insights into what the letter was trying to communicate.

Next, how did the letter gain access to the Osler Library? According to Francis, he found it amongst the papers that Cushing returned. Cushing originally published his biography of Osler in 1925 and then provided his meticulously organized files to the Osler Library, which opened on 29 May 1929. Francis was appointed and arrived in Montreal just before the Library's opening. Why did it take him over 10 years to find this curious letter? Or, if he found it earlier and planned to publish it, why did he wait until November 1940 to publish his short (one column of one page) letter to the editor?

Who put Long Seen's letter amongst Osler's papers? Was it there when Cushing reviewed these materials to write his book? Was it amongst the materials Cushing returned to the Osler Library? Could it have been added to the Osler materials once they were at the Osler Library, and if so, by whom? Cushing never comments on the letter and so he provides no insights into the answers to these questions.

Other suspects who could have written the letter

If the letter was not written in 1880 and is not genuine, who had the means, motive, and opportunity to fabricate it? Because it is a complex "crime," the list of prime suspects is small.

First, it seems unlikely that Shepherd could have written it. While he would have known Osler's sense of humor well and would certainly have known that Osler would have appreciated the gesture of slipping this letter in amongst his papers, it seems unlikely that he would have had the means or opportunity, as he retired in 1912 and spent little time at McGill after that. While he continued to correspond with Osler until Osler's death (29 December 1919) and he did privately publish his *Reminiscences of Student Days and Dissecting Room*[19] earlier that year and sent a copy to Osler, Francis died on 19 January 1929, four months before the Osler Library opened its doors and so it is unlikely that he added this letter to the incoming Cushing collection. Ironically, Shepherd was writing his speech for the first Osler Oration at the annual meeting of the Canadian Medical Association to be held in June when he died.[10]

Could Harvey Cushing have written it? He certainly had means, opportunity, and perhaps motive. Cushing obviously had long-term access to Osler's papers and begrudgingly had to deal with Osler's antics, practical jokes, and EYD. Cushing's biographer Michael Bliss states that although Cushing greatly admired Osler, he did not like Osler's "Rabelaisian (tendencies) as evinced in some of the gag articles that he wrote under the pseudonym Egerton Yorrick Davis."[27, p. 390] Clearly, Cushing found it distasteful having to deal with EYD in his Pulitzer Prize-winning biography of Osler. Possibly, in a weak moment, Cushing decided to exact a modicum of justice by fabricating the mysterious letter—knowing Osler's sense of humor and that Osler would have approved. However, if this did happen, he likely expected that his practical joke would remain buried amongst Osler's voluminous papers at the Osler Library, occasionally being found and serving as mystery to a few Oslerian scholars. If this scenario is true, he undoubtedly never anticipated that Francis would publish Long Seen's letter. As noted previously, the letter is dated the year Cushing claimed EYD first appeared. Is this a coincidence? If Cushing did not write the letter but it passed through his possession, he ignored it in the writing of his encyclopedic biography of Osler, which is perhaps not a surprise, as he had access to a letter describing Osler performing an arm's length autopsy via the anus and he opted to exclude this racy tidbit as well.[9,13] Cushing died on 7 October 1939.

Maude Abbott, by all accounts, revered and worshipped Osler, who had mentored her starting early in her medical career and had helped her advance professionally in an often hostile, male-dominated environment.[28–31] therefore, it is almost inconceivable that that she would have fabricated a letter casting a shadow on her hero.[32] However, Abbott would likely have known whether or not the letter was legitimate, as she helped Cushing collect the letters and reminiscences for his book and for her own, *Sir William Osler Memorial Number: Appreciations and Reminiscences*.[33] If she had found this letter, she, like Cushing might also have found it improper to use; however, she likely could have confirmed or denied its existence prior to being found by Francis in the Osler Library. In fact, Abbott was probably the last living person, except possibly Francis (if he wrote it), to know whether the letter was a fabrication, but she died two months before Francis published it. Unfortunately, the Osler Library does not have the correspondence related to when Francis submitted his letter to *CMAJ*; so, whether it was after Abbott's death is unknown. However, it should be noted that the turnaround time for short entries could often be rapid. For instance, Abbott died on September 2, 1940 and her full obituary appeared in the October *CMAJ* issue. The Osler Warned paper was published in November of 1940.

The final suspect is W.W. Francis; could he have written it? Sir William Osler, Lady Grace Osler (Osler's wife who died in 1928), Cushing, and Abbott were possibly the only people who would have known whether the letter was original, and all were now dead. This could have created a risk-free opportunity for Francis to fabricate the letter and add his personal contribution to Dr. Osler's mischievous opus (or considering the topic, perhaps "corpus" is the better word for this particular body of work)? Francis, in his paper "Osler Warned," is the one who suggested that it might be payback for Osler's practical jokes. While this seems likely, he also suggested that it seemed genuine—which it actually does not. Possibly, knowing his second cousin's love of a good practical joke, he might even have felt that he owed it to him, as Osler had played important enabling roles in his career. What could be a better tribute to Osler, whose alter ego EYD relished writing the occasional fabricated letter to the editor, than to send him off with an original one of his own! According to the author of Francis' obituary, he "retained the spirit of youth and laughter to the end."[34] Finally, Francis was sufficiently proud of his letter to the editor that he even bragged about it to friends, likely because it allowed him to display his own personal sense of humor. In a letter dated 26 January 1941 to retired McGill anesthesiologist, medical historian, and longtime friend Dr. W.B. Howell, Francis tells Howell that he is sending him a copy of "my frivolous "Osler Warned."[35] Francis seems to have had means, motive, and opportunity. On the other hand, as Osler Librarian, Francis is known to have been a stickler for accuracy, and this would seem to be an uncharacteristic departure.

Could Osler have written the letter to himself as a final practical joke?

Finally, my pseudo-investigative reporting should consider whether, late in his life, Osler could have written it to himself, knowing it would be found after his death, as his last practical joke? We have already established that Osler had an impish side which enjoyed practical jokes and he and EYD were not opposed to fabrication of a few facts when it served these kinds of purposes.

Osler had a lifelong love of practical jokes and had already fabricated EYD. Was it beyond him to fabricate a letter accusing himself of grave robbing? Of course not, this was totally in keeping with what we now about the other sometimes perverse, erratic, and ribald side of Sir William Osler. We already have established that he was thinking within a year of his death, about the history of grave robbing at McGill and that he had written Shepherd asking him to write down his recollections on this topic. Perhaps, Osler, having just read Shepherd's account, thought it would be fun to try to insert himself into the story. While a case can be made that Osler had means, motive, and opportunity, it is difficult to explain how the letter existed amongst Osler's highly studied papers for two decades after his death and was not found and mentioned by others. But Osler could have written it and then covertly given it directly to Francis with instructions to hold the accusatory letter until it could neither embarrass his wife nor be immediately discredited by his close colleagues. Therefore, it is possible that W.W. Francis was in cahoots with Osler, allowing him to circumvent any personal guilt associated with the deception. However, if Osler was not the source of the Long Seen letter, there are three certainties—he would have loved the irony of it, he would have wanted to congratulate its perpetrator, and he would totally have appreciated Francis publishing it in *CMAJ*!

Handwriting analysis

I examined multiple examples of Osler's (and also EYD's), Shepherd's, Cushing's, Abbott's, and Francis' handwriting at the Osler Library. None of these resemble Long Seen's highly stylized "copybook hand" handwriting. However, almost certainly, if any of my suspects had written the letter in their own handwriting, Francis, as the Osler Librarian, would have known exactly who wrote it and, if he were still to have published it, would have been complicit. While any of the suspects could have used an accomplice to pen the letter, highly stylized "copybook hand" handwriting might have been an even better way to mask the scribe's identity as there would be no need for an accomplice.

Finally, I sent high resolution photographs of Long Seen's letter and 3–6 handwriting samples obtained from the Osler Library for each of my six suspects to Linton A. Mohammed, Ph.D., a diplomat of the American Board of Forensic Document Examiners, for expert analysis. He was pleased with the quality of the photographic evidence and examined them blindly. Like Francis, he also described the handwriting style as copybook and suggested that the letter was written with a steel-nibbed pen, allowing for the shading in the letterforms. Mohammed concluded:

> There is no evidence of common authorship between any of the S1 (suspect 1)–S6 writers and the " bodysnatching" letter. It is quite possible that the latter document may bear disguised handwriting. That is, the writer deliberately altered their handwriting. You can observe that in the first two sentences, there is a slight forward slant, which then changes to a more upright slant, and then to a backward slant especially in the last two lines. This is a common disguise strategy. . . . The variation in the letter "t" (initial, middle, and terminal" is also of interest. S1-S6 maintained a consistent slant throughout their samples as you would expect. . . . (Linton A. Mohammed, personal communication, 6 March 2018).

Conclusion

Taking all of the above speculation into account, it seems almost certain that the letter was one final practical joke—perpetrator unknown. The quirky publication of the "frivolous" letter in the *CMAJ* was possibly a conspiracy, either involving Francis and Osler or perhaps Francis and at least one of the other abovementioned suspects—all knowing that Osler would have approved of Francis publishing the letter and fully believing that Osler was smiling down from above (and EYD, smiling from somewhere else) at the moment it was published.

However, if it was not a conspiracy between Osler and Francis, my next favorite theory is that Francis simultaneously fabricated both his *CMAJ* letter to the editor and Long Seen's letter (on which it was based) as his personal tribute to Osler's other side, EYD, and that he did this as soon as he knew he could get away with it. If so, his critique of Long Seen's punctuation and grammar (i.e., "not (being) yours or mine") was one additional small deceit—there is no doubt that his mentor would have approved!

While it was not possible to solve the mysteries surrounding the "Osler Warned" letter, my paper represents the only discussion of this 75-year-old puzzle. More importantly, it allows the readership to explore Sir William Osler's other side and to even speculate about his role in resurrectionist activities.

Acknowledgments

I thank Lily Szczygiel, Osler Library of the History of Medicine, McGill University, for archival assistance; Pamela Miller, former Osler Librarian (retired), for reading a draft and providing helpful comments; and Linton A. Mohammed, Ph.D., D-ABFDE, Forensic Document Examiner, Forensic Science Consultants, Inc., Burlingame, CA for handwriting analysis. This research was supported in part by a Scholar-in-Residence Award from The Ohio State University Medical Heritage Center.

References

1. Schulz SM. Body Snatching: *The Robbing of Graves for the Education of Physicians in Early Nineteenth Century America*. MacFarland; 1992.
2. Sappol M. *A Traffic of Dead Bodies: Anatomy and Embodied Social Identity in Nineteenth Century America*. Princeton: Princeton University Press; 2002.
3. Wright JR Jr. The Pennsylvania Anatomy Act of 1883: Weighing the roles of Professor William Smith Forbes and Senator William James McKnight. *Journal of the History of Medicine and Allied Sciences* 2016; 71: 422–446.
4. Hanaway J, Cruess R. *McGill Medicine. Volume 1. The First Half Century 1829–1885*. Montreal & Kingston: McGill-Queen's University Press; 1996.
5. Lawrence DG. The William Osler Medal Essay: "Resurrection" and legislation or bodysnatching in relation to the anatomy act in the Province of Quebec. *Bulletin of the History of Medicine* 1958; 32: 408–424.
6. Cushing H. *The Life of Sir William Osler*. Oxford: Clarendon Press; 1925.
7. Reid EG. *The Great Physician: A Short Life of Sir William Osler*. London: Oxford University Press; 1931.
8. Bensley EH. *McGill Medical Luminaries*. Montreal: Osler Library McGill University; 1990.
9. Bliss M. 1999. William Osler: A life in medicine. Toronto: University of Toronto Press; 1999.
10. Howell WB. *F. J. Shepherd—Surgeon. His Life and Times*. Toronto and Vancouver: J.M. Dent & Sons Ltd.; 1934.
11. Rodin AE. *Oslerian Pathology: An Assessment and Annotated Atlas of Museum Specimens*. Lawrence, Kansas: Coronado Press; 1981.
12. Wright JR Jr., Why did Osler not perform autopsies at Johns Hopkins? *Archives of Pathology and Laboratory Medicine* 2008; 132: 1710 (letter).
13. Wright JR Jr. Sins of our fathers: Two of "The Four Doctors" and their roles in the development of techniques to permit covert autopsies. *Archives of Pathology and Laboratory Medicine* 2009; 133: 1969–1974.
14. Bean WB. William Osler: The Egerton Yorrick Davis alias. In McGovern JP, Burns CR, eds. *Humanism in Medicine*. Springfield, IL: Charles C. Thomas; 1973: 49–59.

15. Nation EF. Osler's alter ego. *Chest* 1969; 56: 531–537.

16. Tigertt WD. An annotated life of Egerton Yorrick Davis, M.D., and intimate of Sir William Osler. *Journal of the History of Medicine and Allied Sciences* 1983; 38: 259–297.

17. Burrow GN. The trial and tribulation of Egerton Yorrick Davis. *Western Journal of Medicine* 1991; 155: 80–82.

18. History 4—Shepherd to Flexner Report. https://www.mcgill.ca/anatomy/files/anatomy/history_4_-_shepherd_to_flexner_report_aug_25.pdf [accessed April 2018].

19. Shepherd FJ. *Reminiscences of Student days and Dissecting Room.* Privately printed; 1919.

20. Osler W to Shepherd FJ, letter dated 11 Jan, 1919. Osler Library of the History of Medicine, McGill University, Acc. 417, Folder 127, 22, January-March 1919.

21. Francis WW. Osler warned! *Canadian Medical Association Journal* 1940; 43: 493.

22. Shakespeare W. *Hamlet.* Reprint edition, New York: Modern Library Classics; 2008.

23. Foolscap. http://www.dictionary.com/browse/foolscap, Accessed 25 November 2020.

24. Foolscap. http://www.merriam-webster.com/dictionary/foolscap. Accessed 25 November 2020.

25. Sappol M. The odd case of Charles Knowlton: anatomical performance, medical narrative, and identity in Antebellum America. *Bulletin of the History of Medicine* 2009; 83:460–498.

26. Shepherd FJ. Osler's Montreal period. A personal reminiscence. In [Abbott ME, ed.] Bulletin No. IX of the *International Association of Medical Museums and Journal of Technical Methods. Sir William Osler Memorial Number. Appreciations and Reminiscences.* Montreal: privately printed [Murray Printing Co., Limited, Toronto]; 1926: 152–158.

27. Bliss M. *Harvey Cushing: A Life in Surgery.* Toronto: University of Toronto Press; 2005.

28. Abbott MES. Autobiographical sketch (dated March 31, 1928). *McGill Medical Journal* 1959; 28: 127–152.

29. MacDermot HE. *Maude Abbott—A Memoir.* Toronto: Macmillan; 1941.

30. Waugh D. *Maudie of McGill: Dr. Maude Abbott and the Foundations of Heart Surgery.* Oxford: Dundurn Press; 1992.

31. Wright JR Jr, Fraser RS, Adams A, Hunter M. Portraying Maude Abbott. *Canadian Medical Association Journal* 2017; 189: E281–E283.

32. Francis WW. Maude Abbott, hero-worshipper. *McGill Medical Journal* 1940; 10: 38–43.

33. [Abbott ME, ed.] Bulletin No. IX of the *International Association of Medical Museums and Journal of Technical Methods. Sir William Osler Memorial Number. Appreciations and Reminiscences.* Montreal: privately printed [Murray Printing Co., Limited, Toronto]; 1926:

34. MacNalty AS. Obituary: W.W. Francis, A.B., M.D. (1978–1959). *Medical History* 1960; 4: 163–166.

35. Francis WW to Howell WB, letter dated 26 Jan, 1941. Osler Library of the History of Medicine, McGill University. Acc 381, box 7, Folder #27 [Howell to Francis 1939, 1940, 1941, 1942, 1943, 1945], 3-103-731-423E.

Osler and Ophthalmology: Additional Insights

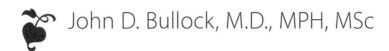 John D. Bullock, M.D., MPH, MSc

William Osler graduated from medical school in 1872 and went abroad hoping to become an ophthalmologist. This plan unraveled in London, first during one or more conversations with Sir William Bowman and later from advice from his Montreal mentor, R. Palmer Howard. The story of how Osler did not become an ophthalmologist has been told by Osler biographers Harvey Cushing and Michael Bliss and by others.[1-5] The purpose of this article is to add details in three areas: (1) Why Osler did not become an ophthalmologist; (2) How Osler may have managed his first paying patient, who had a "spec" in the cornea; and (3) How an Osler Professorship of Ophthalmology came to be endowed at Harvard Medical School.

How Osler did not become an ophthalmologist

Osler's desire to be an ophthalmologist seems at first blush a bit puzzling since he had few immediate role models. During his Toronto period (1868–1870), he was aware of the reputation of William Rawlins Beaumont (1803–1875), the first physician on record to have performed eye surgery in that city. Osler called Beaumont "the highest type of the cultivated English surgeon,"[6] but Beaumont was well past his prime when Osler arrived in Toronto, having lost vision in his left eye. There were no trained eye specialists in Montreal when Osler was in medical school at McGill (1870–1872). Nineteenth-century advances had been

Presented in part at the forty-ninth annual meeting of the American Osler Society, Montreal, Quebec, Canada, on 13 May 2019. Portions of this article have been previously been published in *Sir William Osler: An Encyclopedia* (edited by Charles S. Bryan; Novato, California: Norman Publishing/History of Science.Com; 2020: 103–104, 118–119, 564–565, 578–579), and are reproduced with permission.

much more spectacular in general medicine and surgery than in ophthalmology. There were, for example, the discovery of the anesthetic properties of nitrous oxide (Sir Humphry Davy, 1800), invention of the stethoscope (René Laennec, 1816), a successful blood transfusion (James Blundell, 1818), ether as a general anesthetic (Crawford W. Long, 1842), prevention of childbed fever (Ignaz Semmelweis, 1842), isolation of the cholera vibrio (Filippo Pacini, 1854), identification of microorganisms as the cause of fermentation (Louis Pasteur, 1857), introduction of aseptic surgery (Joseph Lister, 1867), and the germ theory of disease (Robert Koch, 1876). By contrast, ophthalmology could boast mainly about the invention of the ophthalmoscope (Hermann von Helmholtz, 1859), a chart to measure visual acuity (Herman Snellen, 1862), and operative approaches to cataracts and glaucoma (iridectomy) introduced by Albrecht von Graefe (1825–1870) of Germany, who is often considered the founder of ophthalmology as we know it today.

The idea of becoming an ophthalmologist possibly percolated in Osler's mind during his early years. He never met his uncle Edward Osler (1798–1863), his father's older brother, but he would have been aware that Edward practiced eye surgery in Swansea, Wales, and in Truro, Cornwall, before embarking on the literary, poetic, and religious career that made him famous (notably for writing more than 50 liturgical hymns, some of which are still used). William's father, the Reverend Featherstone Lake Osler (1805–1895), dispensed spectacles in the Canadian backwoods, and it is suggested here that he may have learned the rudiments of optical dispensing from his older brother. However, family heritage was not the only reason Osler considered ophthalmology. He perceived that ophthalmology was a potentially lucrative specialty that would afford time "to pursue science rather than to have practice pursue him."[2] With these ideas in mind, Osler went to London in 1872 hoping to secure a position as house surgeon at the Royal Ophthalmic Hospital at Moorfields (later renamed Moorfields Eye Hospital), where his fate would be determined by William Bowman (1816–1892) (Figure 1).[7]

What took place during Osler's interview (or interviews) with Bowman is not known, but Charles Snyder suggests it was a moment of high drama."[3] Bowman advised Osler to prepare himself in "physiology," then a general term

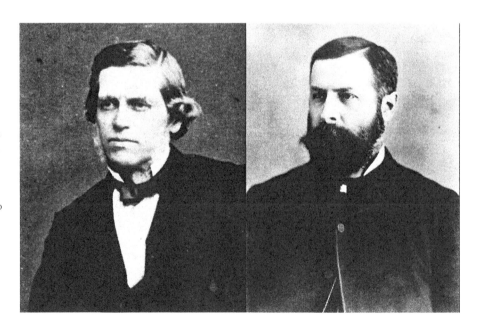

Figure 1.   Sir William Bowman (1816–1892), a pioneering London eye surgeon (left), and his pupil Francis (Frank) Buller (1844–1905), who became Montreal's first trained eye surgeon. *Credit:* National Library of Medicine (Bowman); Osler Library of the History of Medicine, McGill University.

Figure 2.   Ledger showing Osler's fees for his first paying patient, who had a "spec" in the cornea (highlighted in box). On August 21 he received 50 cents for examining the patient, and on August 22 he received $1.00 for removing the spec, apparently after consulting various sources on the proper procedure. Note that between July 26 and August 25, Osler's income (as judged from this ledger) was $205.25, of which only $5.25 came from his practice as locum tenens. The rest consisted of contributions from his father ("from pater"). He then received an appointment at the McGill medical school, where his income derived primarily from student fees ("S.F."). *Credit:* Osler Library of the History of Medicine, McGill University.

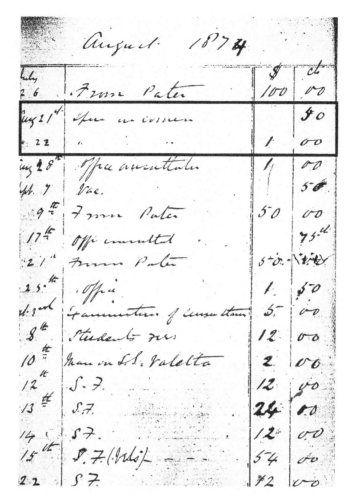

for the basic sciences, and to that end referred him to John Burdon-Sanderson (1828–1905). Under Burdon-Sanderson's tutelage Osler rendered an early observation of the blood platelets. Ironically, Osler's initial research under Burdon–Sanderson involved an animal model of inflammation in the anterior chamber of the eye, using frogs.

Bowman, in advising Osler to prepare in the basic sciences, gave mentoring advice consistent with his own career development. However, there was a stronger reason. We do not know how many applicants Bowman had to choose from, but the strongest applicant was almost surely Francis Buller (1844–1905). Five years older than Osler, Buller had spent four years in Berlin where he not only studied ophthalmology under von Graefe but also pathology under Rudolf Virchow (1821–1894). These credentials clearly made Osler the lesser choice.

Osler received another blow in the form of a letter from his Montreal mentor R. Palmer Howard (1823–1889), who told him that "you will have much more to contend with than we ever thought of when we spoke together on the subject." Two McGill graduates and a British specialist were planning to come to Montreal to practice ophthalmology. Howard advised Osler to concentrate instead on learning as much as he could about the broad field of medicine. Osler answered: "As you may imagine I was not a little disappointed at the blighting of my prospects as an ophthalmic surgeon, but I accept the inevitable with a good grace." We can only speculate whether Osler would have become as famous and influential in ophthalmology as he became in general medicine.

Buller returned to Montreal as the city's first trained eye surgeon. There he became Osler's close friend and, for a while, his landlord. Howard's advice to Osler that Montreal would soon have too many ophthalmologists seems, however, a bit questionable. Joseph Hanaway, writing about the early history of the Montreal General Hospital (MGH), observes:

> Another ongoing problem at the clinic was created by Frank Buller, the first eye doctor at the MGH, who arrived in 1877. Being the first trained eye specialist in Montreal, Buller rapidly had a huge clientele and flooded the clinic with patients. He saw too many patients, took too much time, and encroached upon the time of the other clinics. He was well trained in his work and was given the first Chair of Ophthalmology and Otology at McGill in 1883, with no salary. In 1894, he moved to the RVH [the Royal Victoria Hospital, competitor of the MGH], where he directed the eye, ear, nose and throat department. in Montreal.[8]

If there is a moral, it might be that young persons should pursue their interests irrespective of the job market, since one cannot predict with accuracy where future demands will be.

How Osler managed his first paying patient

After studying abroad for about 18 months, Osler returned home to his family in Dundas, Ontario. He had no job, and therefore spent several weeks as locum tenens for a physician in the Dundas-Hamilton area. On 21 August 1874 he saw his first paying patient, who had a "spec in the cornea." Osler's fee was fifty cents (Figure 2). This event has been noted previously, but without additional comment.[1-5]

Osler's account book further documents that the patient returned to him the next day, 22 August 1874, and received the same diagnosis. Osler's fee for the second visit was $1.00—twice his fee for the first visit. Physicians then as now typically charged more for the first visit, since the second visit would be what we now call a "follow-up visit."

It is suggested here that Osler charged less for the first visit because he did not remove the foreign body on the cornea. It is likely that he did not know the proper method, lacked the proper equipment, or both. It is suggested here that, in the interim, with ample time on his hands (judging from his account book, Figure 2), he (1) researched the proper method, (2) acquired the means; and/or (3) asked a colleague for advice. He then charged double the next day because he successfully removed the foreign body.

But where would he have turned for advice? Perhaps he acquired therapeutic options from one or more books in the library of the physician for whom he was doing locum tenens. Perhaps he turned to a skilled general practitioner since removal of a foreign body from the cornea was (and remains) within the scope of general practice. And what technique did use? Topical ocular anesthesia did not appear until ten years later when, on 11 September 1884, the Austrian

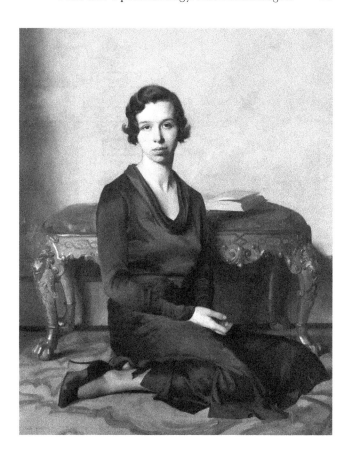

Figure 3. *Susan Toy Morse Hilles* (1931), by Sir Gerald Festus Kelly (1879–1972). *Credit:* Boston Athenæum.

ophthalmologist Carl Koller (1857–1944) performed the first cataract extraction facilitated by the topical anesthetic properties of cocaine. (As an unintended consequence of Koller's innovation, surgeons began self-experimenting with cocaine for peripheral nerve block, which caused many deaths and the addiction of William S. Halsted, who became Osler's colleague in Baltimore.)

How the William Osler Professorship of Ophthalmology came to be endowed at Harvard Medical School

In 1984 the William Osler Professorship of Ophthalmology at Harvard was endowed by Susan Toy Morse Hilles (1905–2002) (Figure 3), who was heiress to an industrial fortune, discriminating art collector, and philanthropist. Previous accounts of this donation mention her distant relationship to Sir William Osler but provide few other details.[9–12]

Susan Toy Morse Hilles was the only child of William Inglis Morse (1874–1952) and Susan Alice Ensign Morse (1873–1951). Her father, William Inglis Morse, was born in Paradise, Nova Scotia, and graduated from Acadia College (1897) and the Episcopal Theological School (1900). While serving as chaplain and instructor in English at the Westminster School in Simsbury, Connecticut, he met Susan Alice Ensign, a member of the town's leading family whose wealth came from manufacture of safety fuses and explosives. Morse continued to serve

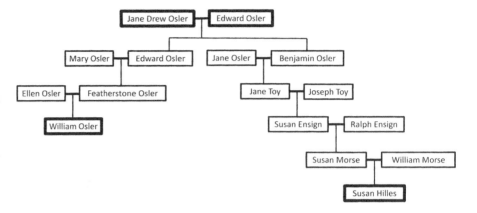

Figure 4. Abbreviated family tree, showing William Osler and Susan Hilles's common ancestors, Edward Osler (1732–1786) and Jane (or Joan) Drew Osler (? –1827).

as a minister in Connecticut and Massachusetts until 1929, when he began to devote his time to historical research.

William and Alice Morse became significant benefactors to Dalhousie University, Acadia College, Harvard, and Yale, where they endowed the Susan A.E. Morse and William Inglis Morse Fund for the Purchase of Canadiana. An account of the Canadiana collection at Yale draws "on the words of encouragement issued by its greatest champion, William Inglis Morse, 'Building up means tearing down & reverse & then some.... Keep up the struggle & never give in!'"[13] Their daughter, Susan, married lieutenant colonel Frederick Whiley Hilles (1900–1975), an intelligence officer with the U.S. Army during World War II in which he served as a code-breaker at Bletchley Park in Buckinghamshire, England. After the war he became Bodman Professor of English Literature at Yale and authority on Sir Joshua Reynolds.

Drawing on this rich legacy of philanthropy, and also on her sophistication in art and literature, Susan Toy Morse Hilles became a benefactress to several institutions, including Radcliffe College (The Susan Morse and Frederick Whiley Hilles Library, now known simply as the Hilles Library at Harvard and a popular student center) and the Massachusetts Eye and Ear Infirmary.[19] Her donation to the Department of Ophthalmology at Harvard Medical School was in all likelihood primarily out of gratitude for successful treatment of her own complex eye condition that began as herpes zoster ophthalmicus.

It is suggested here that Susan Hilles had at least two other reasons to fund a William Osler Professorship of Ophthalmology at Harvard. First, she probably absorbed from her father a keen sense of appreciation for all things Canadian, and Osler was (and remains) Canada's most iconic medical figure. Second, she was aware that she and William Osler had common ancestors in the persons of Edward Osler (1732–1786) of Falmouth, Cornwall, and his wife, Jane (also known as Joan) Drew Osler (1738–1827) (Figure 4). However, it is unlikely that Susan Hilles ever met Osler. She was born in 1905, the same year Osler sailed to England to become Regius professor of medicine at Oxford, and she was only 14 years of age when Osler died. A search that included the Susan Hilles Papers at the Schlesinger Library, Radcliffe Institute, and the records of the Development Office of Harvard Medical School gave no indication that she and Osler ever met.

Osler, if alive today, might appreciate the irony of a professorship named for him, in a specialty he was unable to enter.

Acknowledgments

I thank the staffs of the Osler Library, McGill University, Montreal, Canada, the Howe Library of Ophthalmology, Massachusetts Eye and Ear Infirmary, Boston, the Schlesinger Library, Harvard University, Cambridge, Massachusetts, and the Offices of Development at Harvard University and at Harvard Medical School, and the Boston Athenaeum, Boston Massachusetts.

References

1. Cushing H. *The Life of Sir William Osler*. Oxford: Clarendon Press; 1925L i: 91–94; ii: 252–253.
2. Bliss M. *William Osler: A Life in Medicine*. Toronto: Toronto University Press; 1999: 7, 68–69.
3. Snyder C. Young doctor Osler and the road not taken. *Archives of Ophthalmology* 1965; 73(1): 124–127.
4. Barnes CH. Osler and ophthalmology. *Documenta Ophthalmologica* 1990; 74(1–2): 1–8.
5. Fishman R. William Osler, almost ophthalmologist. *American Journal of Ophthalmology* 2007; 146(3): 368.
6. Osler W. The Master-word in medicine. In Osler W. *Aequanimitas, With other Addresses*.
7. Hanaway J. Early history, 1819–85. In Hanaway J, Burgess H. *The General: A History of the Montreal General Hospital*. Montreal & Kingston: McGill-Queens University Press; 2016: 46.
8. Heath P. Sir William Bowman. *Bulletin of the Medical Library Association* 1936; 24(4): 205–208.
9. http://eye.hms.harvard.edu/professorships/osler. Accessed 20 July 2020.
10. www.legacy,com/obituaries/hartfordcourant/obituary.aspx?n=susan-morse-hilles&pid=181450. Accessed 20 July 2020.
11. https://www.geni.com/people/Sir-William-Osler-MD/6000000007279500132?through=6000000015974576283. Accessed 20 July 2020.
12. https://www.geni.com/people/susan-Toy/6000000029421404887?through=6000000053394442064/ Accessed 20 July 2020.
13. Little G. "I think Canada has a future." William Inglis Morse and the Canadian Collection at Yale University. *Papers of the Bibliographical Society of Canada* 2009; 47(1): 75–91.

The Centenary of William Osler's "The Old Humanities and the New Science"

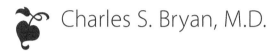 Charles S. Bryan, M.D.

Sir William Osler (1849–1919), the most famous physician in the English-speaking world during the early-twentieth century, continues to inspire through popular aphorisms and various writings, such as the 22 addresses published under the title *AEQUANIMITAS*.[1–3] He gave the *AEQUANIMITAS* addresses before leaving North America in 1905 to become Regius Professor of Medicine at Oxford. Less well-known are his later addresses to British audiences, some of which contain deeply philosophical musings on the human condition.

Osler's last published address, entitled "The Old Humanities and the New Science" and given as the presidential address to the Classical Association on 16 May 1919, is often cited as a paean to the Hippocratic maxim, "Where there is love of humanity (*philanthropia*), there also is love of the art (*philotechnia*)."[4–8] Osler's deeper concern that day, however, was the destructive power of the weapons unleashed during the Great War (1914–1918). He yearns for wisdom (*philosophia*) to secure "the longings of humanity," by which he implies health, prosperity, and world peace. He fires an early shot across the bow against what is now being called the myth of human exceptionalism: "There must be a very different civilization or there will be no civilization at all."

Presented in part as the inaugural Charles S. Bryan Lecture in the Medical Humanities, South Carolina Chapter, American College of Physicians, Charleston, South Carolina, on October 21, 2017, and also at the forty-ninth annual meeting of the American Osler Society, Montreal, Quebec, Canada, on 15 May 2019. This paper was previously published in the *Journal of Medical Biography* (2019; 27[4]: 197–204), and is reproduced with permission.

Background

"The classics" comprise the languages and cultures of Greek and Roman antiquity and, during Osler's lifetime, were virtually synonymous with "the humanities." Grounding in the classics identified the British professional and social elite. Classics teachers reigned in public schools and universities. Oxford and Cambridge required Greek and Latin for entrance.

Around 1870 a push began for greater emphasis on science and technology. In 1873 science professors at Oxford, wanting better-prepared students, motioned to remove the compulsory Greek requirement. They failed but their cause did not go away.[9]

The Classical Association was founded in 1903 partly to defend the pre-eminence of the classics in education and public life, and this *raison d'être* assumed greater importance during and after the Great War.[10] In 1918 its president was Gilbert Murray (1866–1957), Regius Professor of Greek at Oxford, public intellectual, outspoken peace advocate, and friend of William Osler.[11–14] Murray nominated Osler to succeed him.

The Classical Association was not the first organization of British educators to ask Osler to be its president. He had previously been president of the Association of Public School Science Masters. On 4 January 1916, Osler told the science teachers:

> Your society indicates the position which the science master has reached in our public schools, not without long years of struggle. The glamour of the classics lingers, but the shock which the nation has had in this great war will make us realize in the future that to keep in the van we must be in the van intellectually in all that relates to man's control of nature. Science "Heads" at Winchester, Eton, and Harrow would give the death-blow to the old-time Anglican tradition so well-expressed . . . by the late Dean Gaisford [Thomas Gaisford (1779–1855)] that classical learning "not only elevates above the common herd, but leads not infrequently to positions of considerable emolument."[15]

A committee formed and drew up "a strong memorandum on the unsatisfactory position which science occupies in national affairs and particularly in our public schools and old universities." Osler was among 36 "distinguished men of science" signatory to the document published in *The Times*.[16,17]

By late 1916 educational interest groups included a Committee on the Neglect of Science, a Conjoint Board of Scientific Societies, and a Council for Humanistic Studies, whose sections included the Classical Association, the English Association, the Geographical Association, the Historical Association, and the Modern Language Association. There ensued a series of joint conferences, at the center of which was Sir Frederic Kenyon (1863–1952), a classicist, paleographer, biblical scholar, director of the British Museum, chairman of a committee to plan cemeteries for the British Commonwealth war dead, and friend of William Osler.[18–20] In 1917 Kenyon edited a pamphlet for the Council for Humanistic Studies, holding that while science and technology were "essential to our industrial prosperity and national safety," the classics pertained "to the deeper interests and problems of politics, thought, and human life." Moreover, "The scientific method is not the peculiar property of physical science; all good work in all studies is based upon it; it is indispensable to law, history, classics,

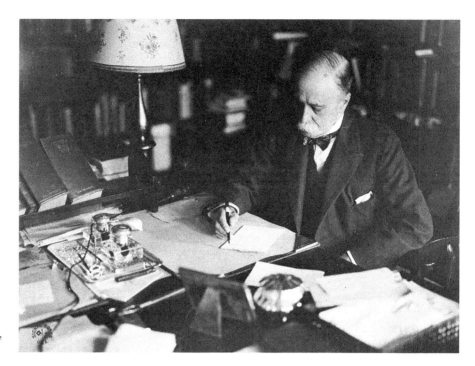

Figure 1. During the last two years of his life, Sir William Osler, shown here at his desk at Oxford, dialogued with other British intellectuals on ways to recalibrate the balance between the humanities and the sciences in British public schools and universities.
Credit: Osler Library of the History of Medicine, McGill University.

politics, and all branches of knowledge rightly understood."[18] Osler and Murray were among the signatories.

Murray, in nominating Osler for president of the Classical Association in January 1918, praised him for his "broad interest in letters of all kinds."[21] Osler was a keen student of the classics. In Baltimore he had enjoyed a playful running debate with the American classicist Basil Gildersleeve (1831–1924) over the worthiness of Eryximachus, the doctor in Plato's *Symposium*.[22] At Oxford he had lectured on "Lessons of Greek Medicine" to one of Murray's classes.[23] In the spring of 1918 Osler wrote a friend, "I have to do a lot of reading for the Presidential Address to the Classical association! . . . . I am the first Doctor, so I take it as a compliment, but a bit of a burden. I shall talk on the 'the classical Tradition in Science.'"[7, ii: 600]

Osler later changed the title, suggesting he changed his mind and revolved to face the curricular controversy head-on. Thus, in April 1918, he wrote another friend, "I am struggling with an address . . . [and] am a bit nervous. I have a good subject, *The Old Humanism & The New Science*."[7, ii: 647] He probably substituted "The Old Humanities" for "The Old Humanism" after reading a paper on "The Humanities" by Percy Stafford Allen (1869–1933), to which Osler refers in his lecture.

In 1917 Percy Allen, an Oxford colleague of Osler and authority on the Dutch humanist Desiderius Erasmus (1466–1536), reviewed ways by which the "subjects of human study" had been grouped through the centuries.[24,25] At one time, for example, there had been the *trivium* (grammar, logic, and rhetoric) and the *quadrivium* (arithmetic, geometry, music, and astronomy). It was not until the Renaissance that scholars commonly spoke of *studia humanitas* (the humanities). Allen asserted that by 1917 most subjects fell into either of two categories, so that "roughly speaking, we may say that on one side is the study of nature, on the other of man." Allen pointed out that "*humanist* has had many senses," and called for revival of "the humanities" as the appropriate term for the classics. Osler's title thus became "The Old Humanities and the New Science."

Osler fretted up to the last hour. On record as an advocate for more science in the curriculum, —–what might he say to the Classical Association, representing nearly 1,500 persons many of whose jobs hinged on the curricular controversy? He told his former Baltimore colleague William Henry Welch (1850–1934), in Oxford for the occasion, that he "had never given so much time and thought to the preparation of an address" as he did to this one.[7, ii: 65] Osler's faults included an excessive desire to be liked. He had even signed petitions both for and against Oxford's compulsory Greek requirement.[29]

Osler and Welch spent the hour before the address reviewing two exhibits Osler had prepared for attendees. At last Osler donned his scarlet robe, joined the academic procession, and mounted the black oak pulpit of the Oxford Divinity School ready to admit to the classicists "such anticipatory qualms as afflict an amateur at the thought of addressing a body of experts."[4-6]

The Address

The literary and cultural critic H. L. Mencken (1880–1956) admired Osler's technical prose but faulted his essays: "He wrote gracefully and charmingly, but I doubt if his compositions will be long remembered. Even today, indeed, they are not much read. A considerable pedantry is in them; they smell of the lamp."[27] The smell of the lamp wafts heavily over "The Old Humanities and the New Science." Few if any other addresses by Osler contain so many references to antiquity, the Bible, English poets, Shakespeare, historical figures, and obscure facts.[28] The address remains of interest because of the continued relevance of its main themes: the relationship of the humanities to the sciences and the destructiveness of modern weapons.

Osler describes himself as "not an educated man in the Oxford sense" and "a mere picker-up of learning's crumbs." Alluding to the Scientific Revolution, he acknowledges the "wonderful privilege" of living through "an epoch matched only by two in the story of the race [the classical period and the Renaissance]." Never before in its long evolution," he continues, "has the race realized its full capacity." He stops short of saying "full capacity for good and evil," perhaps because this was self-evident to an audience recovering from the Great War. Most attendees were probably aware that the Oslers, like so many others, had lost their son, Second Lieutenant Edward Revere Osler (1895–1917) and were still grieving.

Before the war Osler like others during the Progressive Era (roughly, 1896 to 1916), saw science mainly as a force for good. In a 1910 lay sermon at the University of Edinburgh, "Man's Redemption of Man," Osler rejoiced in "the final conquest of nature" and quoted Percy Bysshe Shelley that "Happiness and Science dawn though late upon the earth..."[29] Five years later, as the Battle of Loos raged across the English Channel, Osler acknowledged that "some of us had indulged the fond hope that in the power man had gained over nature had arisen possibilities for intellectual and social development.... We were foolish enough to think that where Christianity had failed Science might succeed." After reviewing the destructiveness of the new weapons one by one, he asked: "And what shall be our final judgment—for or against science?"[30]

Now, the war over, Osler asks his Oxford audience what war reveals about ourselves:

> Enough to say that war blasts the soul, and in this great conflict the inner sense of humanity has been shocked to paralysis by the helplessness of our civilization and the futility of our religion to stem a wave of primitive barbarism.... What a shock to the proud and mealy-mouthed Victorian who had begun to trust that Love was creation's final law.... we stand aghast at the revelation of the depth and ferocity of primal passions which reveal the unchangeableness of human nature.

He confesses: "Two years changed me into an ordinary barbarian," and continues:

> ... it has yet to be determined whether Science, as the embodiment of a mechanical force, can rule without invoking ruin. Two things are clear: there must be a very different civilization or there will be no civilization at all; and the other is that neither the old religion combined with the old learning, nor both with the new science, suffice to save a nation bent on self-destruction.

He observes that "the suicide of Germany, the outstanding fact of the war" occurred despite its strong religious heritage and supremacy in the classics; the proportion of students who studied Greek and Latin had been higher in Germany than in any other Western nation.

Turning now to the title theme and with implied reference to the curricular controversy, Osler starts with the classicists. He compares them to the larvae of an insect hive: "Among academic larvae you have for centuries absorbed the almost undivided interest of the nest, and not without reason, for the very life of the workers depends on the hormones you secrete." Those who teach the humanities "secrete materials which do for society at large what the thyroid does for the individual. The Humanities are the hormones." He reviews the extent to which classicists dominated Oxford. In 1919 only 51 of the 257 Heads and Fellows of the 23 colleges at Oxford were scientists, even including the mathematicians. Osler tells the classicists that their teaching methods were stale and that and they paid insufficient attention to Lucretius (c. 99 B.C.–c. 15 B.C.), the Roman poet and natural philosopher.

As to the scientists, their spiraling specialization risks loss of perspective:

> The extraordinary development of modern science may be her undoing. Specialism, now a necessity, has fragmented the specialties themselves in a way that makes the outlook hazardous. The workers lose all sense of proportion in a maze of minutiae.... Applying themselves early to research, young men get into backwaters far from the main stream. They quickly lose the sense of proportion, become hypercritical, and the smaller the field, the greater the tendency to megalocephaly.

Scientific papers can be almost incomprehensible beyond small spheres of interest. Science must be accessible, for it "will take a totally different position ... when the knowledge of its advances is the possession of all educated men." He asks for "recognition of a new philosophy—the *scientia scientiarum*," which we would now call the philosophy of science. Being intrinsically value-neutral, science needs the humanities for guidance. The old humanities and the new science should be complementary and mutually-reinforcing.

Harking back to antiquity, Osler asks whether cultural flourishing such as occurred during the Golden Age of Athens (480 B.C.–404 B.C.) is even possible "in a civilization based on a philosophy of force." He ends with his frequently-quoted paraphrasing of a Hippocratic fragment (*Precepts*, vi, 6):

> There is a sentence in the writings of the Father of Medicine [Hippocrates] upon which all commentators have lingered . . . the love of humanity associated with the love of his [the physician's] craft!—philanthropia and philotechnia—the joy of working joined in each one to a true love of his brother. Memorable sentence indeed! in which for the first time was coined the magic word *philanthropy*, and conveying the subtle suggestion that perhaps in this combination the longings of humanity may find their solution, and Wisdom—philosophia—at last be justified of her children.

The audience applauded and drifted over to 13 Norham Gardens, where Lady Osler entertained some 200 classicists over tea.

Epilogue

British and American colleagues praised the address for its "well-night perfect example of the union of science and the humanities"; for its "wealth of knowledge, insight, and wit"; for how it "was Osler at his very best"; and for how Osler showed "the best classical men" in England how little they knew about science.[7, ii: 650; 31,32] An American classicist who had not been there in person took offense at Osler's criticism of classicists' teaching methods and carped that Osler said nothing new.[33]

On 29 December 1919, Sir William Osler died from hemorrhage into an empyema cavity after a prolonged lower respiratory infection. Some contemporaries felt grief over his son contributed to his death. Osler's closing paragraph on *philanthropia* and *philotechnia* thus became his farewell valentine to medicine.

In 1920 Oxford and Cambridge dropped compulsory Greek requirements for entrance. However, efforts to recalibrate British education toward more emphasis on science failed. Between 1922–1923 and 1938–1939 the proportion of science students in British universities actually fell.[34]

In 1946 a group of U.S. scientists including Albert Einstein (1879–1955) and J. Robert Oppenheimer (1904–1967), joined by opinion leaders such as Walter Lippman (1889–1974) and the Federation of American Scientists, issued a booklet entitled *One World or None*, reminiscent of Osler's warning that "there must be a very different civilization or there will be no civilization at all."[35] In 1947 an international group of researchers wound up a hypothetical Doomsday Clock.

In 1959 C. P. Snow (1905–1980), in *The Two Cultures and the Scientific Revolution*, called for more integration of science into intellectual life, more interaction between the sciences and the humanities, a rethinking of educational priorities, and public alarm over the still-newer (nuclear) weapons—just as Osler had done 40 years earlier.[36] Snow's title made "the two cultures" a cultural cliché, although Sir Frederic Kenyon, Percy Allen, Osler, and others had expressed the same idea four decades earlier.

In 2009 the developmental psychologist Jerome Kagan (b. 1929) proposed a "three cultures" grouping of the subjects of human study that takes into account

Table.   The Three Cultures Grouping of the Subjects of Human Study*

Area	Natural Sciences	Social Sciences	Humanities
Primary focus	Understanding and explaining natural phenomena	Understanding human behavior and psychological states	Understanding the meaning humans impose on experience as a function of time/place and life history
Chief sources of evidence	Observations of material entities	Behaviors, verbal statements, and (less often) biological measures	Written texts and human behaviors
Extent of control of conditions	Rigorous control is strongly desired.	Control of contexts is often difficult.	Minimum control of the conditions of observations.
Primary vocabulary	Semantic and mathematical concepts	Constructs referring to psychological features, states, and behaviors of individuals or groups	Concepts regarding human behavior, with serious contextual restrictions on inferences
Influence of history	Minimal	Modest	Major
Ethical influence	Minimal	Major	Major
Criteria for beauty	Conclusions that involve the most fundamental components of nature	Conclusions that support a broad theoretical view of human behavior	Semantically-coherent arguments described in elegant prose

*After Kagan (40)

the social sciences, such as anthropology, economics, linguistics, political science, psychology, and sociology (Table).[37] Previous generations looked to the humanities for wisdom—*philosophia*, Osler's ultimate desideratum. Social scientists and natural scientists have begun to take "wisdom" seriously—how to define it, how to measure it, how to promote it. Psychologists, following the lead of Paul Baltes (1939–2006), seek ways to measure wisdom defined as "expertise in the fundamental pragmatics of life."[38,39] Neuroscientists explore the anatomy, chemistry, and physiology of wisdom.[40–42] Artificial intelligence will enhance decision-making capacity, but wisdom will be needed to harness its algorithmic capabilities.

Osler could not have known about artificial intelligence when he alluded to "additional capabilities of mental nutrition, and that increased breadth of view which is of the very essence of wisdom,"[43] but we can safely assume that he would exhort us to glean all we can from the natural sciences, the humanities, and the social sciences to fulfill "the longings of humanity" for the present and future generations. He might remind us of the famous dictum of Rudolf Virchow (1821–1902), "Medicine is a social science and politics nothing but medicine at a larger scale."[44] He might reiterate the sentiment he expressed in one his 1905 farewell addresses to North American physicians: "The profession of medicine forms a remarkable world-unit in the progressive evolution of which there is a fuller hope for humanity than in any other direction."[45]

And, with reference to the classics and to newer approaches to wisdom through the natural sciences and the social sciences, he might echo a sentiment expressed by his Oxford colleague Percy Allen: "The world needs all the knowledge it can get."[25] Physicians and other health care workers, operating at the interface of the natural sciences, the social sciences, and the humanities, are at least as well-positioned as most others to make a difference.

References

1. Osler W. *Aequanimitas, With other Addresses to Medical Students, Nurses and Practitioners of Medicine.* Third edition, Philadelphia: P. Blakiston's Son & Co., Inc.; 1932.

2. Kimbrough RC III. The good gift: A comparison of the Eli Lilly presentation copies of *Aequanimitas. Journal of the South Carolina Medical Association* 1999; 91: 350–354.

3. Silverman ME, Murray TJ, Bryan CS. *The Quotable Osler.* Philadelphia: American College of Physicians; 2003.

4. Osler W. The president's address. *Classical Association Proceedings* 1919; 16; 5–34.

5. Osler W. The old humanities and the new science. *British Medical Journal* 1919; 2(3053): 1–7.

6. Osler W. *The Old Humanities and the New Science.* Boston: Houghton Mifflin Company; 1920.

7. Cushing H. *The Life of Sir William Osler.* Oxford: Clarendon Press; 1925: ii: 648–652.

8. Bliss M. *William Osler. A Life in Medicine.* New York: Oxford University Press; 1999: 460–462.

9. Stray CA. Culture and discipline: classics and society in Victorian England. *International Journal of the Classical Tradition* 1996; 3(1): 77–85.

10. Bryce J. The worth of ancient literature for the modern world. *Classical Association Proceedings* 1917; 14: 8–32.

11. Dodds ER. Introduction. In: Smith J, Toynbee A, eds. *Gilbert Murray: An Unfinished Autobiography.* London: George Allen and Unwin, Ltd.; 1960:13–19.

12. Murray G. Faith, War, and Policy. *Addresses and Essays on the European War.* Boston: Houghton Mifflin Company; 1917.

13. Murray G. *The League of Nations and the Democratic Idea.* Oxford: Oxford University Press; 1918.

14. Wilson D. *Gilbert Murray OM: 1866–1957.* Oxford: Oxford University Press; 1987.

15. Osler W. Intensive work in science at the public schools in relation to the medical curriculum. *The School World. A Monthly Magazine of Educational Work and Progress* 1916; 18(206)(February): 41–44.

16. Daniell GF. Science at educational conferences. *Nature* 1916; 96(2411): 547–549.

17. Unsigned. University and educational intelligence. *Nature* 1916; 96(2414): 639–640.

18. Kenyon FG. *War Graves: How the cemeteries abroad will be designed. Report to the Imperial War Graves Commission.* London: H.M.S.O.; 1918.

19. Kenyon FG, ed. *Education: Scientific & Humane. A Report of the Proceedings of the Council for Humanistic Studies.* London: John Murray; 1917.

20. Kenyon FG. *Education: Secondary and University. A Report of Conferences between the Council for Humanistic Studies and the Conjoint Board of Scientific Societies.* London: John Murray; 1919.

21. Murray G, presiding. Report of general meeting held at King's College, Strand, on January 7th and 8th, 1918. *Classical Association Proceedings* 1918; 15: 41–51.

22. Bryan CS, Wise BK, Briggs WW. William Osler and Basil Gildersleeve on Plato's Eryximachus. *Journal of Medical Biography* 2003; 11: 35–40.

23. Golden RL. *The Lessons of Greek Medicine: William Osler's Cardinal Ethic.* Montreal: Osler Library, McGill University, and the American Osler Society; 2013.

24. Mansfield BE. Anguish of an Erasmian: P. S. Allen and the Great War. *Parergon* 1996; 14: 257–276.

25. Allen PS. The humanities. *Classical Association Proceedings* 1917; 14: 123–133.

26. Garrod A. The power of personality. *British Medical Journal* 1929; 2(3584): 509–512.

27. Mencken HL. Osler [review of Cushing H. *The Life of Sir William Osler*]. *American Mercury* 1925; 5(20): 505–507.

28. Hinohara S, Niki, H, eds. "The Old Humanities & the New Science." In: Hinohara S, Niki H, eds. *Osler's "A Way of Life" and Other Addresses, with Commentary and Annotations.* Durham: Duke University Press; 2001: 65–97.

29. Osler W. *Man's Redemption of Man. A Lay Sermon, McEwan Hall Edinburgh, Sunday July 2nd, 1910.* New York: Paul B. Hoeber; 1913.

30. Osler W. On science and war. *Lancet* 1915; 186(4806): 795–801.

31. Mackail JW. [Remarks]. *Classical Association Proceedings* 1919; 16: 64–65.

32. Viets H. Glimpses of Osler during the war. In: [Abbott ME, ed.]. *Sir William Osler Memorial Number. Bulletin No. IX of the International Association of Medical Museums and Journal of Technical βMethods.* Montreal: Privately printed; 1926: 402–406.

33. [Knapp C]. Sir William Osler on the classics (especially Aristotle and Lucretius). *The Classical Weekly* 1919; 13(12): 89–90.

34. Sherrington G. *English Education, Social Change and War 1911–20.* Manchester, UK: Manchester University Press; 1981: 171.

35. Masters D, Way K. *One World or None. A Report to the Public on the Full Meaning of the Atomic Bomb.* New York: McGraw-Hill Book Company, Inc.; 1946.

36. Snow CP. *The Two Cultures and the Scientific Revolution.* New York: Cambridge University Press; 1959, 19, 54.

37. Kagan J. *The Three Cultures. Natural Sciences, Social Sciences, and the Humanities in the 21st Century.* New York: Cambridge University Press, 2009.

38. Baltes PB, Staudinger UM. Wisdom. A metaheuristic (pragmatic) to orchestrate mind and virtue toward excellence. *American Psychologist* 2000; 55: 122–136.

39. Banicki K. The Berlin Wisdom Paradigm: A conceptual analysis of a psychological approach to wisdom. *History & Philosophy of Psychology* 2009; 11(2): 25–35.

40. Meeks TW, Jeste DV. Neurobiology of wisdom: a literature overview. *Archives of General Psychiatry* 2009; 66: 355–65.

41. Jeste DV, Harris JC. Wisdom—a neuroscience perspective. *Journal of the American Medical Association* 2010; 304: 1602–1603.

42. Williams PB, Nusbaum H. Toward a neuroscience of wisdom. In: Absher JR, Clotier J, eds. *Neuroimaging, personality, social cognition, and character.* London, UK: Elsevier; 2016: 383–395.

43. Osler W. The army surgeon. Osler W. *AEQUANIMITAS, With other Addresses to Students, Nurses and Practitioners of Medicine.* Third edition, Philadelphia: P. Blakiston's Son & Co., Inc.; 1932: 97–113.

44. Mackenbach JP. Politics is nothing but medicine at a larger scale: reflections on public health's biggest idea. *Journal of Epidemiology and Community Health* 2009; 63: 181–184.

45. Osler W. Unity, peace and concord. In: Osler W. *AEQUANIMITAS, With other Addresses to Students, Nurses and Practitioners of Medicine.* Third edition, Philadelphia: P. Blakiston's Son & Co., Inc.; 1932, 425–443.

SECTION II

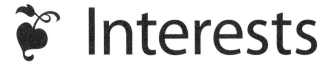 Interests

Sir William Osler and Robert Burton's *The Anatomy of Melancholy,* "The Greatest Medical Treatise Written by a Layman"

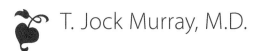 T. Jock Murray, M.D.

In the niche in the Osler Library that holds Sir William Osler's favorite books there are the many editions of Robert Burton's *The Anatomy of Melancholy*, which Osler famously called "the greatest medical treatise written by a layman."[1] Of all the books collected by and associated with Osler, this treatise on depression occupied more of his time than any other book. In a recent publication about the books associated with Osler, I wrote a chapter on Osler's relationship with Burton's *The Anatomy of Melancholy* and suggested we knew more of Osler's views on this book than any other, even Sir Thomas Browne's *Religio Medici*, with which he is famously associated.[2] He spent years searching for the books of Robert Burton in Oxford and he lectured and wrote on Burton, his library and on the text of *The Anatomy of Melancholy*.[3]

At the annual meeting of the American Osler Society in 2012, I outlined my personal search for evidence of Osler's search.[3] When Osler was appointed as the Regius professor of medicine at Oxford he initially stayed in the Old Library at Christ Church and said he was delighted to be in the same rooms as Burton and John Locke. He stayed in room number five, up the old stairs of the building

Presented in part at the forty-second annual meeting of the American Osler Society, Chapel Hill, North Carolina, on 23 April 2012. Portions of this paper have been published in the *Osler Library Newsletter* (2012, number 117[fall]: 2–5) and in *Osler's Bedside Library* (Lacombe MA, Elpern DJ, eds., Philadelphia: American College of Physicians; 2010: 237–248), and are reprinted with permission.

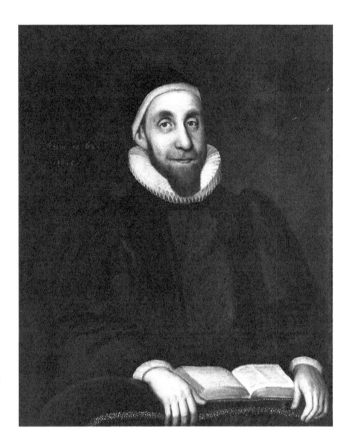

Figure 1. Copy of the Brasenose portrait of Robert Burton commissioned by Osler.

now used as a student residence. He wrote to Daniel Gilman: "I have rooms at Christ Church.... My quarters are in the old [Library] building & I picture to myself that Burton or Locke may have inhabited them."[4]

Soon after, Osler set out on a search for the many editions of Burton's *The Anatomy of Melancholy* and the hundreds of volumes Burton referenced and quoted in this monumental work.[5,6] The copies in the Bodleian were easier to find as the librarian who received the part of Burton's library bequeathed to the Bodleian made a list of the books. It was more difficult to find the books bequeathed to Christ Church Library as they were distributed throughout the collection. Osler, with the assistance of a student, Charles Woolly, later a famous archeologist, and a secretary, searched for books with Burton's name, initials and other marks he made on his books. Osler was disappointed that he didn't find much interesting marginalia or many important medical books among the collection.

Over the next few years Osler lectured to groups about Burton, his great book, and his library. He even planned a new edition of Burton's book. We get a flavor of his love for the book from his Silliman Lectures at Yale University in 1913:

> No book of any language presents such a stage of moving pictures—
> kings and queens in their greatness and in their glory, in their madness
> and in their despair; generals and conquerors with their ambitions and
> their activities; philosophers of all ages, now rejoicing in the power of
> intellect, and again groveling before the idols of the tribe; the heroes of
> the race who have fought the battle of the oppressed in all lands; crimi-
> nals small and great, from the petty thief to Nero with his unspeakable

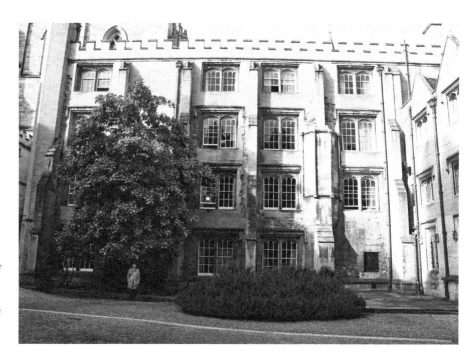

Figure 2. Old Library at Christ Church, Oxford, where Osler stayed in what may have been Burton's former room.

atrocities; the great navigators and explorers with whom Burton traveled so much in map and card, and whose stories were his delight; the martyrs and the virgins of all religions, the deluded and fanatics of all theologies; the possessed of devils and the possessed of God; the beauties, frail and faithful, the Lucretias and the Helens, all are there. The lovers, old and young; the fools who were accounted wise, and the wise who were really fools; the madmen of all history, to anatomize whom is the special object of this book; the world itself, against which he brings a railing accusation—the motley procession of humanity sweeps before us on his stage, a fantastic but fascinating medley at which he does not know whether to weep or to laugh.[7]

Osler initially located 580 volumes in the Bodleian and 429 in Christ Church Library that were referenced by Burton, and felt they should be brought together with all the editions of *The Anatomy of Melancholy* as they "should not and could not be divorced."[4, ii: 113] He arranged for a bookcase on one wall of the Christ Church Library to hold the books and in the middle was a portrait of Burton, a copy of the portrait at Brasenose College, which Osler commissioned. A photo of the wall and portrait can be seen in a photograph in Harvey Cushing's biography of Osler.[4, ii: opposite p. 113] Renovations in this room by the librarian in 1968, to make it more current for undergraduates, resulted in the books being removed to a new bookcase in the Archives Supra up a back stairway, and the portrait being placed above the entrance door, where they remain today.

In the summer of 1907, Osler gave a lecture in the Extension Course at Oxford titled "An Introduction to the Study of Anatomy of Melancholy."[4: ii: 101–102] He then planned a series of three lectures on the man, his book and the library. In November 1909 he spoke to the Biographical Society in Hanover Square, London, on "The Library of Robert Burton," relating his experience collecting the books.[8] He abandoned his plan to bring out a new edition of Burton's work when he heard that W. Aldis Wright of Cambridge, a noted Shakespearian, and Edward Bensley of Aberystwyth were already working on a new edition. A

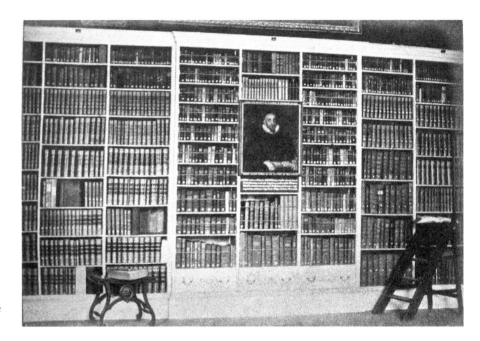

Figure 3. Osler's collection of Burton's reference books and the portrait of Burton.

copy of *The Anatomy of Melancholy* in the Osler Library has a letter from W. Aldis Wright tucked inside. Unfortunately, Wright toyed at this project for years and never completed the task. When the work was passed to Bensley, he decided to completely redo all of Wright's work, and this took so long it was never completed. The dawdling and procrastination of Wright and Bensley prevented us from having a new edition with an introduction written by Osler.

In his introduction to a 1964 edition of *Anatomy of Melancholy*, Holbrook Jackson said, "Robert Burton was a bookman, first and last."[9] This would certainly endear him to Osler, who was the consummate bookman. Like Burton, Osler sprinkled his writings with quotations from many sources in literature, medicine and philosophy. But as Osler said, there is hardly anything in literature like Burton, who had over 1,250 references and quotations in his book, including many of Osler's favorites such as Shakespeare, Montaigne, the Bible, Greek and Latin scholars, ancient philosophers, and many others. Burton had many, sometimes a dozen, quotations and references on every page.

Osler said, "By a profession a divine, by inclination Burton was a physician, and there is no English medical author of the seventeenth century whose writings have anything like the same encyclopedic character of a medical condition."[7]

The Life of Robert Burton

Robert Burton (1577–1640) was born at Lindley, Leicestershire, and educated at the free school of Sutton Coldfield and at Nuneaton Grammar School. He became a commoner at Brasenose College and was elected a Student at Christ Church, Oxford. He took holy orders and became the vicar of St. Thomas, Oxford, and later was rector of Seagrave, Leicestershire, appointed by his patron, Lord Berkeley.

In *The Anatomy of Melancholy* Burton warns of the danger of solitariness for the melancholy, even though he was a solitary person content to stay in his rooms surrounded by stacks of books. He was not a recluse, however, and could be charming and entertaining company and a cheerful and scintillating conversationalist able to discuss on any topic. He never married and suffered long periods of melancholy. He was very self-aware of his emotional state and the influences upon it and even stated that he had become addicted to the condition, which probably explains his long years preparing his great book on melancholy.

Although Burton is mainly associated with this one great book, he also wrote a Latin play, *Philosophaster*, which was thought to have disappeared until a manuscript was uncovered in 1862. Another play, *Alba*, was lost. He also wrote 19 poems for various Oxford miscellanies.

Burton had prophesized to friends that he would die at age sixty-three, and when he did, it sparked rumors that he had entered Heaven by way of the noose. There is no evidence that he committed suicide, however. He was buried in the north aisle of Christ Church Cathedral, and his older brother William Burton, author of a History of Leicestershire, provided a monument with his bust in colour with the epitaph he wrote himself carved underneath: *Paucis notus, paucioribus ignotus, hic jacet Democritus Junior, cui vitam dedit et mortem Melancholia.*

The Text of *The Anatomy of Melancholy*

Osler not only brought together the editions of Burton's *The Anatomy of Melancholy* (Figure 4), he also owned many copies. In the Osler Library at McGill University there is a copy with the inscription "Alexr Boswell/LB 1728," which probably was one of the two copies owned by James Boswell's father. In the Osler Library there is also an unpublished paper by Osler, "The Library of Robert Burton" (*Bibliotheca Osleriana* 4637).

Burton had called his work a "patchwork," but Osler disagreed, saying "it was a great medical treatise, the greatest ever written by a layman, orderly in arrangement, intensely serious in purpose, and weighty beyond belief with authorities . . . The centuries have made Burton's book a permanent possession of literature."[7] He said that if the work had just been a medical text it would have "since sunk in the ooze" like so many other seventeenth-century medical works but it lives on because of the human sympathy of his approach. On that point, Osler noted there were 86 medical texts in the Burton library, none of which are of great importance, and his medical knowledge was based on Galenical teachings, with little attempt in the later editions to keep up with the changing views of the newer science of the day such as the work of Harvey.[7]

Burton's book was published in 1621, a quarto of 900 pages, under the pseudonym Democritus Junior. He took the name from the story of Hippocrates visiting Democritus in Abdera and finding him under a tree, surrounded by dissected animals and reading a large book. Democritus explained that he was attempting to understand the basis of *astra bilis*, or melancholy. Burton explained that he was writing the book in Democritus' lap. The title page illustrates the three kinds of love melancholy—jealousy, heroical love, and superstition; and on the other side solitude, hypochondriasis, and madness. Below are two "sovereign plants," borage and hellebore, remedies for melancholy.

He admitted the book was excessively long and needed further editing, but in each subsequent edition he did little editing and added more material. Revised

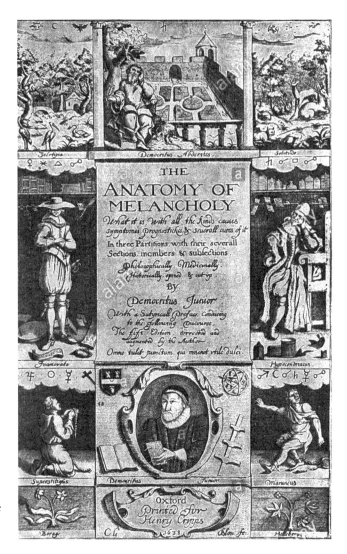

Figure 4. Frontispiece of Burton's *The Anatomy of Melancholy*.

and enlarged several times before his death, the treatise set out to explore the causes and effects of melancholy, but eventually covered many aspects of the human condition, with views from and about science, history, politics and social reform. The work is divided into three main portions: the various kinds of melancholy; the various cures; and an analysis of two specific forms, love melancholy and religious melancholy. The text is rich in quotations and references, excessive even in an age when heavy referencing was common. Burton's prose style is informal, anecdotal and witty, but often rambling.

Burton read hundreds of texts about melancholy and developed, like Samuel Johnson, personal maneuvers to ward off the black dog of melancholy whenever he felt its looming presence. In fact, the writing of this monumental work was a form of therapy. One might expect a work on melancholy by a melancholic man to be particularly depressing reading but readers for centuries have found it an interesting and often humorous work. Samuel Johnson said it was the only book that caused him to arise from bed two hours earlier than he wished.

Burton wrote a lot about medicine, physicians and various remedies. He said he got his love of medicine from his mother, a competent wise woman who had skills in surgery and the cure of many illnesses, who served the poor and destitute of the area, many of whom would attest to her abilities. Burton recognized he was meddling in physic but noted that many physicians were clerics and that melancholy was a compound illness, involving body and soul so clerics had just as much right examining it as did physicians. Burton's portrayal of melancholy and his own melancholy was, "Philosophically, Medicinally, Historically opened & cut-up," he says in the sub-title of *Anatomy*. It is a unique text on the subject. Osler also knew of an earlier book on melancholy, by physician-cleric Timothy Bright, *A Treatise on Melancholy*, which was undoubtedly used by Shakespeare as a basis for the psychology used in *Hamlet*.[10] In the Osler Library at McGill are Osler's copies of Bright's thesis and six of his other works (*Bibliotheca Osleriana* 2128–2134). Perhaps Burton's "addiction" to melancholy may explain some paradoxes in the work. He can be cheerful and witty when speaking of melancholy. He preaches a happy existence but does not practice it. He warns of solitariness but is a very solitary person. He writes of the importance and joys of travel but never traveled. His three-volume work has many apologies for being longwinded, and yet he expanded each edition. He worries that his discussion of love melancholy will go on too long, and then continues for another 200 pages. He expounds on marriage and the importance of a good wife, and of love and a strong family relationship, yet never married.

Why was Osler so interested in *The Anatomy of Melancholy*?

Osler would agree with the central recommendation in Burton's text—keep busy and do your work. Osler wrote an essay on the watchword of medicine, which is "Work," and Burton begins with this admonition and repeats it even more strongly in the last paragraph of the book. Osler would also share his views on illness having aspects of mind as well as body and on the need for physicians to have a priestly as well as a medical role. Osler, often called a therapeutic nihilist, would share Burton's critical acceptance of the physician's medicines, asking that when they are necessary, they should be coupled with mirth and lack of stress. Both believed that "tincture of time" would heal many disorders. But perhaps most important, Osler loved books, especially rare books, and this was a remarkable opportunity to pursue a medical subject through hundreds of texts.

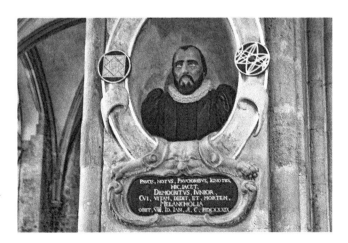

Figure 5. Osler's coffin rested overnight under the bust (effigy) of Robert Burton in Christ Church Chapel.

Epilogue

After Osler's death in 1919, a book of essays was published on Burton (1926) and Osler's tripartite article on the man, his book and his library was "reconstructed" into a chapter with the assistance of Lady Osler, Dr. W.W. Francis and Dr. Archibald Malloch.[11] There is an additional chapter by Osler on Burton as a transmitter.[12] Also included are two of Osler's lists of Burton's books and his will.

On the last page of Cushing's biography of Sir William Osler, he commented that when Osler died, his casket rested overnight in the chapel at Christ Church "with the quaint effigy of his beloved Robert Burton nearby."[13] Although a copy of Thomas Browne's *Religio Medici* was placed on his casket, and was said to be his favorite book, no book occupied Osler's energy and his time more than Robert Burton's *The Anatomy of Melancholy*.

Acknowledgments

I thank my daughter, Dr. Shannon Murray, Professor of English at the University of Prince Edward Island, for her insightful comments on Burton, corrections to the manuscript and for introducing me to Timothy Bright's *Treatise on Melancholy*. My wife, Janet Murray, was a keen-eyed copy editor and improved the work by insightful questioning. Pamela Miller, former head of the Osler Library, helped reference the Osler material on Burton in the Osler Library at McGill University. I also thank the staff at the Osler Library, the Wellcome Library, London, the British Library and the librarians at Christ Church Library, Oxford.

References

1. Osler W. *The Library of Robert Burton. Summary of his presentation to the Bibliographical Society of Great Britain, November 15th, 1909*.
2. Murray TJ. Robert Burton's *The Anatomy of Melancholy*. In LaCombe MA, Elpern DJ, eds. *Osler's Bedside Library: Great Writers Who Inspired a Great Physician*. Philadelphia: American College of Physicians; 2010: 237–248.
3. Murray TJ. Sir William Osler and Robert Burton. *Osler Library Newsletter*, 2012: No. 117 (Fall): 2–5.
4. Cushing H. *The Life of Sir William Osler*. Oxford: Clarendon Press; 1925: ii: 27.
5. Burton, R. *The Anatomy of Melancholy. What it is, With all the Kindes, Causes, Symptomes, Prognostickes, and Severall Cures of it. In Three Maine Partitions with their severall Sections, Members, and Subsections. Philosophically, Medicinally, Historically, Opened and Cut up. By Democritus Junior, With a Satyricall Preface, conducing to the following Discourse*. Macrob. Omne meum, Nihil meum. Oxford, 1621.
6. Burton, R. *Anatomy of Melancholy*. London: Dent. and Co.; 1964.
7. Osler, W. Burton's *Anatomy of Melancholy. Yale Review* 1914 (January): 251–271. Also quoted in Cushing, *Life of Sir William Osler*, ii: 359. Also in Francis WW, Hill RH, Malloch A, eds. *Bibliotheca Osleriana*. Oxford: Clarendon Press; 1919: 419 (entry 4637).

8. Osler W. The Library of Robert Burton. *Transactions of Bibliographical Society* 1910; XI: 4–7 (A summary of Osler's paper presented to the Society on November 15, 1909). Also quoted in Cushing, *Life of Sir William Osler*, ii: 199–201.

9. Jackson H. Introduction. In Burton R. *The Anatomy of Melancholy*. London: Dent. and Co.; 1964.

10. Bright T. *A Treatise of Melancholy, Containing the cavses thereof, & reasons of the strange effects it worketh in our minds and bodies: with the phisicke cure, and spirituall consolation for such as haue thereto adioyned an afflicted conscience.* London: Thomas Vautrollier; 1586.

11. Osler W. Robert Burton—the man, his book, his library. In Madan F, ed. Robert Burton and the *Anatomy of Melancholy*: Papers by Sir William Osler, Professor Edward Bensley, and Others. Oxford: Oxford University Press; 1926: 163–190.

12. Osler W. Burton as a Transmitter. Robert Burton and the *Anatomy of Melancholy*. In Madan F, ed. Robert Burton and the *Anatomy of Melancholy: Papers by Sir William Osler, Professor Edward Bensley, and Others*. Oxford; 1926: 163–190.

Sir William Osler's "Treasure" at Ewelme

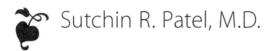 Sutchin R. Patel, M.D.

After deciding to leave Johns Hopkins for Oxford, Osler wrote to his former student, C.N.B. Camac (1868–1939) in 1904, "I leave Baltimore next year, after the session. I have accepted the Chair of Medicine at Oxford. Virtually it is a retirement as there is no clinical school but a purely academic berth, with as little or as much teaching as one likes. I am tired of the strain of the past few years which could only have one end—a breakdown."[1] One of the many aspects of Osler's time in Oxford that helped decrease the stress in his life was his connection to the almshouses at Ewelme.

The almshouses at Ewelme

Osler's appointment as Regius professor of medicine at Oxford also conferred upon him the title of Master of the old almshouses at Ewelme (Figure 1). (The terms "almshouse" and "almshouses" are used interchangeably here; technically, there was more than one building.) William de la Pole, Earl of Suffolk (1396–1450), along with his wife Alice (1404–1475), who was the granddaughter of the poet Geoffrey Chaucer (c. 1343–1400), played a prominent role in the founding of the Ewelme Almshouse which was originally a hospital. The village of Ewelme is situated in the Chilterns between London and Oxford. It is in Oxfordshire approximately 14 miles southeast of Oxford. It is first mentioned in the Domesday Book of 1086 as Lawelme. One story states that "Ewelme" means "spring" or "source of a river" describing the clear water that gushed from the hillside near the church.[2] An engraving describing the founding of God's House

Presented at the forty-fourth annual meeting of the American Osler Society, Oxford, United Kingdom, on 12 May 2014.

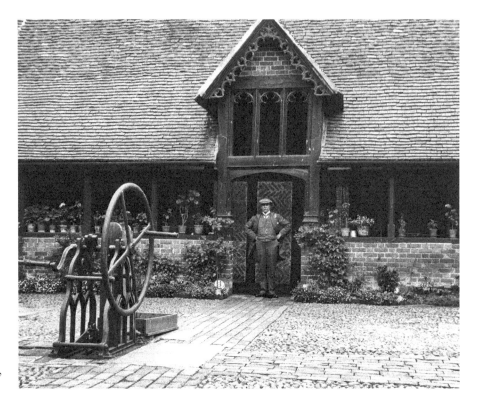

Figure 1. William Osler standing in the cloisters at the entry to the master's quarters, Ewelme almshouses. *Credit:* Osler Library of the History of Medicine, McGill University.

states that Ewelme was named so because of the "number of elms" in the area and because it was formerly called "New Elm."[3] Sir Charles Sherrington (1857–1952), a colleague of Osler at Oxford, describes Ewelme as a "small village which in itself was old-world, rural, and intersected by little running streams or 'freshets' full of watercress grown for the London market."[4]

The de la Pole family has been associated with Ewelme and the surrounding region for centuries. William de la Pole succeeded his father in 1415 as Earl of Suffolk when his father was killed at the battle of Agincourt. He subsequently became Duke of Suffolk. He married Alice Chaucer, the granddaughter to the poet Geoffrey Chaucer. Alice's father, Thomas Chaucer (c. 1367–1434), was Lord of the Manor of Ewelme. Both William and Alice were responsible for the founding of the Ewelme almshouse that was a hospital at the time. On 3 July 1437, King Henry VI granted to William, Duke of Suffolk and Alice "that they found a Hospital at their Manor of Ewelme, in the County of Oxford, and settle a sufficient endowment, not exceeding the yearly value of 200 marks, for the maintenance of two chaplains and thirteen poor men, to be incorporated and to have a Common Seal." One of the chaplains was to be called "Master of the Almshouse" who was to govern it and administer the affairs of the almshouse. The other chaplain was to be the "Teacher of Grammar" and in charge of the school. Each chaplain was to receive ten pounds each year, each of the thirteen almsmen was to receive three pounds, eight pence in a year and were given an allowance of coal and free medical and nursing care. In 1513 the de la Pole possessions were forfeited to the Crown and the three manors originally designated remained in a trust to support the almshouses. In 1617, James I annexed the Mastership held by one of the chaplains to the Regius professorship of medicine at Oxford to enhance the professor's meager income.[2, 5-6]

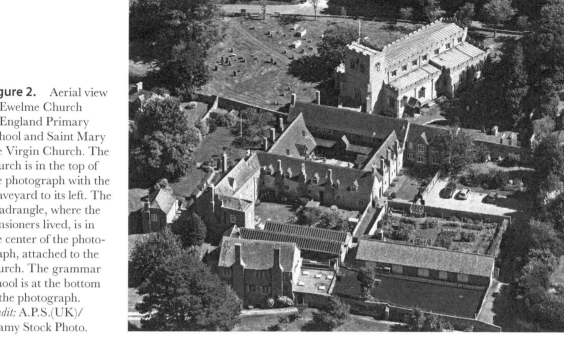

Figure 2. Aerial view of Ewelme Church of England Primary School and Saint Mary the Virgin Church. The church is in the top of the photograph with the graveyard to its left. The quadrangle, where the pensioners lived, is in the center of the photograph, attached to the church. The grammar school is at the bottom of the photograph. *Credit:* A.P.S.(UK)/ Alamy Stock Photo.

Shown in Figure 2 is a recent aerial view of the almshouses, St. Mary the Virgin Church and the Ewelme Church of England Primary School. In the almshouses, each of the almsmen had two rooms, an upper and lower room with a fireplace. The connected "cottages" opened into the center of the quadrangle. The master's rooms were located on the second floor at the southern end. A common hall existed on the upper floor of the northern end of the east range. The Master of Grammar's living quarters extended off the western aspect of the almshouses and was close to the grammar school. It is still a functional church primary school and is the oldest school building in the country to be in use as a state primary school. The upper classroom is known for its magnificent roof beams made from ship's timbers. The almshouses had gardens north, south and west of the quadrangle and it was amongst the almsmen's daily tasks to "keep clean the cloister and the quadrate about the well from weed and all other uncleanness and their gardens and alleys." The almshouse was named "God's House in Ewelme" and that remains to this day as the formal name of the charity which administers the trust and charity activities.[2,5]

The church at Ewelme is dedicated to St. Mary the Virgin and has a general likeness to East Anglican churches as it is a mixture of flint and stone. The church was built in 1437, the same year that Alice and the Duke of Suffolk built the school and founded the almshouse. It has no chancel arch, which adds to the lightness of the interior, nave and chancel. In the church, Alice the Duchess of Suffolk lies buried in an alabaster tomb (Figure 3). It is a two-story design. At the top, she wears a wedding ring on her right hand and the Order of the Garter on her left wrist. This is a distinction granted few women and marks the friendship between Suffolk and his wife and Henry VI and Margaret of Anjou. Queen Victoria, before her coronation is to have sent to Ewelme to ascertain the correct way to wear the garter. The tomb is flanked on either side by eight angels that

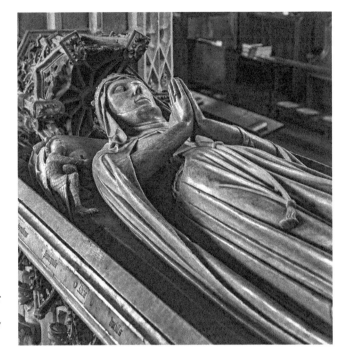

Figure 3.   Effigy of Alice de la Pole, Duchess of Suffolk and granddaughter of Geoffrey Chaucer. On her left arm is the Order of the Garter.
Credit: Charles O. Cecil/ Alamy Stock Photo.

bear the coat of arms of the many great families that the marriage of the de la Poles to Alice could claim a connection to. Beneath the tomb is a grating, or open crypt, which bears the effigy of the Duchess in graveclothes. Her tomb bears the inscription: "Pray for the soul of the most serene Princess Alice, Duchess of Suffolk, patron of this church and first foundress of this Almshouse, who died the 20th day of May in the year 1475."[2, 5]

The Oslers at Ewelme

It was in this quaint, pastoral village that the Oslers would become an important part of the community. On 19 June 1905, Mrs. Osler wrote: "Saturday Willie and I paid a visit to the much talked-of Almshouse at Ewelme. It is a most interesting place . . . there are rooms for the Master, but they have been altered and look painfully modern. The building nearly 500 years old is very picturesque and looks its age. The surgeon who looks after them [referring to the Almsmen] met us and we visited each member—it was most amusing. We carried tobacco and illustrated papers for each, and they were enchanted. I am sure Willie will make them all fond of him and be good to them."[3, ii: 6] By July 1906 Osler was moved into his master's quarters. Osler's biographer Harvey Cushing later wrote that "during the last two weeks of July, for the first time in man's memory the master's room were actually occupied by their rightful owner."[3, ii: 56]

Osler found peace and happiness in the village. Cushing wrote: "He was fascinated with the serene beauty of the place, knew the pains and aches of the old inmates and was generally adored by the villagers, among whom he played the part of antiquarian, physician, country gentleman and lover of nature. Enjoying everything and enjoyed by all."[3, ii: 56] Cushing's description illustrates the symbiosis between Osler and the villagers and pensioners at Ewelme. Osler took great pleasure in the connection to the almshouses at Ewelme and its thirteen elderly pensioners, who became a focal point of his interest and leisure time.

Both he and Lady Osler became a revitalizing part of the village and almshouses. They regularly picnicked with the families and children of the surrounding area in addition to the old pensioners. Osler's personal interest and love for children has been documented in many vignettes. Cushing describes one such story in Ewelme, "late in the afternoon a child of ten who had been missed by her mother was found wandering hand in hand with an unknown man she was calling 'William.' He had been devoting himself to her, and she was carrying a new doll."[3]

The "treasure"—the safe and its contents

In 1906 Osler discovered an ancient safe in one of the master's rooms at Ewelme. Both Cushing and Sherrington describe the episode where the safe was opened.[3, ii: 57–58; 4] A photograph entitled "Ewelme Muniments" shows Osler's second cousin, Dr. W.W. Francis (1879–1959), spreading the documents out at the graveyard on the North side of the church to dry in the sun.

Beneath the picture, Osler had written: "The photograph was taken on the day [July 28] we opened the safe in 1906. The safe had rusted and we had tried in every way to open it and at last had to get Chubb's man from London. The interior was coated uniformly with mold and the documents were reeking with damp. We took them into the graveyard and the photograph shows my nephew Dr. W.W. Francis of Montreal spreading them to dry in the sun. I then took them to the Bodleian where Maltby put them in order and bound them. William Osler Master"[3, ii: 57–58]

The contents of the safe included a document from 1359 a grant of various manors in England to Thomas de la Pole. Ancient title-deeds, indentures, audit accounts, conveyances, court rolls--some of them from the fourteenth century. The endowing of the almshouse at Ewelme with the manors of Marsh, Connock and Ramridge. The earliest document was a parchment roll of receipts, with direction for making Saltpeter—or gunpowder—it was then unknown to warfare but was useful for making a horrible noise.[3, ii: 58–59]

The documents could be divided into four sources: (1) documents relating to the administration and ownership of the almshouse estates—the earliest were passed on to the foundation by the de la Poles at the time of its establishment; (2) documentation generated by the Almshouse administration from William Marton's ascension to the mastership in 1455 onwards; (3) a collection of documents relating to the de la Pole's family concerns dating to between 1460 and 1467 which were in the possession of Alice's chaplain, Simon Brailles; and (4) the remaining documents included a set of documents including letters written by Alice to a favored member of the household, Robert Bilton. The muniments of Ewelme are currently housed in the Bodleian Library.

Cushing describes Osler's reaction to the muniments, "This was all very exciting and naturally enough when the muniments, having been restored by Maltby, were returned to their proper quarters there were many visitors to see them. The Master of the Hospital once invited the Oxford Architectural and Historical Society to hold a meeting at Ewelme, when he 'learnedly discoursed on the foundation, respecting which he exhibited interesting munimentary information."[3, ii: 58–59]

Sherrington described what happened when Osler noticed the strong box in his bedchamber: "The key when inquired for was not to be found and Osler, thoroughly intrigued wired to Chubb's of London, for an expert to pick the ancient lock. The expert when he came, looked at the chest, then taking a small wooden mallet from his travelling-bag, tapped the sides of the lid and almost at once lifted it.... The box contained deeds, many of them on vellum with seals attached, each seal in its little case fixed to the ribbon belonging to the document. Osler was enchanted. All the way home he could speak of nothing else."[4]

Earl Nation had a letter dated October 31, 1906 from Osler that further described his enthusiasm regarding the muniments. Osler wrote "I have been looking over the farm records of an old Hospital of which I am ex officio the Master and for which our farm accounts go back to 1393. If you wish to know the price of a pig in 1400 or of a calf in 1505, I can tell you to a farthing."[2]

The Oslers' later years at Ewelme

Sir William and Lady Osler entertained many guests at Ewelme. One such guest was John Brett Langstaff. His father and Osler were classmates in Toronto (at Trinity College and then at the Toronto Medical School) and when young Langstaff enrolled as a student of divinity at Magdalen College in Oxford in 1914, the Osler's invited him to spend a four-month vacation in the master's lodging at Ewelme writing his thesis on the English translation of the Latin Liturgy, entitled "The Holy Communion in Great Britain and America."[7, 8]

The last years of Osler's life involved the Great War and the death of the Oslers' son, Revere (1895–1917). Visits to Ewelme became less frequent. Lady Osler wrote in August 1914, "We went to Ewelme for church yesterday. Thirty men have gone from the village and hardly any left in the choir." Cushing later wrote that the men had gone from Ewelme "just as they had gone with the husband of Alice of Suffolk from Ewelme to Agincourt." After Sir William's death, Lady Osler would slowly resume her visits to Ewelme, likely finding solace in its tranquility.[2]

Caroline Ticknor visited Ewelme in 1924 and wrote: "It was a special privilege to visit Ewelme last summer in the company of Lady Osler, who is regarded by the villagers in this picturesque spot as 'Lady Bountiful,' she having endeavored in every way in her power to supplement her husband's work for the betterment of the village folk as well as the old pensioners."[9] On the south wall of the church in Ewelme, there is a memorial tablet with the names of Sir William, Lady Osler and Revere and under their names is one word: "Aequanimitas"

What were the true treasures of Ewelme?

Reflecting back on Sir William Osler's time at Ewelme, one might ask: What was the true treasure of Ewelme?" The muniments found in the strong box in the master's quarters brought Osler much excitement. They were a time capsule that allowed Osler a direct connection to the rich history of the village. However, the true treasures of Ewelme were the almshouses, the pensioners and the village. Ewelme gave Osler a refuge. It brought him peace and tranquility and helped rejuvenate his spirit.

Acknowledgments

I thank the late Earl Nation, who wrote about Osler as Master of Ewelme, and Michael E. Moran, who introduced me to the subject of Osler and Ewelme.

References

1. Nation EF. The influence of Osler on his students. *Journal of the American Medical Association* 1969; 210(12): 2226–2232.
2. Nation EF. Sir William Osler, the Master of Ewelme. *Canadian Medical Association Journal* 1973; 109(11): 1128–1132.
3. Cushing H. *The Life of Sir William Osler.* Oxford: Clarendon Press; 1925; ii: 57.
4. Sherrington C. Osler at Oxford. *British Medical Journal* 1949; 2(4618): 43–45.
5. Goodall JAA. *God's House at Ewelme: Life, Devotion and Architecture in a Fifteenth-Century Almshouse.* United Kingdom: Ashgate Publishing Limited; 2001.
6. Ward R. Ewelme, almshouses at, William Osler as Master of. In Bryan CS, ed. *Sir William Osler: An Encyclopedia.* Novato, California: Norman Publishing/HistoryofScience.com; 2020: 242–244.
7. Langstaff JB. Youthful recollections. *Journal of the American Medical Association* 1969; 210(12): 2233–2235.
8. Ward R. Langstaff, John Brett (1889–1985). In Bryan CS, ed. *Sir William Osler: An Encyclopedia.* Novato, California: Norman Publishing/HistoryofScience.com; 2020: 424–425.
9. Ticknor C. Sir William Osler and the thirteen pensioners of Ewelme. *Scribner's Magazine* 1925; 77(April): 417–422.

Christ Church and the Oslers

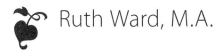 Ruth Ward, M.A.

Before William Osler attended the 1904 conference of the British Medical Association in Oxford he received an invitation from Dr. Thomas Banks Strong, Dean of Christ Church, to be his guest.[1] In November of that year he wrote to Herbert Warren (later Sir Herbert), President of Magdalen College, where his predecessor, Sir John Burdon-Sanderson, was a fellow, "I have accepted a Professorial Studentship at Christ Church ... I had invitations from Oriel and Lincoln and New. I hope I have not made a faux pas in accepting at Christ Church but I had no time for consultation with anyone. ..."[2] Warren reassured him, "remembering your speech in the Hall at Christ Church, it seems to be very happy and appropriate that you should belong there, to the House of Locke and Burton, and of course it is one of our very greatest foundations. I think you are, in every sense of the word, 'well housed.'"[3]

Christ Church is the largest and most famous of Oxford's 39 colleges. St. Frideswide, Oxford's patron saint, founded a nunnery on the site in the eighth century. Rebuilt in 1002, it was established a century later as an Augustinian Priory. In 1525 Cardinal Wolsey suppressed the priory and began the building of a new college of Oxford University, naming it Cardinal College, but he fell from power four years later. King Henry VIII took it over, initially naming it King Henry VIII College. By 1545 he had made the college chapel Oxford's cathedral, and the college was renamed "Aedes Christi," the House of Christ.[4] It is often referred to as "The House" hence Warren's pun. A fellow, or senior faculty member, is known as a student in this college. "Undergraduate" or "junior member" are terms for people known elsewhere as students.

Oxford colleges are traditionally built in monastic style with a chapel, dining hall, library and accommodation arranged in quadrangles, known as quads. Christ Church has Oxford's largest quad, built by Wolsey and named Tom Quad after Great Tom, the bell which was moved from the cathedral tower and rehung in 1684 in the magnificent Tom Tower, designed by Christopher Wren. This

Presented in part at the forty-fourth annual meeting of the American Osler Society, Oxford, United Kingdom, on 13 May 2014.

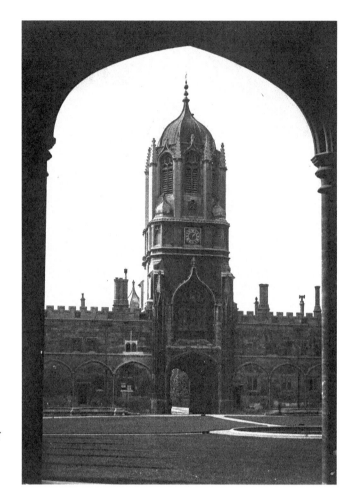

Figure 1. Tom Tower as seen from the door of Christ Church Cathedral.
Credit: Osler Library of the History of Medicine, McGill University.

tower completed the Tudor gateway, unfinished at the time of Wolsey's fall. It is one of Oxford's most iconic buildings.

Three sides of the priory cloisters survive today. The refectory, on the south side, served as the college library till 1775, when it was converted into apartments for 'students' after a new library was built. Osler had rooms here, set (apartment) 5 on the first floor, which provided a base for him in college, but he sometimes used it to house guests when the Open Arms was unavailable. Grace wrote to her mother, "he has a sitting room there and a wee bedroom; he can put up any man friend there any time he wants."[5] (Co-education was still seventy years away). Osler's idea that Locke and Burton had occupied these rooms could not be literally true since the building was still a library in their time, but they would undoubtedly have worked there.

The Great Hall, built by Cardinal Thomas Wolsey in 1525, is the largest in Oxford. Osler often dined there on Sunday evenings during term time. He would have sat at the high table and frequently brought a guest. The rules allowed only one guest, and although he often ignored this, he always got away with bringing two.[6] After the first two courses everyone adjourned to the senior common room for fruit, nuts and port. Osler always claimed he could never do justice to the port.[7]

Two special events here deserve mention. Lady Osler had worked tirelessly on behalf of refugee Belgian academics, many of whom were accommodated in Christ Church. On Friday, July 16, 1915, she wrote to her sister, "The Duchess

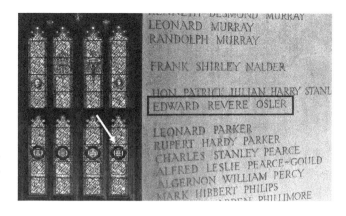

Figure 2. Stained-glass window in the Great Hall of Christ Church, showing the coat of arms of Sir William Osler (arrow). The other coats of arms on this row are (from left) those of Thomas Willis (1621–1675), Sir Henry Acland (1815–1900), and Sir Archibald Garrod (1857–1936). On the north wall of the cathedral porch are tablets commemorating Christ Church men that died in World War I, including Edward Revere Osler (box).
Credit: Christ Church, Oxford.

of Vendome, Belgian Princess, has announced to pay a visit to Oxford to see the Belgians. She comes next Wednesday and sleeps at Mrs Max Mueller's. The Magdalen people have a luncheon for her. And the Oslers have all the Belgians to tea in Christ Church. It is a fearful nuisance but . . . we cannot say no."[8] There is no record of this visit in the Christ Church archives, but Brett Langstaff, an American student at Magdalen College who was a frequent visitor at the Oslers', wrote to his parents that "the sister of the Belgian king, the Duchess of Vendome, will lunch in College this week. Lady Osler says she is doing good work in grouping the refugees from her country in a sort of colony." And later he recorded, "Lady Osler told of having brought the sister of King Albert of the Belgians to lunch at Magdalen with Sir Herbert Warren several days ago . . . The Oslers also invited all the nice Belgians to meet Her Highness in the Great Hall of Christ Church. The 'Belgiums' mistook Lady O for the Duchess and were funny and businesslike."[9]

The other event was the visit of the Harvard Medical Unit on December 3, 1915. Sir William organised a day of visits to Oxford hospitals and laboratories for 30 members of this unit, with lunch at Christ Church. Lady Osler wrote that "the hall and pictures never looked more wonderful, 64 places and all the Imperial old silver and gold vases, tankards etc, with chrysanthemums, oak colour, to harmonise with the wood, and two huge fires sputtering and snapping."[10] Flowers were always very important to her, and she found the college silver so impressive that she admitted "Paul Revere would have had to take a back seat."[11]

The Hall windows date from 1983. They are the work of Patrick Reyntiens who made the Baptistry window in Coventry Cathedral. Each one contains four family coats of arms of famous men connected with Christ Church. The one above the fireplace on the north side commemorates four great medical men. The first three were Christ Church alumni: Thomas Willis, neurologist and royal physician; Henry Acland, Regius professor and founder of Oxford's Natural History Museum; Archibald Garrod, Osler's successor in the regius chair, and then Osler himself. The crests are in the order in which these men entered Christ Church, and thus Garrod, who entered the college in 1876 as an undergraduate, precedes Osler who arrived in 1905.

The splendid library building of 1772 replaced the old monastic one in the cloister and formed one side of Peckwater Quad. Osler made a significant contribution here. Robert Burton had left about 500 books to Christ Church, but as Osler wrote to C.N.B. Camac on 5 January 1908, they were scattered indiscriminately. He reassembled them and had a copy made of Burton's portrait at Brasenose College which was inserted between the bookshelves. The books are now housed in a room in the upper library and the portrait now hangs in the senior common room.[12]

By the autumn of 1914 huge numbers of Oxford undergraduates had volunteered for military service. Lady Osler wrote to her sister in September of that year that "Willie was opposed to Revere joining anything at once, so it is decided for him to come to Christ Church. They are to wear uniform—no games—form the new company of Officers' Training Corps, and work hard at that."[13] He was allocated a room in Peckwater Quad, on the first floor of Staircase 4, opposite the library, but on a temporary basis since the former occupant was away at the front. Grace helped him to move in, giving him linen and some pieces of family silver.[7, p. 405] With so many absent on the battlefields, the college was depleted but the Dean, Thomas Strong, believed in business as usual so there was little change in the ordered life of the college and the cathedral.

The chapel of Christ Church is also the cathedral of the city of Oxford, unique in being the only cathedral in the world which stands inside the walls of a private institution. It is also England's smallest medieval cathedral since it was originally the priory church, raised to cathedral status by Henry VIII in 1545. The Oslers arrived in Oxford on Saturday, May 27, 1905, and the following day they attended morning service in the cathedral, which they came to love, especially Grace, who wrote enthusiastically to her mother about the services. In October that year both Oslers wrote to Campbell Howard from Christ Church. Grace wrote that "we have just come from the service at the cathedral and Reggie has gone into his own stall arrayed in surplice and hood." Osler was more irreverent: "These old fools have put me in a surplice and I had to go to chapel, but I wish I had been in the pulpit instead of the regius prof of divinity, who is a dry old stick."[14] These attitudes continued. Grace wrote to her sister on 15 September 1914, of a wonderful sermon in Christ Church, but added, "Poor dear Reggie can't go to church. He really says he can't endure the prayers and hymns."[15]

Brett Langstaff, whose letters and journal of his time in Oxford, published in 1965, contain many affectionate reminiscences of the Oslers, records a delightful story about the cathedral. "He (Osler) had long felt that there was an historic importance in certain wooden chandeliers in the Lady Chapel of Christ Church where his son, Revere, was an undergraduate. They were both interested in doing cabinet work. And when they learned that I had done something along that line, nothing would have it but that I should make a replica of this remnant of the first lighting of Oxford Cathedral. The three chandeliers were hung very high and a slender ladder which I had to climb to ascertain the exact measurement of the oak triangles with their tapering arms might have seemed precarious except that Sir William placed himself at the base of the ladder and directed my work." Some years later these chandeliers were replaced by electric lighting. Langstaff kept his replica for the rest of his life and had copies made for his church in Walden, New York.[16]

Revere only stayed one term at Christ Church. He felt the pressure to do his bit for the war effort, and, as Grace wrote to her sister on January 5, 1915, "It would be hard for him to stay on another term . . . all his friends except two medically unfit ones are leaving. Today he brought home his books and belongings and went to work for the Canadian Red Cross at Cliveden, and his lovely room must be dismantled."[17] The room was reserved for him for one more term, but even in September Grace had wondered ominously if there would be any "next term" since there were fewer than seventy undergraduates in the college. By December that year Osler wrote to Henry Jacobs, "Revere longs to be back at Christ Church with his books. Oxford is empty—we have 20 men at Christ Church instead of 280."[18] Services for the fallen were now held in the Cathedral on the third Sunday of each month, and the Oslers, like all parents, experienced the anxiety of waiting for news, eventually learning what they had dreaded most of all.

The cathedral is entered via a porch on Tom Quad, on the opposite side from Tom Tower. The walls of this porch are engraved with the names of members of Christ Church who fell in the two great wars, and Revere's name is one of 239 on the World War I memorial. Each year on Remembrance Sunday a book containing all the names on this memorial is placed on the high altar.

On New Year's Day 1920, Osler's funeral was held in the Cathedral which was packed to overflowing. The *Oxford Times* devoted two columns to a report on this, listing the best known guests. In Cushing's elegant description, "Of the many historic services this ancient cathedral has heard, few could have been more simple or more moving than that of the afternoon of January 1st, 1920, over the body of one of the most greatly beloved physicians of all time."[6, ii: 685] The hymns "O God our help in ages past" and Peter Abelard's "O Quanta Qualia," both favourites of Osler and Revere, were sung. After the service the coffin rested overnight in the Lady Chapel, near the memorial to Robert Burton and the shrine of St. Frideswide (which has now been moved to the adjacent Latin Chapel). Lady Osler wrote to the Jacobs, "On Jan. 1st as we followed him into the Cathedral I raised my eyes to say 'Thank God the Christ Church Student and the Christ Church undergraduate are together.' I saw the mass of faces—men representing all that he most loved—men who had come to do him honour—I felt the proudest of women—it was all so beautiful and as he liked. The mediaeval gowns of the University Marshalls standing at head and foot of the coffin—which was covered with an old purple velvet pall—there he stayed all night in the Lady Chapel—near his friend Burton."[19]

Lady Osler maintained her links with Christ Church. On November 12, 1922, she wrote to Archibald Malloch, "A really good sermon at Christ Church this morning—and Sir William's hymn which tore my heart nearly in two."[20] Since this was Armistice Sunday, the hymn was probably 'O God our help in ages past'. On a happier note, she was occasionally invited to dinner there, and after one such occasion she wrote to Malloch, "I more than ever feel the extraordinary aliveness of Sir William's memory here. There is always something said or done."[20, p. 64]

Her funeral took place in Christ Church Cathedral on September 3, 1928, and the same hymns were sung on that occasion. Her affection for the College was manifested in her will in which she bequeathed 13 Norham Gardens to the Dean and Chapter of Christ Church as an official residence for the regius professor of medicine at Oxford University.

At the 2014 AOS meeting in Oxford many members attended an evensong in the Cathedral where John Mason Neale's English translation of "O quanta qualia" (O what their joy, what their glory must be) was sung and a prayer for physicians was offered. On January 26, 2020, a centenary symposium on Osler's life and influence was held in Christ Church, followed by a commemorative evensong at which both hymns from the funeral were sung and the Dean, the Very Reverend Martyn Percy, preached a sermon reflecting Osler's humanity.

Acknowledgments

I thank Lily Szczgiel, Osler Library of the History of Medicine, McGill University, Montreal; Judith Curthoys, Archivist, Christ Church, Oxford; Jim Godfrey, Cathedral Verger, Christ Church, Oxford; and my husband, John Ward, for unfailing support and advice.

References

1. Osler Letter Index, CUS417/100.104, Osler Library of the History of Medicine, McGill University.
2. Osler Letter Index, CUS417/101.98, Osler Library of the History of Medicine, McGill University.
3. Osler Letter Index, CUS417/114, Osler Library of the History of Medicine, McGill University.
4. Butler C. *Christ Church, Oxford, A Portrait of the House*. London: Third Millennium Publishing; 2006: 10–11, 22, 48, 79–80.
5. Osler Letter Index, CUS417/58.31, Osler Library of the History of Medicine, McGill University.
6. Cushing H. *The Life of Sir William Osler.* Oxford: Clarendon Press; 1925; ii: 3.
7. Bliss M. *William Osler: A Life in Medicine.* Oxford: Oxford University Press; 1999: 343.
8. Osler Letter Index, CUS417/55.51. Osler Library of the History of Medicine, McGill University.
9. Langstaff JB. *Oxford 1914.* New York: Vantage Press; 1965: 156–167.
10. Osler Letter Index, CUS417/120.97, Osler Library of the History of Medicine, McGill University. Also in Cushing H. *The Life of Sir William Osler.* Oxford: Clarendon Press; ii: 503–504.
11. Muirhead A. *Grace Revere Osler: A Brief Memoir.* London: Oxford University Press; 1931: 30.
12. Osler Letter Index, CUS417/106.5, Osler Library of the History of Medicine, McGill University.
13. Osler Letter Index, CUS417/55.15, Osler Library of the History of Medicine, McGill University.
14. Osler Letter Index, CUS417/103.58, Osler Library of the History of Medicine, McGill University.
15. Osler Letter Index, CUS417/55.15, Osler Library of the History of Medicine, McGill University.
16. Langstaff JB. Youthful recollections. *Journal of the American Medical Association* 1969; 210(12): 2233–2235.
17. Osler Letter Index, CUS417/55.32, Osler Library of the History of Medicine, McGill University.
18. Osler Letter Index, CUS417/120.106, Osler Library of the History of Medicine, McGill University.
19. Osler Letter Index, CUS417/41.23, Osler Library of the History of Medicine, McGill University.
20. Wagner FB. *The Twilight Years of Lady Osler: Letters of a Doctor's Wife.* Canton, Massachusetts: Science History Publications USA; 1985: 52.

"So Good a Man"— James Edmund Reeves and his Mysterious Gift to Dr. Osler

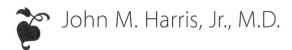 John M. Harris, Jr., M.D.

This story begins in a Philadelphia bookshop where, in 1976, I purchased a copy of the 1824 edition of *A Treatise on Indigestion* by the Scottish-born physician and physiologist A.P.W. Philip (1770–1851).[1,2] It was inscribed, "To Dr. Wm. Osler, with love, James E. Reeves, Chattanooga, Tenn. Oct 17th '95" (Figure 1). Osler had apparently donated the volume to the Medical and Chirurgical Faculty of the State of Maryland, of which he was president in 1896, and it eventually made its way to the Philadelphia bookseller. Philip's book sat on my shelf as part of my small collection of Osleriana until 2013, when the American Osler Society (AOS) came to Tucson and asked the University of Arizona's Continuing Medical Education Office if it could furnish continuing medical education (CME) credit for the annual meeting. I was director of the CME office and happy to work with the AOS. This was also a perfect excuse to attend a meeting I had only heard about and, soon enough, it brought me into the group.

I dusted off my 37-year-old acquisition and asked AOS members if they knew anything about James Reeves from Chattanooga and why he might have given a collectible book to Osler, "With love," in 1895? None had heard of Reeves or could even speculate on the book's history. Later, Chris Lyons of the Osler Library of the History of Medicine at McGill, whom I had met in Tucson, searched in Montreal along with Lily Szczygiel. They found nothing in Osler's notes, but did locate one odd tidbit: there were two other books in the Osler library with exactly the same inscription: Blackmore's *Dissertations on a Dropsy* (1727) and Cheyne's *Essay on Cynache Trachealis* (1813), which were *Bibliotheca Osleriana* numbers 2049 and 2307.[3] Now there was a genuine mystery. James Reeves was obviously a

Presented at the forty-fourth meeting of the American Osler Society, Oxford. United Kingdom, on 13 May 2014.

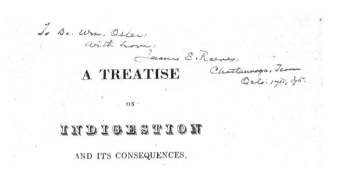

Figure 1.   Inscription by James Reeves to William Osler in A.P.W. Philip's *Treatise on Indigestion* (1824). It was this inscription that prompted the present author to seek more information about Reeves, which led to a biography of Reeves and clarification of the Osler connection.

well-read medical man and a close friend of Osler, but who was he and why did he give Osler three books in October 1895?

Ann Reeves Jarvis, the "Mother of Mother's Day"

The first thread emerged shortly after the 2013 meeting from a Website dedicated to Ann Reeves Jarvis (1832–1905), the West Virginia Sunday school teacher widely known as, "The Mother of Mother's Day." Ann Jarvis has that distinction because her daughter, Anna Jarvis (1864–1948), started a campaign on Ann's death in 1905 for a national holiday to honor mothers. With the help of Philadelphia department store magnate John Wannamaker, Anna got her wish. President Wilson signed the proclamation making Mother's Day a national holiday on May 9, 1914, the ninth anniversary of Ann Jarvis' death. The Mother's Day Websites and histories recount that Ann Jarvis' legacy was built around her Civil War work in rural Virginia and West Virginia, where she tended to the wounded from both sides, often with the help of her brother, Doctor James Edmund Reeves.[4,5] With some rhetorical license, we might say that Osler's unknown Chattanooga admirer, James E. Reeves, was, thus, the Uncle of Mother's Day.

Given that he was a West Virginia physician, whom the Mother's Day literature credited with a number of accomplishments, including (erroneously) a trip to England at Queen Victoria's request, there should have been some mention of Reeves in contemporary or later medical biographies. But there wasn't. Reeves did not show up in Atkinson's 1878 or 1880 physician directories.[6,7] He was not mentioned by Howard A. Kelly in his 1912 and 1920 compendia of American medical biographies.[8,9] Fielding H. Garrison did not include him in his *History of Medicine*.[10] And, despite his seemingly close relationship to William Osler, he is not mentioned in any of the biographies of Osler, nor elsewhere in Osler's records.

Who was James Reeves?

This question has recently been addressed by two books. Medical-legal historian James Mohr argues in *Licensed to Practice—The Supreme Court Defines the American Medical Profession* (2013) that Reeves was a central figure in regular physicians' takeover of medical licensure as a means of eliminating sectarian competitors.[11] It is hard to argue with Professor Mohr because regular physicians *did* use medical licensure to enhance their market position. The question that bothered me

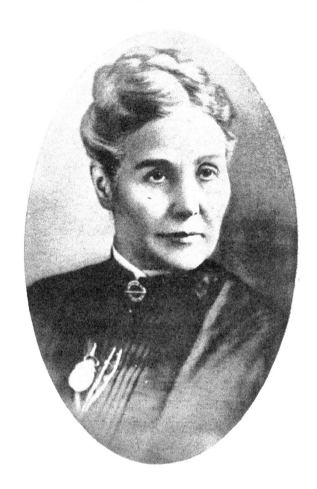

Figure 2.   Ann Reeves Jarvis (1832–1905), younger sister of James E. Reeves and known as "the Mother of Mother's Day" since her daughter, Anna Reeves (1864–1948) launched the campaign for Mother's Day in her honor.

was motive. Did all physicians approach medical licensure as if driven by this goal? Stimulated by the 2013 AOS meeting in Tucson, I have completed a full-length biography of Reeves presenting an alternative view of Reeves as a physician guided by his Methodist morality, who followed less self-interested motives in his pursuit of medical licensure. Indeed, Reeves often clashed with the guild mentality of his professional peers, which explains, in part, why he was forgotten by them.[12–14] He was an outstanding physician of his day and a leader in public health, and in these capacities, he came to know Osler well.

James Edmund Reeves was born in Amissville, Virginia, on 5 April 1829, the oldest child of Josiah and Nancy Reeves. His younger sister, Ann Maria, later Ann Reeves Jarvis, was born in 1832. Their father was a tailor and Methodist lay preacher who moved the family across the Alleghenies in 1843 to the new town of Philippi, Virginia, now West Virginia.

James was a bright boy who had no use for the rural tailor's life his stern father planned for him. Against his father's wishes, he began teaching himself medicine. He apprenticed with two local physicians, beginning in 1848, and took one course of studies at Hampden-Sidney (*sic*) Medical College in Richmond during the winter of 1850–51. Reeves married in 1851 and hung up his shingle in Philippi, just in time for a typhoid fever outbreak. He had only two years of apprenticeship and no diploma, but he was better educated than most of his competitors—Virginia had no licensure law at the time.

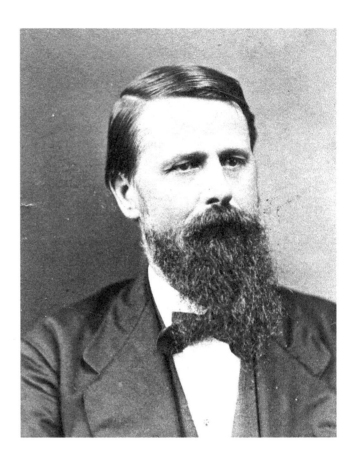

Figure 3. James Edmund Reeves in 1860, age 31, when he was living in Fairmont, Virginia. *Credit:* Joan Webb.

From the beginning, Reeves was remarkably connected to the outside medical world. It is a testimonial to his energy and America's growing transportation infrastructure to see what he achieved, so far removed from the medical mainstream. He published his first book in 1859, *A Practical Treatise on Enteric Fever*, which was a compilation of 130 consecutive typhoid fever cases and distilled guidance on how to manage the disease.[15] *The Boston Medical and Surgical Journal* loved it: "Dr. Reeves's book is both interesting and valuable and we heartily recommend it to the profession."[16]

Reeves polished off his medical education with a series of courses at the University of Pennsylvania in 1859–1860, where he finally received his medical diploma. Returning home, he moved his family to the busy railroad town of Fairmont, Virginia in 1860, just in time for the Civil War. As serious Methodists, neither Reeves nor anyone else in his family took sides. Ann was particularly stubborn and made a point of saying a prayer over the first soldier killed by hostile action in the war, Union Scout Thornsberry Brown, shot near Grafton, Virginia on May 22, 1861. At the time of her prayer, Ann was surrounded by Confederate sympathizers. For his part, Reeves wanted to preserve the Union, but also favored reconciliation with the South. When Virginia began to sunder into Confederate Virginia and Union West Virginia in 1863, he kept his opinions to himself, which, if known, would have branded him a Copperhead in Fairmont, West Virginia.

Medically, Reeves was ahead of his times. Like the medical elite in New York, Boston, and Philadelphia, he accepted that most therapies of the day simply did not work. Florence Nightingale's well-known writings from the Crimean War

(1853–1856) and the medical experiences on both sides of the Civil War pounded the message home. If diseases could not be cured, they must be prevented. This led Reeves into public health.

Reeves as a crusader for licensing standards and public health

Reeves remained a busy family doctor, but he sought to mobilize his fellow physicians, which led him to organize the Medical Society of West Virginia in 1867. This did not go well. He moved to West Virginia's biggest city, Wheeling, later that year and ran into its well-entrenched Republican old guard, whose members tolerated the outsider, but had no use for his ideals. Reeves wanted to remove one of Wheeling's oldest physicians, Archibald Todd, from the state society for selling a secret nostrum. This was precisely what the AMA demanded, but Wheeling's regular physicians were happy to look the other way. Reeves soon drifted from the organization he launched into a career as a public health officer.

Reeves became Wheeling's first permanent health officer in 1869, cleaning streets and vaccinating for smallpox. He became a Wheeling booster, preparing two books on Wheeling's climate, topography, and public health,[17,18] which got him known. When Stephen Smith organized the American Public Health Association in 1872, Reeves was named a founding member. He would become the APHA's president in 1885.

West Virginia's political winds began to shift in Reeves's favor during the 1870s, as its "Bourbon Democrats" regained political control and sought to restore the old order. Reeves was generally removed from daily politics, but the shift favored his engagement and he successfully ran for a seat on the city council in 1877, which he held until 1881. His diligent and generally non-partisan council work, plus his respected position as Wheeling's public health voice, set him up for his 1881 state-wide legislative accomplishment, one for which every physician today owes Reeves a small nod.

After a considerable number of false starts by others, Reeves took on the task of getting a statewide health board law enacted in 1881. He wrote the bill, found sponsors, lobbied the legislature and worked the newspapers. The law sailed through. For the first time anywhere a state health board was totally under physician control and the law included physician licensure. However, unlike Illinois, which also had a strong licensing authority, Reeves was more interested in public health than chasing down physician miscreants. Reeves was appointed Board secretary and he licensed almost every practicing physician in West Virginia in the first six months.

But Reeves still argued that basic standards had to be met. When the physician son of a colleague tried to submit a diploma from a fraudulent medical college, and then refused to take a licensing exam in 1882, Reeves had the man, Frank Dent, arrested for violating the law. It was the only arrest Reeves made during his four years as secretary.

Frank's cousin, lawyer, and future West Virginia Supreme Court judge, Marmaduke H. Dent, challenged Reeves's law. The Dents lost their appeal in West Virginia, whose Court of Appeals upheld the law's constitutionality in 1884. But Marmaduke Dent did not give up. Finally, in 1889, the US Supreme Court ruled that West Virginia's law was constitutional (*Dent v West Virginia*, 129 US 114), establishing the precedent for all professional licensure laws.

Reeves as a microscopist and pathologist

Although Reeves advocated for higher medical education and licensing standards, it was not these aspects of Reeves's career that brought him to Osler's attention. The Osler connection developed during Reeves's late-life career as a medical microscopist. Reeves was fascinated by the microscope, which he may have first seen during his 1860 studies at Penn. By the mid-1880s, after Koch's discovery of the tubercle bacillus, the microscope was a part of public health and this only reinforced Reeves's interest. After 1885, he moved away from public health and began thinking of retirement. He mastered the microtome, taught himself how to stain, and launched a new career as a microscopic pathologist. He became something of a medical microscopy evangelist. He encouraged physicians to use the microscope for bedside diagnosis, and he eventually wrote a well-regarded how-to-do-it handbook.[19]

These interests brought Reeves into the orbit of America's new generation of European-trained, laboratory-oriented physicians, such as William H. Welch and Osler, leaders of the newly formed Association of American Physicians, which invited Reeves to membership in its second year, 1887. That same year, 1887, Reeves left smoke-filled Wheeling for healthier and warmer Chattanooga. By now he was a grand old man of public health and pathology (at age 58) and he fit comfortably into the role. He also clearly knew and respected Osler. When Reeves spoke to the Association of American Physicians in 1890 about the power of microscopy in diagnosis, he quoted Osler, "In the language of Dr. Osler, 'the

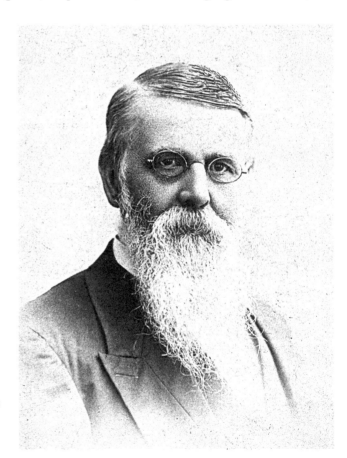

Figure 4.   Reeves in 1893, age 64, when he was living in Chattanooga at the time of the Amick affair.
Credit: Joan Webb.

characteristic changes in malaria are as distinctly determined in the blood as are those of tuberculosis of the lungs in the sputa.'" Reeves was given the honor of presenting the first paper at that meeting, which was on typhoid fever and prompted considerable discussion.[20,21]

Reeves and the Amick Affair

Reeves had one more medical contest in front of him, which also put his name in front of Osler. In 1893, two Cincinnati doctors, William and Marion Amick, took over Chattanooga's major newspaper, the *Times*, to market a phony consumption cure. The Amicks had devised a relatively novel scheme of using newspapers to stage tests of their drugs, with language usually reserved for medical journals. They had recently run their scheme in New York, where a struggling daily, the *Recorder*, breathlessly announced that William Amick had found a cure for mankind's greatest killer, verified by the *Recorder*'s careful and scrupulously monitored tests. Wire services sent the story as news, not advertising, across the country. Medical journals and societies were furious, but seemingly powerless to stop the scam.

As soon as the Amicks announced that they were testing their product in Chattanooga, Reeves called them out, not in a medical journal, but in the pages of the *Chattanooga Times*. If their product was so good, why didn't they study it in the Cincinnati Hospital? Besides, the *Times* was no place to evaluate a medical therapy. Reeves announced that he would test the Amick cure himself and he had the credentials for the job. The *Times*' publisher, Adolph Ochs, loved the controversy and urged him on. The AMA's *Code of Ethics* mandated that physicians not disparage each other publicly, which had allowed the Amicks to progress as far as they had, but Reeves could not have cared less. The Amick brothers were making a frontal assault on medical science that he intended to stop.

And he did. The Chattanooga ruckus dampened the Amicks' game plan and they tried to have Reeves arrested for sending defamatory postal cards. The arrest went nowhere, so they sued Reeves for $25,000 in civil damages. This was a commonly used tool for quack medicine purveyors and any kind of win would have been more than enough to get the Amicks back on track.[22] The suit came to trial in April 1895 and the jury took ten minutes to find Reeves not guilty. Medical journals that had either watched from the sidelines or impotently railed against Amick from lofty pulpits, heralded Reeves's courage and called for a fund to pay his legal expenses. In short order the effort raised $225, more than enough. Osler was one of the bigger contributors at ten dollars.[23] The Amick Cure for consumption soon disappeared.

"So good a man"

Shortly after the win, Reeves began to lose strength. He had trouble entertaining his son and daughter in September 1895 and his personal doctor worried it might be liver cancer. In October, Reeves took the train to Baltimore to see Osler and Osler felt the nodules that confirmed the fatal diagnosis. Reeves handled the news stoically. During his final months several of his closest friends, George Gould in Philadelphia and James Baldwin in Columbus, stayed in contact with Reeves

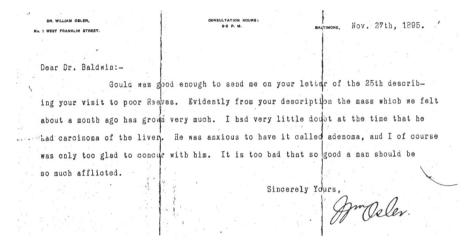

Figure 5. Letter from Osler to James F. Baldwin, Osler's Ohio surgeon, and their mutual friend. *Credit:* Barbara Boren.

and Osler. Osler wrote Baldwin on November 27, 1895 about the discouraging news, gracious as always, "It is too bad that so good a man should be so much afflicted."[24]

Reeves understood he had an unusual disease and specified that his internal organs be shipped to Osler after his death. He died on 4 January 1896 and the mayor and Chattanooga's leading physicians turned out for his funeral the following day. His body was shipped by train to Wheeling and the scene was repeated there on January 7. He was interred in Wheeling's Greenwood cemetery.

Osler received Reeves's remains and studied them on 8 January 1896. Based on the gross appearance, he diagnosed carcinoma of the gall bladder with spread to the liver. According to a letter he sent to Reeves's physician, Osler thought the case so unusual that he forwarded the specimen to Welch for the Johns Hopkins Medical School Museum.[25] Like almost every other connection between Reeves and Osler, except for three books, it has not been seen since.

The mysterious gift explained

What about the books? The timing tells the story. Reeves visited Osler in early October 1895. According to a letter from his friend, George Gould in Philadelphia, Reeves was on his way home from Baltimore on October 15.[26] On October 17 he sent the books to Osler from Chattanooga. Osler would not have charged Reeves for his consultation and the books were certainly Reeves's way of thanking Osler for the professional courtesy.

References

1. McMenemey WH. Alexander Philip(s) Wilson Philip (1770–1847), physiologist and physician. *Journal of the History of Medicine* 1958; 13: 289–328.
2. Unsigned. Alexander Philip Wilson Philip (1770–1851), experimental physiologist. *Journal of the American Medical Association* 1969; 209: 554–555.
3. W.W. Francis, R.H. Hill, and Archibald Malloch, eds., *Bibliotheca Osleriana* (Oxford, UK: Oxford University Press; 2000.

4. Sheets LW. *Mother's Day—The Legacy of Anna Jarvis*. Parsons, West Virginia: McClain Printing Company; 1913.

5. Wolfe HW. *Mothers Day and the Mothers Day Church*. Kingsport, Tennessee: Privately printed; 1962.

6. Atkinson WB. *Physicians and Surgeons of the United States*. Philadelphia: Charles Robson; 1978.

7. Atkinson WB. *A Biographical Directory of Contemporary American Physicians and Surgeons*. Philadelphia: D.G. Brinton; 1880.

8. Kelly HA. *A Cyclopedia of American medical Biography* (two volumes). Philadelphia: W.B. Saunders Company; 1912.

9. Kelly HA, Burrage WL. *American Medical Biographies*. Baltimore: The Norman Remington Company; 1920. [Reeves was ultimately noted in the final edition, *Dictionary of American Medical Biography* (New York: D. Appleton and Company; 1928).]

10. Garrison FH. *An Introduction to the History of Medicine*. Fourth edition, Philadelphia: W.B. Saunders Company; 1929.

11. Mohr JC. *Licensed to Practice—The Supreme Court Defines the American Medical Profession*. Baltimore: The Johns Hopkins University Press; 2013.

12. Harris JM Jr. *Professionalizing Medicine: James Reeves and the Choices that Shaped American Health Care*. Jefferson, North Carolina: McFarland & Co., Inc; 2019. [Unattributed information in the present essay comes from this book.]

13. Harris JM Jr. Medical ethics, Methodism, and a nineteenth-century West Virginian's battles with quackery. *West Virginia History* 2016; 10 (Spring): 27–44.

14. Harris JM. James Edmund Reeves (1929–1896) and the contentious 19th century battle for medical professionalism in the United States. *Journal of Medical Biography* 2015; 23(3): 158–169.

15. Reeves JE. *A Practical Treatise on Enteric Fever; Its Diagnosis and Treatment: Being an Analysis of One Hundred and Thirty Consecutive Cases Derived from Private Practice and Embracing a Partial History of the Disease in Virginia*. Philadelphia: J.B. Lippincott & Company; 1859.

16. [The editor]. Book Review: *A Practical Treatise on Enteric Fever; Its Diagnosis and Treatment: Being an Analysis of One Hundred and Thirty Consecutive Cases Derived from Private Practice and Embracing a Partial History of the Disease in Virginia*. *Boston Medical and Surgical Journal* 1859; 61(4): 84.

17. Reeves JE. *The Physical and Medical Topography, Including Vital, Manufacturing, and Other Statistics of the City of Wheeling*. Wheeling, West Virginia: Daily Register Book and Job Office; 1870.

18. Reeves JE. *The Health and Wealth of the City of Wheeling—Including its Physical and Medical Topography; Also General Remarks on the Natural Resources of West Virginia*. Baltimore: The Sun Book and Job Office; 1871.

19. Reeves JE. *Hand-Book of Medical Microscopy*. Philadelphia: P. Blakiston, Son, & Co.; 1894.

20. Reeves JE. Some points on the natural history of enteric or typhoid fever. *Transactions of the Association of American Physicians* 1990; 5: 1–20.

21. Harvey AM. *The Association of American Physicians, 1886–1986*. Baltimore: Waverly Press; Inc; 1986: 84.

22. Young JH. *The Toadstool Millionaires—A Social History of Patent Medicine in America Before Federal Regulation*. Princeton: Princeton University Press; 1961.

23. "Dr. Reeves Honored—His Brethren of the Medical Profession Remember Him." *The Chattanooga Times*, 1 September 1895.

24. William Osler to James F. Baldwin, 27 November 1895. Personal papers of Barbara Boren, Reeves's great-great-granddaughter.
25. William Osler to P.D. Sims, 10 January 1896. Personal papers of Barbara Boren, Reeves's great-great-granddaughter.
26. George M. Gould to James E. Reeves, 15 October 1895. Personal papers of Barbara Boren, Reeves's great-great-granddaughter.

The Charaka Club: Origins and its *Proceedings*, with Reference to the Contributions of William Osler

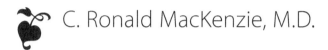 C. Ronald MacKenzie, M.D.

> *The Charaka Club was ... conceived by an Irishman, gestated by a Puritan, delivered by a Yankee, and baptized or, better said, named by a Jew. They were the Four Horses of the Apocalypse and their names were, respectively Collins, Dana, Holden, Sachs.*[1]

The Charaka Club was founded in 1898 by five distinguished New York physicians with interests beyond the usual boundaries of their profession (Figure 1). By 1902 their expectations were sufficiently realized, a name had been designated, and Volume I of the *The Proceedings of the Charaka Club* had been published. William Osler was officially admitted to the club in 1905, the year of his departure from North America. He gave five presentations to the club, only one of which was published in the *Proceedings*. Presented herein is a brief history of the club, an introduction to its *Procedings*, and an account of Osler's contributions.

Presented in part at the forty-sixth annual meeting of the American Osler Society, Minneapolis, Minnesota, on 2 May 2016, and scheduled for presentation in part at the fiftieth annual meeting of the American Osler Society, Pasadena, California, April 2020, which was canceled because of the Covid-19 pandemic.

Charles Loomis Dana: The guiding spirit of the Charaka Club was the professor of nervous disease at Cornell. A prolific writer, his *Textbook of Nervous Disease* extended through 10 editions.

Joseph Collins: Founder of the Neurologic Institute of New York, he was remembered for his red beard, cutting tongue, and energy. Osler nicknamed him the "silver-tongued Alcibiades" after the Athenian orator and general. One obituary began: "Joseph Collins was a strange and interesting personality."

Bernard Sachs: Of the Goldman Sachs family, "Barney" is best remembered today for his description, along with the British ophthalmologist Warren Tay, of Tay-Sachs Disease. He was considered the dean of American neurology.

Frederick Peterson: A neurologist with an interest in psychoanalysis, he was professor of psychiatry at Columbia. An accomplished poet, he was also interested in Chinese art and culture

Figure 1. Founding members of the Charaka Club.
Credits: National Library of Medicine.

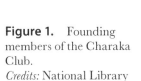

Ward Holden: An ophthalmologist, he was said to be squeamish about profanity, ribald stories, and the sight of blood; hence he never performed surgery. He edited the *Archives of Ophthalmology* and wrote books on the embryology of the eye and the eye in neurologic diseases. His major pastime war art.

Origins of the Charaka Club

The first meeting of the Charaka Club, then nameless, was held on an unrecorded date in November of 1898 at the home of Charles Loomis Dana (1852–1935), who is considered its founder. "Fed up with the regular medical meetings with their case and post-mortem reports," the founding members wished to meet in order to discuss "in an intimate way... "the literary, artistic, and historical aspects of medicine." Four of the founders were neurologists, and the fifth was an ophthalmologist. Discussions concerning the purposes of the proposed organization were conducted along with a reading of the paper "*Qu' on it de Medicine*" by Dana, a contribution on ethics by Joseph Collins (1866–1950) and a poem (*Postumous Diplopia*) read by Frederick Peterson (1859–1938). Five other meetings, under the moniker "Medico-Historical Club" were held that year. The name Charaka was adopted two years later after a presentation on Hindoo medicine by Bernard Sachs (1858–1944). According to Sachs the naming came about extemporaneously at the home of Arpad Gerster (1848–1923), a new member and eminent surgeon. Sachs wrote: "As soon as I brought out the fact that Charaka was the oldest medicine man and priest whose works were still extant, I heard someone whisper, 'We have a name for the Club.'"

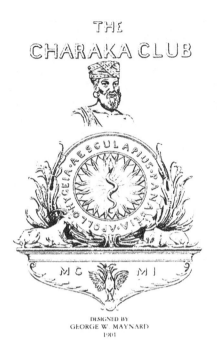

THE
CHARAKA CLUB

DESIGNED BY
GEORGE W. MAYNARD
1901

Our Seal.

A serpent salient, 'mid encircling flames,
'twixt sheaves of lilies (I don't know their names)
With powdered pollen pushing proudly forth,
faces Charaka as the needle, north.

Some gobonated gods of high degree
the border fill—medicinal I see.
Though not Olympic, neither are they small;
their names are needless for you know them all.

This scutcheon silly is upheld below
(as Aesculapian attributes, you know)
By bearded goat, and dog with tail aslant,
in terms heraldic, affronté couchant.

A rooster, rampant, spreading helpless wings
(the field about him strewn with mystic things)
Beneath the platform whence he can't take flight,
a globus pallidus is clutching tight.

The world on which I stand is mine, he crows,
although m.c.m.i. he little knows,
To students of Hippocrates and such,
means

Consultations Many Income Much

Figure 2. Seal of the Charaka Club and descriptive verse. *Credits:* Charaka Club.

The members agreed upon a format for the meeting and stipulated that dress would be black tie—a tradition that continues although on special occasions members have dined in Hindoo garb, Japanese fashion, or *a l'Italienne*.[2] Reports of unique and personal experiences were permisable as were the showing of drawings, prints or illustrations. The reading of poems (not exceeding two verses) were encouraged. The founders, men of serious mien, also sought consultation concerning such matters as the creation of a seal (Figure 2), the final design being the work of George W. Maynard, a well-known painter, illustrator and muralist and friend of Dana's. Abraham Valentine Williams Jackson (1862–1937), a Columbia Universtiy authority on Indo-European languages, advised on correct pronunciation of "Charaka": accent should be on the first syllable, the first two letters should be soft as in the first two letters of "church," the first "a" should be sounded as if "u" and the second and third "a's" should be pronounced as in "Canada." Sachs commented "So far as I can interpret all this, the correct pronunciation would be "Chur-a-ka," but "Char-a-ka" somehow comes easier." Much later, as a gesture of gratitude, George L Walton (1854–1941), a Boston neurologist and ardent club member (known to the group as "Pa-pa") had a signet ring made bearing the Charaka Club insignia which he donated to the organization.[3,4]

In its early years, meetings were held in the members homes, a practice that would eventually wane as it was found preferable to entertain at the local New York establishments. From 1911 through 1923, meetings were held at the Century Association or other facilities. From 1923 to 1984 meetings moved to the Coffee House Club. The club then renturned to the Century which remains its home to the present.

An additional tradition, the brainchild of Karl M. Vogel (1877–1969) and Jerome Webster (1888–1974), is the "safari," a fall excursion and dinner that includes significant others and guests. In 1951 the first such event was a social afternoon and evening hosted by Charakans living in Riverdale. In the early years safaris included visits to Boston, Philadelphia, Cooperstown and Baltimore to name a few locations. Recently Charakans have toured the New York Academy of Medicine's Library and the Ancient Musical Instruments Collection of the Metropolitan Museum.

Proceedings of the Charaka Club

The *Proceedings of the Charaka Club* is perhaps the organization's most enuring legacy. The twelve-volume series presents a vantage point from which to examine the intersection of medicine and the humanities. At the time of the publication of Volume I, the membership stood at ten with an additional hononary member, William Osler, whose first contribution ("On Linacre") was one of 27 presentations during the first four years of the club's existence. Although it was not chosen for the inaugural volume, this distinction was reserved for the founding members with the initial offering that of Bernard Sachs. Entitled "On Hindoo Medicine," this was not the first talk given to the club; indeed it was the eighth and presented under another title ("The Medicine of Ancient India"). It nonetheless serves well as an introduction to the collection as in it Sachs introduces the ancient Hindoo physician Charaka, a figure whose works are amongst the oldest extant treatises on medicine, preceeding those of Hippocrates. Further, as discussed, it was this commentary that suggested the name of the club, a recommendation approved unanimously. By Volume II, a publication of particular interest to Oslerians, another 27 presentations had been given. As will be discussed shortly, two were by William Osler as well as one by his co-inductee Silas Weir Mitchell ("Books and the Man"). One offering from each would be the first presented in Volume II of the *Proceedings*. A description of the Charaka Club dinner in honor of Osler's departure to England (1905) closes the volume. In Volume III, two additional papers by Osler are listed but neither are included amongst those eventually published.

Since its inception over 700 presentations have been made to the society and by the year of the last installment of the *Proceedings* (1985), 214 papers, the contributions of 78 authors, had been selected for includion in the archive. George L Walton holds the record with 11 contributions chosen for publication during his association with the club. A review of the *Proceedings* suggests that the club reached its peak membership in the 1930s with 35 active members listed in Volume VIII (1934).

Through the first half century publication continued at a rate of roughly every four years after which the pace slowed with 38 years elapsing between Volume 11 and the last installment, Volume 12 (1985). A history of the club was published in 1978, edited by Grant Sanger, a Columbia Presbyterian-affiliated surgeon who practiced in Mount Kisco in Westchester, north of New York City, and dedicated to Archibald Malloch, the chief Librarian of the New York Academy of Medicine and the Club's secretary for twenty-one years. During Malloch's tenure he gave eight presentations and was editor of Volumes 7–11 of the *Proceedings*. Sanger's history reviews the Club's origins, membership, chronicles its various activities, and includes memorials of influential members. Papers read and those chosen for inclusion in the club's publication (from its 1898 inception through 1978) are also included.[4]

William Osler and the Charaka Club

Owing to his professional stature and varied interests (clinical medicine, medical history, the humanities, great books), William Osler was an ideal candidate for membership. Listed in the *Proceedings* as an "Honorary Member" in Volume I (1902), he was accepted as a full member three years later, inducted with along with a close friend, the neurologist Weir Mitchell of Philadelphia. During his association with the Charaka Club, Osler was "*an enthusiastic out-of-town member, brought us many books from his rare library, and enlivened many meetings until he was called to Oxford.*" He would give five presentations amongst which include two familiar pieces. The first, a talk recalling a profession hero *Thomas Linacre*, anticipated Osler's *Linacre Lecture* at St John's College, Cambridge (1908); it would eventually be published as a separate monograph. His second presentation "Fracastorius," is well-known to Oslerians for its inclusion in *An Alabama Student and Other Historical Essays.*[6] Osler's contributions were to subsequently include a presentation entitled *Oxford*, given in 1906 a year after his assumption of the Regius professorship, and two others highlighting his interest in libraries, the *Imaginary Libraries* (1907) and *Libraries of France and Italy* (1909), the latter his last Charakan appearance. Although he would not attend another meeting, Osler is recorded as an active member through Volume V of the *Proceedings*, published in the year of his death (1919).

Of the five Charaka presentations only *On Linacre* and *Fracastorius* appear in Osler's bibliography, a somewhat surprising observation given Osler's penchant for publication. Of these only *Fracastorius* would be chosen for publication in the club's *Proceedings* (Volume II).[7] As such it merits specific comment in this review.

Hieronymous Fracastorius (1478–1553) was an important figure of the Italian Renaissance. Born of well-to-do parents he was free to study the stars, read the classics, write poetry, following his varied interests primarily philosophy, mathematics, and medicine. Except for a seven-year period of study at nearby Padua, Fracastorius lived his entire life in Verona, where he was born. An historically tumultuous time, Fracastorius experienced several major disruptions in his life including a prolonged occupation by the German emperor Maximilian (1490–1516) and the plague (1511–1512) resulting in the loss of 13,000 Veronans.

It was in this agitated social and political milieu that he took up the practice of medicine and wrote the major works for which he is remembered 500 years later. Of his seven works, two are noteworthy for their relevance to medicine. *Syphilides, sive Morbi Gallici* (1530), presented in poetic form, describes a shepherd boy (Sifulio) who, having offended Apollo, is punished with a terrible illness which would, for evermore, be called Syphilis. Retiring from medicine after the completion of this work, Fracastorius subsequently wrote six more books, his last the influential *De Contagione et Contagious Morbis* (1546). A product of his experience with both syphilis and typhus, in this work he anticipates what would later be the germ theory, postulating that such epidemics were caused by minute factors, spread either by direct contact, by carriers (fomites), or through the air.

Fracastorius lived a long, happy, studious, and productive life. As Osler writes, "*Poetry, astronomy, cosmography, and natural philosophy, shared with medicine his time and labors*"—just the sort of historical medical figure that would capture Osler's interest. Osler begins his piece with a brief personal history, an analysis of *De Contagione* reproducing the title page of this seminal work in which Fracastorius discusses the problems of contagion and infection, recognizes typhus fever as a distinct clinical entity, and delineates the three classes of infection (infection by contact, by an intermediate agent introducing the term fomites, or infection acquired at a distance such as through the air). Osler closes with the observation that the two most enduring historical contributions concerning syphilis were made by poets (von Hutten, and Fracastorius) thereby connecting this seminal medical discovery with the humanities.

Finally, mention should be made of the Charaka-sponsored dinner held in Osler's honor, an event fondly recalled by Oslerians and Charakans alike. This was a farewell for Osler prior to his departure for Oxford and the assumption of the regius professorship. Held on 4 March 905 at New York's University Club, it was a grand affair for which a ten page "Folia" and an inscribed (*"Medico illustri, litterarum cultori, socio gratissimo"*) bronze medallion were created. Poems (including Weir Mitchell's "Books and the Man") were read, songs were sung, and laudatory speeches given. Reported at the time in the *British Medical Journal*[8] and the *Proceedings of the Charaka Club* (Volume II), the event has been previously reviewed by Truman in the *Persisting Osler* series (Volume III).[9]

In closing, the Charaka Club is one of the longest-standing medical societies of distinction, its membership inclusive not only of its decorated founders but also by such names as Osler, Mitchell, Dock, Rous, Whipple, and Barondess, to name only a few. Its *Proceedings* offer a broad array of topics, consistent with the founders' mandate to promote discourse concerning the literary, artistic and historical aspects of medicine. The twelve volumes present a fascinating but underappreciated resource concerning the history of medicine and the medical humanities.

References

1. Collins J. The past, present and future of the Charaka Club. *Proceedings of the Charaka Club*, volume XI. New York: Richard R. Smith; 1941: 63–69.
2. Emerson H. The first half-century of Charaka, 1898–1949. In Sanger G, ed. *The Charaka Club, 1898–1978: A History*. New York: Charles C. Morchand Co., Inc.; 1978: 4–14.
3. Walton GL. Our seal. *Proceedings of the Charaka Club*, volume VI. New York: Paul B. Hoeber; 1925: 140–145.
4. Sanger G, ed. *The Charaka Club, 1898–1978: A History*. New York: Charles C. Morchand Co., Inc.; 1978.
5. Osler W. *Thomas Linacre*: Cambridge: Cambridge University Pres; 1908.
6. Osler W. Fracastorius. In Osler W. *An Alabama Student and Other Biographical Essays*. Oxford: Clarendon Press; 1908: 278–294.
7. Osler W. Fracastorius. *Proceedings of the Charaka Club, Volume II*. New York: William Wood and Company; 1906: 278–294.
8. Unsigned. The Charaka Club and Professor Osler. *British Medical Journal* 1905; 1(2309): 728–729.
9. Truman JT. A dinner for Dr. Osler. In Barondess JA, Roland CG, eds. *The Persisting Osler—III. Selected Transactions of the American Osler Society, 1991–2000*. Malabar, Florida: Krieger Publishing Company; 2002: 231–237.

William Osler and Dr. Johnson's Club

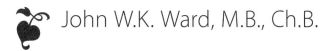 John W.K. Ward, M.B., Ch.B.

In 1919 William Osler received a letter, dated March 5th, from Hubert Burge, Bishop of Southwark, informing him of his election to "The Club"[1] which Cushing was to call "the most famous of the dining clubs of the world"[2] and whose members Bliss would call "the cream of the cream."[3] A less formal letter of the same day from the bishop expressed how much he anticipated seeing Osler at the dinners, recalled earlier correspondence regarding Revere's schooling, and sympathised with him on the death of Revere.[4] Osler also received best wishes from Sir Frederic Kenyon, whose dazzling career as a classical and biblical scholar was well known to Osler. Kenyon noted that the two new members just elected, Osler and Francis W. Pember, were both also members of the Oxford Club, which shared the same motto as "The Club"—"*Esto Perpetua*, May it last for ever."[5] Pember was a distinguished barrister and Fellow of All Souls, Oxford, who later became Vice-Chancellor of Oxford.

To these letters Osler replied enthusiastically, telling the bishop that he had not heard of his proposal and that he would attend the next dinner on March 18th,[6] and sending Kenyon a banker's form and a cheque for "the volume of the *Annals* which I should like to have in my library."[7] This book appears in *Bibliotheca Osleriana* as item number 6144 and is based largely on Sir M.E. Grant Duff's *The Club 1764–1905*,[8] which had been printed privately in 1905 for the Roxburghe Club.[9]

Presented at the forty-ninth annual meeting of the American Osler Society in Montreal Canada on 13 May 2019.

Early history of "The Club"

"The Club," also known as the Literary Club, Dr. Johnson's Club, and the Turk's Head Club, was a dining society dating from February 1764, with nine members. Its birth is best described in James Boswell's *Life of Samuel Johnson* (1791) which states that it was Sir Joshua Reynolds who proposed the project with Johnson's support.[10] Boswell tells us that "they met in the Turk's Head in Gerrard Street in Soho, one evening in every week, usually Tuesday, at seven, and generally continued their conversation till a pretty late hour." Apart from Johnson and Reynolds, the other members were Edmund Burke, Topham Beauclerk, Bennet Langton, Anthony Charmier, Sir John Hawkins and two doctors, namely Oliver Goldsmith and Christopher Nugent.

Oliver Goldsmith (1728–1774) is best known to us as a writer, essayist, poet and playwright, and his works, such as *The Vicar of Wakefield*, *The Deserted Village*, and *She Stoops to Conquer* endure, but his medical career was not sparkling.[11] He had a B.A. from Trinity College, Dublin, and though he half-heartedly studied medicine in Edinburgh between 1752–1755 and in Leiden, he never acquired a medical degree, and his attempts to make his way as a physician in England were unsuccessful. While working on his literary output he took a variety of jobs to earn money, such as an apothecary's assistant and school usher. His title of doctor was assumed. He was an advocate of Robert James's fever powders, and in the story "Goody Two Shoes," which he probably wrote, the death of the heroine's father from fever is attributed to him being in a "place where Dr James's Powder was not to be had." Ironically, Goldsmith's own unfortunate death in 1774 was ascribed by the apothecary William Hawes to his being in a place where Dr. James's powders could be had all too readily! The powder contained one part of the oxide of antimony and two parts of calcium phosphate.

Christopher Nugent (c.1698–1775) was also born in Ireland.[11, p. 275] He gained his M.D. in France and practised initially in the south of Ireland, and then successfully in Bath. In 1753 he published *An Essay on the Hydrophobia* in which he recounted his successful treatment in 1751 of a servant girl who had contracted rabies after being bitten in two places by a turnspit dog. His treatment consisted mainly of a powder of musk and cinnabar. Later parts of the essay discussed the mental and physical aspects of the disease and its resemblance to hysteria, along with proposed treatments. In 1764 he moved to London, and the following year was admitted a licentiate of the Royal College of Physicians as well as a Fellow of the Royal Society. His daughter married Edmund Burke in 1757. A regular attendee of the Club, he was popular. As a Catholic at the Club, Nugent had an omelette at Friday dinners, and on his death in November 1775 Johnson exclaimed, "Ah my dear friend, I shall never eat omelette with thee again."

In his recent book on the Club, Leo Damrosch, Emeritus Professor of English Literature at Harvard University, points out that by 1778 Johnson felt that the whole point of the group had been lost and he attended only occasionally. He attended meetings nine times that year and subsequently never more than three times in any year since he had lost interest and attendance for most members had become sporadic. Damrosch notes that in 1777 Johnson wrote in a letter to Boswell, "It is proposed to augment our club from twenty to thirty, of which I am glad; for as we have several in it whom I do not much like to consort with, I am for reducing it to a mere miscellaneous collection of conspicuous men, without any determinate character.[12] Bruce Redford, the editor of *The Letters of Samuel Johnson* notes that, according to Boswell, Johnson's unwillingness to consort with some members was "on account of their differing from him as to religion and politicks." Redford says that the several to whom Johnson took exception included Charles James Fox (elected 1774), Edward Gibbon (elected 1774) and Adam Smith (elected 1775).[13]

Damrosch's contention of Johnson's loss of interest from 1778 merits further consideration. Johnson had been opposed to the gradual extension of the membership advocated by Reynolds for some years, though attendance had often been poor, and along with others had feared for the group's survival. Indeed, as early as 1768 and 1772 Thomas Percy, the churchman and antiquarian reported that there were occasions when only he and one other member were present. Johnson's attendance was poor particularly in later life. His health problems included bouts of severe depression in which he became idle and unenthused by activity. He himself commented that these led to a state of "Nil but dismal vacuity; much intended but little done." He could be lifted in spirits by regular lengthy visits to Henry and Hester Thrale at their country house in Streatham where he had much of the conversation he could have had at The Club. Additionally, his mood was lifted when the much younger James Boswell was in London; this was an added incentive to attend The Club. Some of the great descriptions in Boswell's *The Life of Samuel Johnson* are of Johnson's contributions to Club discussions at eight detailed meetings.

The Club had grown to thirty-five members by 1792 and after about ten years it met fortnightly, usually on Fridays, during the parliamentary session. In 1783 the Turk's Head closed and meetings moved to multiple locations, including Prince's, Baxter's and venues in St. James's Street. A rule introduced in 1780 had limited membership to forty. The main activities were wining, dining, and debating informally along with discussing possible new members. This entailed proposing candidates, and then "blackballing" those considered inappropriate. Johnson had once remarked that the membership numbered professors in all the main branches of study. Whimsically, Boswell, while accompanying Johnson on their Scottish trip, fantasised of the creation of a university by club members.

Later Charles Burney, the musicologist and father of Fanny, Madame d'Arblay, wrote that Johnson wanted a club "composed of the heads of every liberal and literary profession" and "having somebody to refer to in our doubts and discussions, by whose Science we might be enlightened."

The club thrived over the next century and numbered the cream of British academe, literary, scientific, and political figures, but time restraints prevent me from relating and examining that membership and the various changes. It must be noted though that the rise of professional society in the nineteenth century led to the election of more representatives from the intellectual middle class.

Osler's election to "The Club"

Osler was delighted to have been elected to the club in 1919. Dr. Archibald Malloch's journal entry of Friday, 15 November 1918 recounts that Osler told him he had been proposed for membership in 1915 but had failed to be elected. He had not known of this.[14] In fact he had missed it by one vote.

In a letter to Mabel Brewster on 24 April 1919 he wrote, "Did you ever hear of The Club founded by Reynolds and Johnson in 1764, a dining club? It has been going all these years, and the other day I had the delightful surprise of my election as a member. Members chiefly political and literary. I knew nothing of it—I suppose as Rosebery proposed me I went through."[15] Rosebery was Archibald Philip Primrose, 5th Earl of Rosebery, 1st Earl of Midlothian (1847–1929) and Liberal Prime Minister 1894–1895, and like Osler was a fine book collector.

Osler was a keen member and founder of clubs and societies and felt that "a man misses a good part of his education who has not got knocked about a bit by his colleagues in discussion and criticism." His delight at election to Dr. Johnson's Club was many-faceted. His wide knowledge of literature and its authors included Johnson and his contemporaries. Although most of his knowledge of Samuel Johnson came from his readings of Boswell's magisterial biography, he was sufficiently informed to have included many Johnsonian references in his addresses and lectures. These are covered in my submissions on "Johnson and Osler" and "William Osler and Dr. Johnson's Club" in the new Osler encyclopedia.[16,17]

In the case of the Club, Osler's wide knowledge of science, medicine, the humanities, and literature made him confident to be accepted in disparate circles of knowledge.

Physicians who belonged to "The Club"

In March 1919 Osler wrote, "There have only been six doctors in the club since its foundation—Paget the last—Goldsmith, Nugent & Fordyce were the early ones, Banks, Vaughan, Holland the others."[2; 8, p.45] Apart from the arithmetical error he was incorrect on two other counts. Firstly, Sir Joseph Banks was not medically qualified, and secondly my research through club records identifies eleven others with medical or surgical training, including six with major careers and five others who made their reputations in different fields.

I shall quickly review Osler's named doctors: we have already dealt with Goldsmith and Nugent and deleted Banks. George Fordyce (1736–1892), an Aberdeen graduate, was a successful medical science lecturer in London who wrote treatises on digestion and fever.[19] Sir Henry Halford ne Vaughan (1766–1844) an Edinburgh graduate, had the largest practice in London and became president of the RCP and physician extraordinary to the King.[20] Sir Henry Holland (1788–1873) studied medicine in London, had an enormous practice, was medical attendant to the Princess of Wales, later Queen Caroline, and president of the Royal Institution.[21] Osler's most recent medically qualified club member was Sir James Paget (1814–1899), the great English surgeon and pathologist, regarded with Virchow as a founder of scientific surgical pathology.[22] His career included the presidency of the Royal College of Surgeons, the Hunterian Oration and multiple papers and books. He is remembered eponymously in Paget's disease of nipple, Paget's abscess, and extra mammary Paget's disease.

I shall now survey the six "Club" members with major careers that Osler omitted. Sir Charles Blagden (1748–1820) gained an M.D. from Edinburgh, served as an army surgeon in the American War of Independence (1776–1779), then worked as a physician before becoming Physician to the British forces in Paris in 1814.[23] A close friend of Henry Cavendish, the chemist, and of Sir Joseph Banks, he did much scientific work and became secretary of the Royal Society.

Richard Warren (1731–1797) read classics and mathematics before gaining an M.D. from Jesus College, Cambridge in 1762. He became physician to the Princess Amelia and succeeded his father, Peter Shaw, a physician to George III.[11, p. 425; 24] He attended both Johnson and Boswell and had an enormous medical income. His willingness to learn from his mistakes invited the somewhat dubious compliment, "Dr Warren never killed in vain."

Sir William Flower (1831–1899) trained at University College, became an assistant surgeon in the army then at the Middlesex Hospital before being conservator at the Royal College of Surgeons Museum, then Professor of Comparative Anatomy and Physiology.[25]

Thomas Young (1773–1829) was a polymath who was educated at Edinburgh, Göttingen, and Emmanuel College, Cambridge. Professor of Natural Philosophy at the Royal Institution and physician to St. George's Hospital, he established his practice in London from an inheritance from the death of his mother's uncle, Dr. Richard Brocklesby, who was a friend and physician to Samuel Johnson. He is remembered as the "father of physiological optics."[26]

Sir Richard Owen (1804–1892) graduated from Edinburgh and in 1826 set up practice in London. He was briefly a surgeon in Birmingham before becoming assistant conservator of the Hunterian Museum in Lincoln's Inn Fields, and in 1836 was appointed Hunterian Professor in the Royal College of Surgeons. A great comparative anatomist, he wrote multiple books and conceived the idea of the Natural History Museum.[27]

Sir Prescott Hewett (1812–1891) studied art in Paris but abandoned art for surgery. He entered St. George's, London, and was a pupil and friend of Sir Benjamin Brodie, whose work he helped. He progressed to becoming surgeon to the hospital. In a glittering career he became president of the Clinical Society of London in 1873, president of the Royal College of Surgeons in 1876, and in 1884 sergeant-surgeon to Queen Victoria. Awarded a baronetcy in 1883, he became an FRS in 1874. His lectures on "Surgical Affections of the Head" appear in Holmes's "System of Surgery."[28]

I shall now deal with the five doctors who had medical or surgical training but who made their reputations in other fields.

Sir Humphry Davy (1778–1829), best known to us today as the inventor of a safety lamp and a major chemist, was originally apprenticed at the age of seventeen to a surgeon-apothecary in Penzance. This developed his love of chemistry and he became assistant to Thomas Beddoes' Pneumatic Institution in Bristol. His later career culminated in the Directorship of the laboratory in the Royal Institution and in the Presidency of the Royal Society where he succeeded Banks.[29]

Sir James Mackintosh (1765–1832) studied medicine at Edinburgh before entering the Bar and becoming a legal scholar.[30]

Sylvester Douglas, Lord Glenbervie (1743–1823) studied medicine at Aberdeen and Leiden, where he graduated but subsequently entered the Bar and entered politics.[8, p75]

William Hyde Wollaston (1766–1828) was educated at Caius, Cambridge, and practised as a physician in Huntingdon and then London. From 1800 he became a scientist distinguished in optics and was secretary of the Royal Society.[8, p75]

Thomas Henry Huxley (1825–1895) learned from the teaching of Mr. Wharton Jones, who lectured on physiology at Charing Cross School of Medicine. He had wished to be a mechanical engineer but was overruled and he became an assistant surgeon in the army. Later he became a biologist specialising in comparative anatomy. He became known as "Darwin's Bulldog" for his advocacy of Charles Darwin's theory of evolution, particularly in the famous 1860 debate with Samuel Wilberforce, Bishop of Oxford. He became president of the Royal Society.[31]

Now, why did William Osler make a mistaken tally of doctors in "The Club"? As a Johnsonian he might well joyfully recall Dr. Johnson's reply to a lady rebuking him for his mistaken definition of a pastern as a horse's knee in his great dictionary: "Ignorance, Madam. Pure ignorance." Much more likely is his lack of research on the matter. In 1919 he was sickening with lung disease; probably had not read his newly acquired copy of the "Annals"; could hardly be expected to know the early careers of men distinguished in other fields, and finally, despite his prodigious memory his note was written on the spur of the moment, not as a piece of diligent scholarship.

Osler's participation in "The Club"

Osler did not attend the March 18th dinner of "The Club." His first meeting was on 1 April 1919 at Princes Hotel, Jermyn Street, London, and he recorded his impressions of the evening in handwriting on the back of the menu card.[32] Here he recorded that the Archbishop of York (Cosmo Gordon Lang) was to have been in the chair, but in fact Sir Henry Newbolt (1862–1938, poet, novelist, and historian) took this role. Osler sat between him and Herbert Fisher, historian, and the Minister of Education. The others present were Rudyard Kipling, John Buchan, Francis W. Pember (Lawyer, Fellow and Warden of All Souls, Oxford), John Bailey (writer on literature), Charles Oman (military historian) and Frederick Kenyon. All but Bailey and Newbolt, Osler had known previously. He liked the dining room which the club had used for 20 years with paintings and lithographs of old members on the walls and noted that the dining table was round and set for the ten or twelve members who usually attended. The conversation was good, and Osler described it as a "very good evening." Kipling, whose relationship with the Oslers has been elegantly described by our old friend and colleague Alex Sakula, said "he would not be surprised if in a few years the monastic life was revived—as men were seeking relief from the burdens of a hard world and turning more and more to spiritual matters. . . ."[33]

The evening concluded with the voting in of two new members out of seven candidates.

It is not known if Sir William attended any other meetings of The Club in his final year.

Acknowledgments

I thank Lily Szczygiel, Document Technician, Osler Library of the History of Medicine, McGill University; The Johnson Society of London Forum; and my wife, Ruth, for her unfailing help.

References

1. Hubert M. Burge to William Osler, 5 March 1919. Osler Letter Index, CUS417/127.149, Osler Library of the History of Medicine, McGill University.

2. Cushing H. *The Life of Sir William Osler.* Oxford: Clarendon Press; 1925; ii: 639.

3. Bliss M. *William Osler: A Life in Medicine.* Oxford: Oxford University Press; 1999: 459.

4. Hubert M. Burge to William Osler, 5 March 1919. Osler Letter Index, CUS417/127.150, Osler Library of the History of Medicine, McGill University.

5. Frederick G. Kenyon to William Osler, 5 March 1919. Osler Letter Index, CUS417/127.1512, Osler Library of the History of Medicine, McGill University.

6. William Osler to Hubert M. Burge, 7 March 1919. Osler Letter Index, CUS417/163, Osler Library of the History of Medicine, McGill University.

7. William Osler to Frederick G. Kenyon, 7 March 1919. Osler Letter Index, CUS417/127.164, Osler Library of the History of Medicine, McGill University.

8. Grant Duff ME. *The Club, 1764–1905.* London: Ballantyne Press; 1905.

9. Ward J, *Roxburghe Club, William Osler and: Sir William Osler, An Encyclopaedia.* Novato, California: Norman Publishing; 2020: 703.

10. Boswell J. *Life of Samuel Johnson.* London: Folio Society; 1968; i: 296–298.

11. Rogers P. *The Samuel Johnson Encyclopaedia.* Westport, Connecticut: Greenwood Press; 1996: 162–163.

12. Damrosch L. *Johnson, Boswell and the Friends Who Shaped an Age.* New Haven: Yale University Press; 2019: 274–275.

13. Letter from Samuel Johnson to James Boswell, 11 March 1977. In Redford B, ed. *The Letters of Samuel Johnson.* Oxford: Clarendon Press; 1992; iii; 11–12.

14. Dr Malloch's Journal, 15 November 1918. CUS417/126.135, Osler Library of the History of Medicine, McGill University.

15. William Osler to Mrs. Robert Brewster, 24 April 1919. CUS417/128.38, Osler Library of the History of Medicine, McGill University.

16. Ward JWK. Johnson, Samuel (1709–1784), William Osler and. In Bryan CS, ed. *Sir William Osler: An Encyclopedia.* Novato, California: Norman Publishing/HistoryofScience.com; 2020: 399–400.

17. Ward JWK. "Club, The" (Dr. Johnson's Club), William Osler and. In Bryan CS, ed. *Sir William Osler: An Encyclopedia.* Novato, California: Norman Publishing/HistoryofScience.com; 2020: 154–155.

18. Rogers P. *The Samuel Johnson Encyclopaedia.* Greenwood Press; 1996: 148.

19. George Fordyce, M.D. In Munk W, ed. *The Roll of the Royal College of Physicians of London, Volume II, 1701 to 1800.* London: Royal College of Physicians; 1878: 373–376.

20. Sir Henry Halford, Bart., M.D., G.C.H. In Munk W, ed. *The Roll of the Royal College of Physicians of London, Volume II, 1701 to 1800.* London: Royal College of Physicians; 1878: 427–435.

21. Sir Henry Holland, Bart, M.D. In Munk W, ed. *The Roll of the Royal College of Physicians of London, Volume III, 1801 to 1825.* London: Royal College of Physicians; 1878: 144–149.

22. Peterson MJ. Paget, Sir James, first baronet. In *Oxford Dictionary of National Biography* (online), 2006.

23. Cannadine D, Hennessy P, Saumarez Smith C. *New Annals of the Club.* London: Modern Art Press; 2014: 66.

24. Richard Warren, M.D. In Munk W, ed. *The Roll of the Royal College of Physicians of London, Volume II, 1701 to 1800.* London: Royal College of Physicians; 1878: 242–247.

25. Fletcher K. Flower, Sir William Henry. In *Oxford Dictionary of National Biography* (online) 2007.

26. Cantor G. *Young, Thomas.* In *Oxford Dictionary of National Biography* (online) 2004.

27. Eminent Persons, Biographies reprinted from *The Times.* London: Macmillan and Co. Ltd: 1896; v: 291–299.

28. Hewett, Sir Prescott Gardner (1812–91). In *Plarr's Lives of the Fellows of the Royal College of Surgeons England* (online).

29. Knight D. Davy, Sir Humphry, baronet (1778–1829). In *Oxford Dictionary of National Biography* (online) 2004.

30. Finlay C. *McIntosh, Sir James of Kyllochy (1765–1832).* Oxford Dictionary of National Biography (online) 2004.

31. Desmond A. Huxley, Thomas Henry (1825–95). In *Oxford Dictionary of National Biography* (online) 2004.

32. Osler Letter Index CUS417/127.152 ½, Osler Library of the History of Medicine, McGill University.

33. Sakula A. Rudyard Kipling, Sir William Osler and the history of medicine. *Kipling Journal*; 1983: 56(226) (June): 10–24.

The Persistent Unintended Effect of a Footnote in Osler's Last Published Work

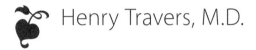 Henry Travers, M.D.

In the preface to the first edition of *The Persisting Osler* the editors expressed the hope "that these essays will serve to stimulate ... further exploration of those timeless issues" in which Sir William Osler was interested.[1] One of those topics was astrology, and today answers to persisting questions about whether Confederate General Thomas J. (Stonewall) Jackson practiced astrology trace back primarily to Osler.

A typical Google search (Figure 1) regarding Jackson's beliefs returns, on the first page of results, William Osler's *The Evolution of Modern Medicine* which claimed that Jackson had, indeed, believed in astrology.[2] Osler's assertion, made in a footnote, was of doubtful provenance. The background of the footnote's inclusion is the subject of this paper.

Unfinished at the time of his death in December 1919, Sir William Osler's *The Evolution of Modern Medicine* was based on his April 1913 Silliman lectures on the history of medicine at Yale University. The lectures' galleys were sent to Osler for revision in 1913, but by mid-1915 Osler had returned his author's fee to Yale and considered himself free of further editorial obligation.[3] The incomplete galleys were edited by Dr. Fielding Garrison, Dr. Harvey Cushing and others, and *The Evolution of Modern Medicine* was posthumously published in 1921.

In the book, Osler, the Regius professor of medicine at Oxford, presented a history of medicine from ancient times through triumphs over malaria and

Presented at the forty-fifth annual meeting of the American Osler Society, Baltimore, Maryland, on 28 April 2015.

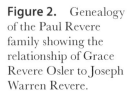

Figure 1. Sample of results on the first page of a Google search on the terms "Stonewall Jackson, Astrology."

yellow fever in Cuba. He included a section on "Astrology and Divination" which illustrated the impact of astrology on medieval medical practice. Reproducing the title page of Culpepper's 1658 treatise, *An Astrological Judgment of Diseases,* Osler detailed astrology's effect on medical prognostication.

Not part of his original lecture at Yale, but included in the book, was a startling footnote about Confederate General Stonewall Jackson, an inclusion that, as noted above, came to serve as a modern basis for asserting that Jackson practiced astrology. The footnote repeated, as fact, a story authored by General Joseph Warren Revere, grandson of Revolutionary War hero Paul Revere and first cousin once removed to Osler's wife, Grace (Figure 2).

In comparison to other footnotes in the text, this footnote was different (Table 1). It added nothing to the topic at hand, came from an unlikely and suspect source and seemed placed there as a sensational revelation.

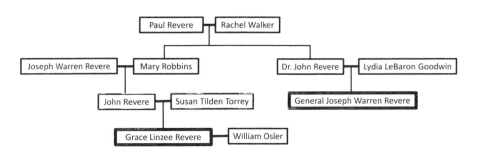

Figure 2. Genealogy of the Paul Revere family showing the relationship of Grace Revere Osler to Joseph Warren Revere.

Table 1. Footnote Comparison

Jackson Footnote	Typical Osler Footnote
Unrelated to text; text describes an astrologer-patient who forecast stocks	Extended text information directly related to subject
Unsubstantiated story	Verified information
Sensational assertion	Lack of sensationalism

The footnote and Its origin

The footnote was added by Osler probably soon after he received the galleys in 1913.[4] His handwritten note on the galley page differs from the text eventually printed. The latter represented editorial changes of fact, suggesting the editors had a copy of the note's source in hand. Below are the two versions with the changed or deleted text <u>underlined</u> and added text in **bold**. His original hand-written text read:

> It is not generally known that Stonewall Jackson practiced astrology. Col. JW Revere in "Keel and Saddle" tells of meeting Jackson in 1852 on a Mississippi steamer and talking with him on the subject. Some months later Revere received a letter from Jackson enclosing his (Reveres) horoscope. There was a "culmination of malign aspect at or during the first days of May 1863—both will be exposed to a common danger at the time indicated." At the battle of Chancellorsville 1863 Revere saw Jackson's death!

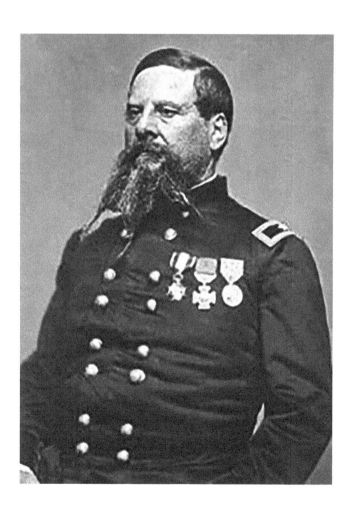

Figure 3.   General Joseph Warren Revere.
Credit: Wikimedia Commons.

The published text read:

> It is not generally known that Stonewall Jackson practiced astrology.
> Col. JW Revere in "Keel and Saddle" (**Boston, 1872**) tells of meeting
> Jackson in 1852 on a Mississippi steamer and talking with him on the
> subject. Some months later Revere received a letter from Jackson enclos-
> ing his (Revere's) horoscope. There was a "culmination of malign aspect
> <u>at or</u> during the first days of May 1863—both will be exposed to a com-
> mon danger at the time indicated." At the battle of Chancellorsville, on
> 2 May 1863, Revere saw Jackson **mortally wounded**!

Keel and Saddle, a book written in 1872[5] by Joseph Warren Revere (Figure
3), included Revere's 20-year service in the Navy until 1850 and two subsequent
years as a colonel in the Mexican army. Returning from military service in
Mexico, Revere related meeting Lieutenant Thomas J. Jackson on a steamer
bound from New Orleans in early 1852 (Figure 4). Over a two-day period, the
two men spent considerable time discussing metaphysics. Part of their conversation, quoted by Revere in detail, was this summary of Jackson's astrologic
philosophy: "Not a living being, not even a flower, but has its patron and guide

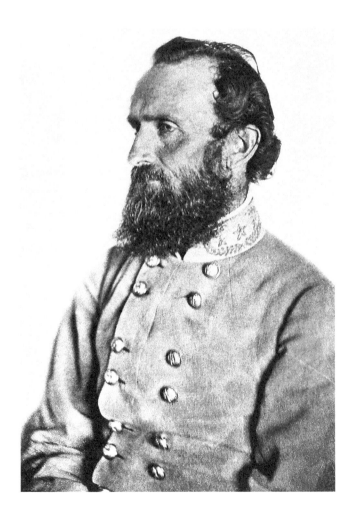

Figure 4.   General Thomas J. (Stonewall)
Jackson April 1863.
Credit: Wikimedia Commons.

on high in one of those orbs suspended in ether."[5, p. 256] The two men parted at Pittsburg, Mississippi with Jackson promising Revere a horoscope. The latter, according to Revere, was duly conveyed by letter after a few months and contained an ominous prediction: "It is clear to me that we shall both be exposed to a common danger at the time indicated."[5, p. 257] The "time indicated" by Jackson's calculations: May 1863.

Later in *Keel and Saddle* is an account of the evening of May 2, 1863 on the Chancellorsville battlefield in which Revere, then a Brigadier General commanding the Excelsior Brigade, described following on horseback the sounds of musketry, encountering a riderless horse, and coming upon a gravely wounded Confederate soldier surrounded by several officers. Revere concluded: "These left no doubt in my own mind that the person I had seen lying on the ground was that officer [Stonewall Jackson], and that his singular prediction—mentioned previously in these pages—had been verified."[5, p. 277] On the page following this statement, Revere paradoxically appeared to disavow astrologic predictions, observing: "Jackson's death happened in strange coincidence with his horoscopic prediction made years before: but the coincidence was, I believe, merely fortuitous; and I mention it here only to show what mysterious 'givings-out' we sometimes experience in life."[5, p. 278]

How did Osler come to insert the footnote?

It appears that Osler had only a passing familiarity with the American Civil War. There is no evidence, at least in Osler's writings,[6] of an interest in American military topics other than some aspects of military medicine. This notwithstanding, it is quite likely that a copy of *Keel and Saddle* had its place on the Osler family bookshelves.

The author of the footnote's source document was cousin to Osler's wife, Grace Revere Osler, and Lady Osler's father had a deep interest in the Civil War.[7] Warren Revere had gifted copies of *Keel and Saddle* to many, among them George Brigham Revere, her father's distant cousin.[8] Moreover, Osler, in a letter to Weir Mitchell on 21 November 1913,[9] acknowledged Grace's specific interest in Civil War events involving Revere descendants.

It is also likely that a member of the household, most probably Lady Osler or Revere Osler, pointed Osler to the story as he revised the astrology section of his manuscript. While Osler's friendship with Fielding H. Garrison suggests Garrison as a source of information, there is no direct record of it. Garrison, the lead editor of *The Evolution of Modern Medicine*, was a colonel in the Army, and a close friend of John Shaw Billings, himself an internationally known bibliophile, who was "warmly attached" to Hunter McGuire, Stonewall Jackson's surgeon.[10] Even though Osler knew Billings and wrote fondly of him after his death,[11] this association, too, contained nothing to suggest Osler's knowledge of the Revere tale came from that quarter.

Osler may not have questioned the veracity of Revere's account out of respect for the Revere family, his interest in spiritualism[12] and the possibly impulsive nature of its inclusion in the manuscript. The latter seems a reasonable inference because the footnote was so unique among his writings.

The veracity of the Revere account

Revere's story, however, was very likely untrue. His tale of events surrounding Jackson's death contained a quotation he said was from the *Richmond Enquirer* of May 12, 1863, a newspaper he reported seeing two weeks after the events at Chancellorsville. According to Revere, the newspaper article described Jackson's wounding and death and mentioned an unknown horseman (which Revere implied was himself) in the clearing where Jackson lay wounded. Revere's newspaper quotations, however, are suspect: the *Richmond Enquirer* did not publish an edition on May 12, 1863; the closest dates were May 8th and May 15th where there is respectively a mention of Jackson's injury and an account of Jackson's wounding, but without the detail Revere supplied.[13] The *Richmond Dispatch* of 14 May, 1863[14] and the *Daily Richmond Enquirer* of the same day[15] quote an article in the *Enquirer* "of yesterday," but that, too, does not match the lengthy quotation that Revere offered.

Some authors, contemporaneous with General Revere, accepted Revere's account. Sarah Randolph's biography of Jackson[16] records the Revere tale as "too curious and too authentic to be omitted from a life of Jackson …" Nonetheless, aside from her biography and one or two book reviews in 1873,[17] Revere's story of Jackson does not seem to have gained much historical traction. It does not appear in any of several biographies of Jackson.[18–21]

In 1873, the year after the publication of *Keel and Saddle*, retired Confederate General Jubal A. Early published a refutation of Revere's story.[22] Early produced a letter from General Francis H. Smith, superintendent of the Virginia Military Institute (VMI) who confirmed Stonewall Jackson's joining the VMI faculty in 1851 as professor of natural and experimental philosophy and artillery tactics. Smith confirmed that, at the time of Revere's alleged encounter with Lieutenant Thomas J. Jackson, Stonewall Jackson was an active member of the VMI faculty and did not travel further south than Charlotte, North Carolina until the commencement of the Civil War in April 1861.

Concerning the scene of Jackson's shooting, Early provided eyewitness documentation that only two individuals attended the fallen Jackson, not the group of "several persons" reported by Revere. The eyewitness, R.E. Wilbourn, pointed out that the solitary rider in the newspaper story was "…changed, however, so as to make it appear more like a romance than reality."[22] Wilbourn here does not mention the specific newspaper and may be referring to Revere's description of its contents. Of the lone horseman, Wilbourn said he appeared to be a courier and Wilbourn directed him to investigate the identity of Confederate troops in the vicinity. The man rode off with these instructions and his identity was never determined.[23]

Neither Early nor contemporary Jackson biographer Robert Dabney[24] provided any evidence that the devoutly Presbyterian Stonewall Jackson harbored beliefs in astrology. Smith, writing to Early, stated: "I never heard General Jackson allude to astrology, nor have I been able to find any one among his former associates who had."[22]

William Chemerka's recent biography of General Revere mentions Early's critique.[8,p. 154] He agreed with Early that Revere was "mistaken" in both the 1852 encounter on the Mississippi and in the Wilderness at the Battle of Chancellorsville in 1863 but declined to suggest the mistakes were intentional. Chemerka mentioned the possibility, found in Early's refutation, that the "Jackson" Revere encountered at New Orleans was Lieutenant Thomas K. Jackson, an army officer who graduated from West Point two years after Stonewall Jackson. The 1852 letter from Jackson to Revere is not referenced in Chemerka's exhaustively researched book and Mr. Chemerka did not find it during his research.[25]

Why would Revere have written this account?

After the battle of Chancellorsville, Revere was court-martialed for marching his command "an unnecessary distance to the rear" while it was engaged with the enemy. He was found guilty of the specification, but not of the specific charge itself (misbehavior before the enemy). He was also found guilty of "conduct to the prejudice of good order and military discipline."[26] The court sentenced him to be dismissed from the military service of the United States and on 10 August 1863, by General Order 282 of the War Department, the sentence was carried out.[27]

The court's judgment was controversial. Revere supporters harshly criticized the factual findings of the court martial and the legality of its proceedings, testifying to Revere's virtues as a soldier. Revere himself wrote a lengthy rebuttal. Many of those who fought in the campaign, though, were inclined to agree with the court. In a history of the Excelsior Brigade,[28] Bruce Sutherland observes:

> It [dismissal from the army] came as a severe blow to the man who had entered the United States Navy in 1828 as a fourteen-year-old midshipman, who had raised and organized the Seventh Regiment of New Jersey Volunteers at the beginning of the war and had fought with them since Williamsburg, who had two brothers in the Federal service and who was a descendant of the Revolutionary War hero, Paul Revere, yet the verdict could hardly have been otherwise.

Efforts by Revere, his relatives and highly placed friends to reverse the court-martial's sentence were unsuccessful[29–33] until late in 1864 when Lincoln approved the War Department's Special Order 30 revoking Revere's dismissal from the Army and accepting Revere's resignation effective August 10th 1863.[8, p. 147] Revere, for the rest of his life, actively tried to remove the stain on his reputation whenever the matter was discussed.

Revere was not a braggart and genuinely believed in the truth of what he had written.[25] Nonetheless, he had not been entirely forthcoming about aspects of his life that would adversely affect his reputation. He omitted from *Keel and Saddle*, for example, the reason for his 1850 resignation from the Navy: a love affair with another man's wife that would have led to a court martial. His autobiography may have been a response to the disgrace of dismissal from the armed forces of the United States, particularly for an act that could be interpreted as cowardice. Through a celestially ordained connection with the highly respected Jackson, he may have sought to claim supernatural sanctification as a warrior.

Could the story have been simply the union of two "mistakes," Revere confusing an amateur astrologer named Jackson on a Mississippi riverboat for Stonewall Jackson and then a wounded soldier encountered during his twilight ride in the bewildering circumstances of the Wilderness battlefield for the same person? Simple confusion is plausible as *Keel and Saddle* contained other inaccuracies attributable to inexact recollection. On the other hand, the book's descriptions of two days with Jackson on the riverboat, detailed quotations from Jackson's letter to him and his quotations of a newspaper account seem too precise for unassisted memory. Were documents not readily at hand during the writing—and they do not seem to be among Revere's personal papers—the story recounted in the book would appear created out of whole cloth.

The persistent Osler

The content of the Osler's persistently influential footnote was almost certainly fictitious. In inserting it, perhaps an inspiration honoring his wife, Osler could not have foreseen its modern citation to support, with the gravitas associated with Osler's reputation, the nonexistent astrological beliefs of Stonewall Jackson. In any case, as Osler himself would likely remind us given his well-known sense of humor, the whole affair illustrates the Hippocratic maxim that experience is fallacious and judgment difficult, even among those generally revered.

References

1. Barondess JA, McGovern JP, Roland CG, eds. *The Persisting Osler: Selected Transactions of the First Ten Years of the American Osler Society.* Baltimore: University Park Press; 1985.
2. Osler W. *The Evolution of Modern Medicine.* New Haven: Yale University Press; 1921: 124.
3. Letter, Osler to Cushing, 29 January 1916 and Letter, Osler to Stokes, uncertain date, but probably 1915. Osler Library of the History of Medicine, McGill University, P417 Harvey Cushing fonds.
4. Unpublished manuscript pertaining to *The Evolution of Modern Medicine.* In Francis WW, Hill RH, Malloch A. *Bibliotheca Osleriana.* Oxford: Oxford University Press; 1926: 689 (item number 7652).
5. Revere JW. *Keel and Saddle: A Retrospect of Forty Years of Military and Naval Service.* Boston: James R. Osgood and Company; 1872.
6. McGovern JP, Roland, CG, eds. *The Collected Essays of Sir William Osler.* Birmingham: The Classics of Medicine Library; 1985.
7. Harrell G. Lady Osler. *Bulletin of the History of Medicine* 1979; 53: 81–99.
8. Chemerka WR. *General Joseph Warren Revere: The Gothic Saga of Paul Revere's Grandson.* Duncan, Oklahoma: Bear Manor Media; Nook eBook Version, 2013.
9. Cushing H. *The Life of Sir William Osler.* Oxford: Clarendon Press; 1925; ii: 386.
10. Mayer E. Dr. John Shaw Billings, An Appreciation. *The Medical Pickwick* 1916; 2: 53–55.
11. [Osler W]. John Shaw Billings, M.A., M.D. (Obituary). *Lancet* 181(4673) (March 22): 859–860.
12. Rudyard Kipling to William Osler, 20 November 1909. CUS417/35.10, Harvey Cushing fonds, Osler Library of the History of Medicine, McGill University.
13. *Richmond Enquirer,* 8 May 1863, page 1; 15 May 1863, page 1. The detail that Revere quotes is found in Wilbourn's letter to Faulkner (reference 23).
14. *Richmond Dispatch,* 14 May 1863, page 1.

15. Andrews JC. *The South Reports the Civil War*. Princeton: Princeton University Press; 1970: 300.
16. Randolph SN. *The Life of Gen. Thomas J. Jackson ("Stonewall Jackson")*. Philadelphia: J.B. Lippincott & Co.; 1876: 326–328.
17. Book Review. *Appleton's Journal: A Magazine of General Literature* 1872; 7(185) (25 May). The author of the review states: "General Revere's life has been a checkered one, and the record of it is more readable than most novels."
18. Robertson RI. *Stonewall Jackson: The Man, The Soldier, The Legend*. New York: Macmillan; 1997.
19. Fritz J, Gammell S. *Stonewall*. New York: GP Putnam's Sons; 1979.
20. Davis B. *They Called Him Stonewall*. Ithaca: Burford Books, 1999.
21. Farwell B. *Stonewall: A Biography of General Thomas J. Jackson*. New York: W.W. Norton & Company; 1992.
22. Early JA. Stonewall Jackson—The Story of His Being an Astrologer Refuted. *Southern Historical Society Papers* 1878; 6: 261–282, 1878 (Originally published in *Southern Magazine* 1873; 12: 537–555).
23. Captain Richard Eggleston Wilbourn to Colonel Charles J. Faulkner, May 1863. Virginia Historical Society Manuscript Collection (https://www.virginiahistory.org/collections-and-resources/virginia-history-explorer/general-orders-no-61/eyewitness-account).
24. Dabney RL. *Life and Campaigns of Lieut.-Gen. Thomas J. Jackson, (Stonewall Jackson)*. New York: Blelock & Co; 1866.
25. William Chemerka, personal communications, 31 July and 1 August 2013.
26. Revere JW. *A Statement of the Case of Brigadier-General Joseph W. Revere*. New York: C.A. Alvord; 1863. This pamphlet, prepared by General Revere, included the transcript of the court martial in its entirety as well as additional explanations and alleged exculpatory evidence.
27. General Order 282. General Orders of the War Department Embracing the Years 1861, 1862 and 1863. New York: Derby & Miller; 1864: 355–356.
28. Sutherland B. Pittsburgh Volunteers with Sickles' Excelsior Brigade (Part 4). *Western Pennsylvania Historical Magazine* 1962; 45(4) :309–310.
29. Joseph Revere to Abraham Lincoln, 15 November 1863. Lincoln Papers, Library of Congress.
30. Relatives of Revere to Abraham Lincoln, 15 November 1863. Lincoln Papers, Library of Congress.
31. Andrew J. Rogers to Abraham Lincoln, 29 January 1864. Lincoln Papers, Library of Congress.
32. Joseph W. Revere to Abraham Lincoln, 4 February 1864. Lincoln Papers, Library of Congress.
33. Thomas D. Eliot to Abraham Lincoln, 1 February 1864. Lincoln Papers, Library of Congress.

SECTION III

❧ Friends, Family, Colleagues

Marian Francis Kelen's Memories of Oxford and of her Father, W.W. Francis, the First Osler Librarian

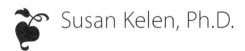 Susan Kelen, Ph.D.

These two short reminiscences were written by my mother, Marian Francis Kelen (1922–2014). The reminiscences are about Osler's Oxford home and her father, W.W. Francis, and their early family life. W.W. Francis catalogued and edited Osler's books and he was the first Osler Librarian. W.W. Francis was Osler's first cousin once-removed.

The first reminiscence was written up after an impromptu speech given at the 1984 American Osler Society Meeting held in Oxford and included a tour of 13, Norham Gardens. 13 Norham Gardens was my mother's first home and a place she would know for her first 6 years. My mother grew up immersed in the stories, teachings, and spirit of Osler. She moved with her parents to Canada on the ship S.S. *Montclair* with the books for the Osler Library. The Captain would tease W.W. Francis that crates of books and a baby grand piano were spotted off the port side of the ship!

The second reminiscence of her father was found in our family papers, dutifully typed up by my father. This was probably written around the same time. It gives some insight to my grandfather's personality.

Presented in part at the forty-ninth annual meeting of the American Osler Society, Montreal, Quebec, Canada, on 13 May 2019.

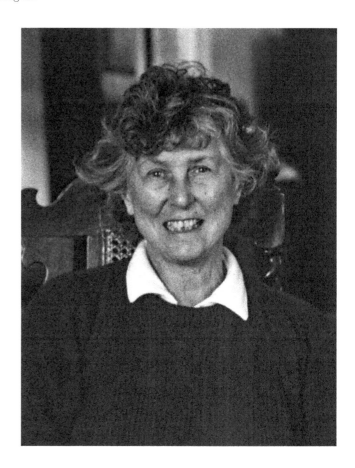

Figure 1.   Marian Francis Kelen at about age 60, in 1982.
Credit: Kelen Family Collection.

What is missing in my mother's reminiscences are references to Maude Abbott. My grandfather knew Maude Abbott from McGill and attended many events she sponsored, such as at least four vernissages [private showings of artwork] for an artist with failing eyesight.

My mother grew up roller-skating on the McGill sidewalks. Years later she entered medical school at McGill. In her university years she cross-country skied with the legendary "Jack Rabbit" Smith-Johannson. It was during these ski trips that she met a fellow medical student who became her husband of sixty years. Their honeymoon started with a canoe strapped to the side of a float-plane. They had five children.

She practiced medicine in a group practice, with my father, in rural Quebec. They offered affordable medical care in the days before Medicare. She was the first female doctor in the region. She was an excellent diagnostician and much appreciated by her patients.

She had an encyclopedic memory and could be counted on for an appropriate quotation from Shakespeare or Winnie the Pooh. Family dinners often ended with her reading aloud from a reference book appropriate to the dinner table discussion. She was a voracious reader and a humorous poet writing about events in family life, such as when one of her children left for Nigeria.

In her final years, her daily routine included reading from Osler's copy of the *Fireside Encyclopedia of Poetry*, which was kept on her dining room table, the same table where Osler's books were catalogued. She was always cheerful and accepting with what life brought her. She died at age 92.

Memories of Oxford (dictated by Marian Francis Kelen, January 1985)

This is Marian Francis Kelen, of Ormstown, Québec, a short 34 miles from the Osler Library at McGill University. Margaret Dewey and Mrs. Philippe Shubik both asked me to record some of my memories at 13, Norham Gardens when my husband and I came to the Osler Revisited (AOS) Conference in September 1984. My visit to 13, Norham Gardens was Tuesday, September 25 and it brought back vivid memories.

I remember a lot about 13, Norham gardens and its inhabitants, the Upstairs family and the Downstairs family. The reason I was there was because my father, W.W. Francis, had been working on the library with Sir William Osler [WO] before WO's death and came to Oxford in order to prepare the Catalogue, later published as the *Bibliotheca Osleriana*. My family arrived from Switzerland just before my birth on January 10, 1922 at the Acland Home in Oxford. We stayed at 13, Norham Gardens until I was three, when we moved out to a house in Kingston Road and later Bainton Road. I remember Lady Osler at work at her desk in her bedroom writing letters on paper with a black margin. When we came down the stairs my father had a ritual. I would hold his hand and he would look at the big etching of a lion on the stairway and say," It's a ROARING lion!" And (when we came) to that corner and he would say, "It's a BAD corner!" And I would reply, "It's a GOOD corner!" At the foot of the stairs there was a grandfather clock which showed the faces of the moon. He would pick me up to look at the moon and its face. He had the job of winding it every week.

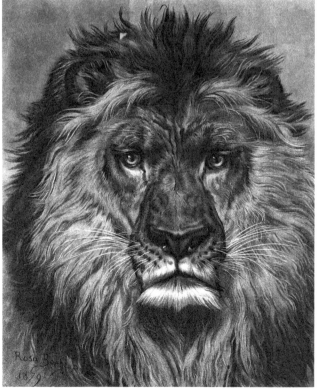

Figure 2. The lion in the stairwell at 13 Norham Gardens. This version of *The Old Monarch* was painted by the French artist Rosa Bonheur (1822–1899) and engraved by the British printmaker William Henry Simmons (1811–1882). The engraving that hung in the stairwell and would therefore have been seen by William Osler several times each day remains with the Francis family. When the print was restored, a newspaper from the *Philadelphia Evening Standard* was found in the back—suggesting that the print moved with the Oslers from the United States to Oxford.
Credit: Kelen Family Collection.

On entering 13, Norham Gardens again in September 1984 I saw the door, which was locked on the left side of the hall, leading to the "consulting room." Osler's consulting room was the room in which my father had worked with Dr. Archie Malloch and Mr. Reg Hill and others on the Catalogue. I remember the hall because there was a telephone in it, and my father had telephoned every day to Reg Hill when he was a worried about the Hills' little son, Alan, who was very ill and died in hospital.

The first room on the right as you go was the drawing room. The baby grand piano was there, a German piano bought at a bargain price, because it was German, during the war. Here, Aunt Grace poured the tea at tea parties. There were many students and visiting friends, some of them were John and Lucia Fulton and Harvey Cushing. I remember them particularly well because we saw them later in Canada and in New Haven, Connecticut. The things that were served at tea included plates of a very thin, very soft white bread and butter, and round, flat, lemon- or almond-flavored sugar cookies. The library let into the dining room where there were pictures of Edward Jenner and Heinrich Heine; I think they were both engravings. Either in this room or the dining room had a picture of Atlanta, stooping down to pick up a golden apple in her race with Hippomanes. There was the door leading out to the terrace and the garden. The dining room table and chairs in the library all shone so beautifully. Florence Ivings kept everything beautiful and shiny. She swept up the breadcrumbs at dinner with the curved brush between courses. She let me help her sweep the carpet with my little dustpan and brush, but I was annoyed that she did it over again after I'd done it! The dinner table conversation was usually about Osler. Another thing they talked about at dinner were the people they knew who had "gone down in the *Lusitania*." This caused me some concern because our ship that would soon take us to Canada might also sink! (Of course, when I saw how enormous and unsinkable it looked at the dock in Liverpool, I did not worry.)

The kitchen and service hall downstairs were below the dining room. The kitchen was in front of the house and the servants' dining room was on the north side. I only remember one window on that side. You entered by a door to

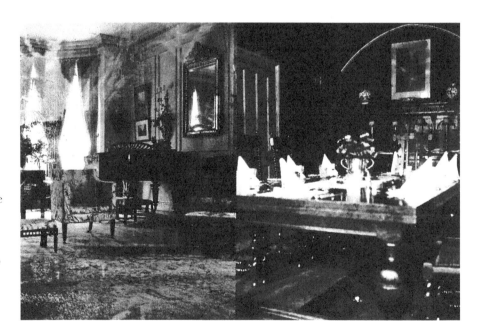

Figure 3.   *Left:* The drawing room of 13 Norham Gardens where Lady Osler served tea. Note the baby grand piano against the wall. *Right:* The dining room, with the table set for dinner. *Credit:* Kelen Family Collection.

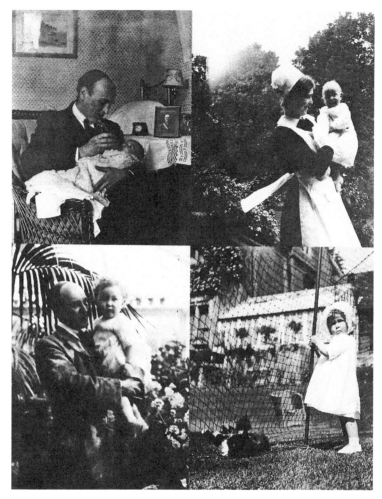

Figure 4.   Photographs of Marian Grace ("Maisie") Francis as a child in Oxford. *Clockwise from upper left:* W.W. Francis bottle-feeding Marian at three months; Florence Irvings, the parlor maid, holding Marian at three months (April 1922); Marian at 17 months with Michael, the cat, rolled up in the tennis court net with the greenhouse behind them; W.W. Francis holding Marian at 14 months in the greenhouse at 13 Norham Gardens. *Credit:* Kelen Family Collection.

the right of the stove. Each of the servants kept her sugar in their cupboard in a large individual jam jar with her name on it. I don't know why, as there was no more sugar rationing. The war had been over for years. Mrs. Parsons, the cook, was the chief executive of the servants' hall. She came from Birmingham and she probably lived at 13, Norham Gardens, but I'm not positive about this. Florence Ivings, the parlor maid, waited on the table and was assisted by Ethel, the chambermaid. Florence set the fireplaces and lit the fires. Ada was the scullery maid. The one I loved best was Mrs. Cleaver, known to me as "Dids." She was the sewing woman, and her sewing room was on the very top floor above the servants' hall, up two flights of stairs. It was a rather dark corridor up there, and it had an S-shaped Iron bracket holding a bare light bulb. I had to close my eyes and run past it to get up to visit her. Mrs. Cleaver lived at 9, Ship St. with her daughter, Elsie. We visited her in her old Tudor house with a narrow stone spiral staircase. Once Mrs. Parsons make the most beautiful Christmas cake with a robin on top. The reason I remember was that I was not allowed to have any!

Figure 5. *Left:* Marian Grace ("Maisie") Francis at 17 months with W.W. Francis and Susan Torrey Revere Chapin ("Aunt Sue"). Sue Chapin figures prominently in the biographies of William Osler, but photographs of her seldom appear in the Osler canon. *Right:* W.W. Francis with Marian Grace Francis on the handlebar of a bicycle. *Credit:* Kelen Family Collection.

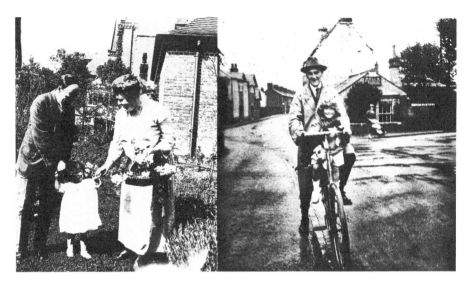

One important member of the household was Michael, the black and white fluffy cat. He was the most gracious cat. He welcomed visitors to the house and on the terrace. Sometimes he played in the tennis net, rolling up in it.

The garden was beautiful. My parents play tennis on the courts which were directly below the terrace. They were big cedar trees and several clumps along the wall that leads to the University Gardens. And they were beautiful roses. Once Henry, the gardener, annoyed me very much by cutting off the rosebuds! He explained that he wanted one or two big roses instead of a lot of little ones. I pleaded with him, but he wouldn't listen to me. He grew the best little tomatoes in the greenhouse. There were two of the nicest smells I've ever known connected

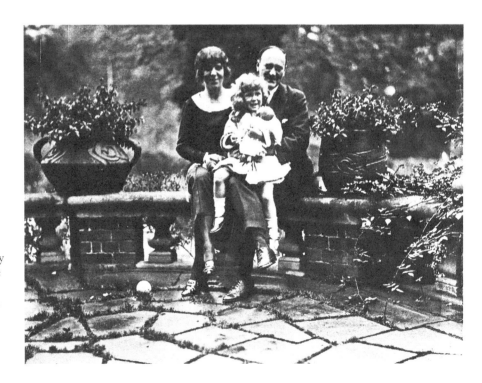

Figure 6. Family portrait of Hilda Colley Francis, Marian Grace Francis at about three years of age, and W.W. Francis at 13 Norham Gardens, Oxford. *Credit:* Kelen Family Collection.

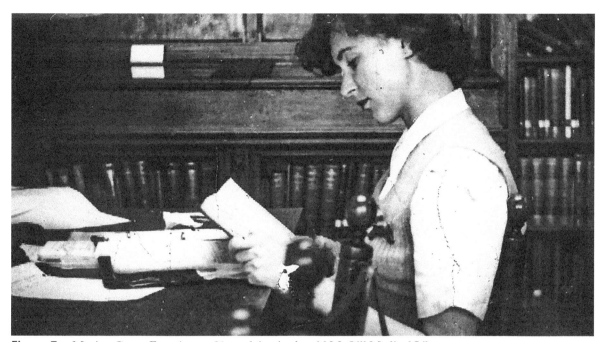

Figure 7.   Marian Grace Francis, age 21, studying in the old McGill Medical Library.
Credit: Kelen Family Collection.

with this house. One was in the greenhouse. I think it was the mixture of geraniums and tomatoes and moist warm earth. The other smell was the garage, strangely enough. It contained the "motor car." Perhaps the chauffeur put some special polish on it. We went for rides in it, especially when Mrs. Sue Chapin, Aunt Sue, Lady Osler's sister came to visit.

I learned to ride my bike on the soft green lawn in the garden. On the road I was afraid to stop in case I fell. My mother ran holding the saddle all the way from Bainton Road to 13, Norham Gardens, a long way! Then as soon as I got on the grass, I could go by myself.

The servants were quiet and very gracious group of ladies. I remember the deep respect that they showed on the day that Aunt Grace died. My parents and I had ridden over on our bikes. I ran in first into the servants' hall and finding no one there I ran to the upstairs hall outside Aunt Grace's room where Mrs. Parsons, Mrs. Cleaver, Florence, Ethel, and Ada were standing in a circle with their heads bowed and their hands folded in front of them. "She's gone," Mrs. Parsons told me.

"Gone where?" I said. She explained. This was the end of an era for me.

Addendum

The Kingston Roadhouse had a garden path leading to the canal. Families with children live on the barges that were pulled along by cart horses who plotted along the tow path very slowly. The two Bainton Roadhouses that we lived had the nicest back gardens surrounded by a long brick wall where the kittens could play safely and where my rabbit dug himself a comfortable bed under the sunflowers.

We've bicycled all over Oxford. My mother and I had a favourite destination, a restaurant called The Candied Friend, where they sold cherry tarts. On special occasions we took a bus up to Boar's Hill Hotel which had swings and a very big rocking horse. Not far from Payton Road there was Port Meadow, which had a very exciting floods in the spring. When the floodwaters receded, I could go and collect frog spawn and find newts. The frocks spawn hatched out in the garden into little pollywogs with legs and then turned into frogs.

The only thing wrong with Oxford was that my father had to go to work! He was home for part of the morning as he preferred to work late at night. We did go on some very nice picnics, in bluebell woods and to Wytham Hill where we found primroses growing. My mother and I often walked to The Trout Inn for tea where they had peacocks strutting in the garden.

Life with Willie [W.W. Francis]

I don't I don't know how early I can remember him, but I certainly remember going down the stairs at 13, Norham Gardens where we would pass a big engraving of a lion and he would say, "It's a ROARRING lion!" with a loud roar! And he claimed he used to say, holding my hand "it's a bad corner!" (referring to where the lion hung) and that I would reply, "it's a good corner!"

After we moved to a little house near the Canal in Oxford when I was three, Goggy" was so much fun I did not want him to go to work ever! He got up later than we did and he sang to our maid Ruby, "Hey Ruby, love-a-duck, will you fetch some hot water for a Gogs?" He drove me around Oxford on the bar of his bike and when I was 4 my mother was brave enough to take me on her bike carrier which was much more comfortable.

Goggy read me lots of stories and played English and French nursery rhymes on the piano. Pooh and Alice in Wonderland were two of our favorite stories. He must have suggested the name for my hobby horse "Pegasus" and my purple and gold elephant "Hathi." He said Indians call their elephants "Hathi." He loved astronomy and pointed out the constellations to me. He went off in search of an eclipse of the sun once to Giggleswick (in Wales) which occasioned some mirth, and another time he went to Holland on a similar search and brought me back a book of adventures of an ape called Jocko, in Dutch, with great pictures.

He was stubborn about a lot of things, like animals. Perhaps this was because he knew we would soon leave Oxford and did not want to have to find a home for a dog, cat or rabbit when we left. My mother believed animals were very important and got around his stubbornness by the technique of "fait accompli." This meant to getting something done without further discussion! Somehow, she managed to bring home "Mummy Pussy" in her bicycle basket one day. This cat had two kittens, Romulus and Remus, who were the delight of my life. I was given at charming chinchilla rabbit who was free to run in the garden all day. The three of us rounded him up at sunset and put him in his hutch for the night.

Later, in Montréal, my mother and I had trouble with him over the animal question. "You can't keep a dog or cat in an apartment!" he would exclaim. "That cat leaves by Wednesday or I'll move to the club!" Once he came back from an historical meeting to celebrate the quadrennial of Vesalius to find a black-and-white fluffy kitten called Vesalius had moved in who insisted on helping him unpack! On another occasion I brought home an abandoned part-German Shepherd who soon improved and grinned on one side of his face when he wagged his tail. Only my father got the two-sided grin from the dog, a mark of highest esteem!

He would not own a car or let my mother get one. Nor would he buy house. He thought real estate values would go right down. A house my mother wanted to buy in 1934 for $14,000 is now worth far more than $140,000! He managed to live within walking distance of the library. He thought it was much safer, and it simplified life to have a janitor look after the maintenance of our apartment. This way he had time to read and write to his friends and play tennis on the courts on Mount Royal, a 15-minute walk from home.

Every July, we went to Hubbards, Nova Scotia, to a small hotel with excellent food and the beach with relatively warm water. It took 22 hours to get there on the train and car ferry across the Bay of Fundy. We all played baseball on the beach and had shuffleboard matches. At the concerts at the hotel, Willie played the piano and sang his two favorite songs, "On the Road to Mandalay," and "Way down yonder on the Yankety Yank, a bull frog jumped from bank to bank."

Willie was a good swimmer, having been brought up on "The Island" in Toronto every summer. My mother, Hillie, was not. We would tease her from the raft in Como, Québec where we went each August, by pointing at her and saying "Mrs. Hippo" and she would get the giggles and sink, finally struggling to the surface and grabbing the ladder on the raft! Willie was the clown when swimming and he loved to do handstands and show off his slim legs in the shallow water.

At the boarding house we stayed at in Como there were two old ladies who were terrified of cats. They could sense if a very small kitten was even thinking of leaving the kitchen or going into the lounge. People laughed at them on account of this peculiarity. The boarding house always had a mother cat and at least one kitten so they were always in trouble. Willy made him feel much better by explaining that they suffered from a well recognize condition known as Aleurophobia, and that they couldn't help it!

Another of his medical achievements long after he given up practice, was reducing the hotel chef's dislocated shoulder by the Hippocratic method, with the heel in the axilla. He said it was so easy that he suspected the chef of putting his shoulder out on purpose so people would buy him a drink.

At Como I was given a 14-foot sailing dingy by my Uncle Arthur who lived in England and Willie tried to teach me to sail. The second day out I jibed by mistake and the thick boom rammed him into the gunwales breaking a couple of ribs. After that he said I could teach myself to sail.

He was very popular with the little girls of Grade 3 and 4 in the Montréal High Junior School. The kids would all ambush him, leaping down from the wall as he passed the school with shouts of "Willie!" When I had Halloween parties he dressed up as a ghost and chased them around our circular apartment. I was so proud of him when teachers at our school took us to the McGill campus to watch the convocation parade. The faculty were in their gowns and hoods, looking very distinguished. Willy would grin and wave at his little friends.

Addendum—"Blessed BooBoo"
(another of his many family nicknames)

We found a little field mouse when we went on a picnic near Oxford. I put him in Willie's trouser cuff so he'd be safe while some noisy boys passed by. He must have been a very young mouse as he didn't move or try to escape. We set him free in the field hoping he'd find his family.

Willie, Hillie and I had a big job chasing my rabbit, "Bun" or "Bunrab" as Willie called him, at sunset every evening as he was safest in his hutch night. The garden was completely enclosed by brick wall at Number 8 Bainton Road. We got him cornered and into his hutch he went.

Willie made us laugh! He had a good story about Hillie's friend who was the spiritualist, telling her how the spirit hovers around the dead person for five days after death. "Dear Mrs. Francis," she said, "keep Dr. Francis for five days!" At that point, the subject in question, Willie, arriving home from work, raised his hat, and made a funny face at the window. This caused Hillie to collapse with laughter. I'm sorry I missed this!

Willie and Hillie played cards every evening. Hillie swore she'd never play with him again as he got so cross if he didn't win, but they played anyway: Rummy, Cabosse, a kind of solitaire and Snap. Hillie shrieked whenever she was Rummied which livened up the evening.

Willie and I like to tease "Little Hillie." She was not a good swimmer and when swimming around the raft at Como she would sink like a stone with the giggles when Willie and I pointed and said "Mrs. Hippo" or even just pointed. She came up sputtering.

Como was 30 miles from Montréal. Willie knew Como because his old friend, Dr. Frank Shepherd, had lived there, and his two daughters were good friends. We stayed at the boarding house or "Willow Place" every August and he commuted by train to the library every day. He arrived back in time for swimming and some tennis.

His tennis was accurate and reliable. Hillie's was impulsive and sometimes brilliant (but) often the ball was out. Many sets finished 7-5 or 8-6. There were junior tournaments so I played with mostly with my friends but sometimes the three of us played a round-robin.

Once when I was four or five, I was given a long box full of about a dozen little jars of jam all different flavors. I didn't want to share them. Willie warned me what would happen if I did not share them: "Thy jam with turn IP!" he said, waving his hand over them in a magic spell. To my horror, the next morning, my favorite kind looked and smelled a lot like Vaseline—or was it Turnip Jam. Willy hated turnips, and this was an awful thing to do to jam! When I agreed to share the rest, this spell was removed, and the nasty brown jam turned into the bright red raspberry variety.

He and I played scary game. I would be under the bedclothes, well tucked in by Hillie and he would cry, "Sphyxie will get you!" holding down the sheet so I couldn't escape.

Willy's religion was a problem to Hillie. She would have liked it if at least one of us would go to church with her. Willie only went on St. Luke's Day when Archdeacon Gower Rees called upon the McGill faculty of medicine to read the lesson and deliver the sermon. Several of the faculty came in solemn procession in their gowns and hoods. Willie read, "Though I speak with the tongues of men and of angels" one year, and about the sick of the palsy the next (from St. Luke). Once he even delivered the sermon, Uncle Willie's "Man's Redemption of Man." Hillie and I really liked the services and we were so proud of him! After the St. Luke's Day services, we often had dinner or sherry at Dr. and Mrs. Birkett's. Dr. B. was Willie's former Colonel-in-Chief from No. 2 Canadian General Hospital.

As he grew older, he went to more and more funerals and always enjoyed them.

"Dear-old-Dick-everybody-loves-him!" was his name for one of his old pals. He met his old friends at funerals, and they were a time of mixed sadness and happiness.

I attended the Christ Church Cathedral Brownies near where we lived. Two of the Brownies were going to be confirmed, in beautiful white dresses like little brides. I studied the catechism on my own and taught it to my stuffed animals and I wanted to be confirmed. But Willie said," Let the Pet wait till she's grown up and then decide."

Why was he so disillusioned with his mother's and Little Auntie's (Jennette Osler) religion? Was it because God did not stop the Germans from bombing the poor patients at Number 2 Canadian General Hospital. "The poor devils were in traction." he said. Perhaps he felt that the death of Revere and so many others should have been prevented by Little Auntie's God.

Willie loved *Rubaiyat of Omar Khayyam* and collected many editions. He never indulged in wine like Omar—only a glass of sweet wine like Muscatelle before supper. He was worried if we gave our children sips of beer they would turn into alcoholics.

Willie enjoyed having the Osler Library in the medical building and knew all its staff. If one of the staff retired, he would compose a poem for the occasion. Even when the janitor retired an appropriate poem was read. He was the poet laureate of the medical building. The library was a place to share the books with old and new friends. If there were new visitors to the library, he demonstrated the books with what he called "Showman's Patter" finding books he felt would interest them most.

About the grandchildren he had mixed feelings. When we arrived for Sunday dinner Willie would kiss them all and then retreat to the faculty club, returning in time to kiss them all goodbye. The children were born in 1948, 1949, 1951, 1952, and 1956, so the succession of fights and general lack of manners were too unnerving for him as much as he loved them. The little ones often stayed with him one at a time for several days and became good friends.

Willie's heart attacks may have had some connection with his serious addiction to cigarettes. He gave them up without complaint after his first attack in 1946. Hillie, however, continued to smoke.

After his eighteen-month as a patient with TB in Ste-Agathe, "The Cure" became a way of life for him. "The Cure" included rest in bed, good food, and lots of sleep. He married the right girl! Hillie, who had nursing experience as a V.A.D. (Voluntary Aide Detachment) during the war, was a real expert at making a patient comfortable in bed. She would bring us lovely things to eat and drink. If we had a cold, aspirin and Vaseline in and on the nostrils and around the entire nose was one of Willy's favorite remedies. And he would put on his warm sweater, a woollen nightcap that he'd worn at Ste-Agathe. Friar's Balsam mixed in boiling water inhaled from a jug with a towel over the patient's head was one of Hillie's favorite remedies.

Thus, Willie survived five of his heart attacks. Only the sixth one proved fatal. Once in the Ross pavilion of the Royal Victoria Hospital (in Montreal) a maid came to change the water in the flowers. He sang, "*Il reviendra le temps des roses*" to her. She was delighted. (It will come again, the time of roses.)

Editorial note

Marian Francis Kelen (1922–2014), born Marian Grace Francis, was an honorary member of the American Osler Society (AOS). She was the only child of William Willoughby Francis (1878–1959) and Hilda Colley Francis (c. 1886–1962). W.W. Francis, "Bill" or "Billy" to his friends, was the son of George Grant Francis, II (d. 1907), and Marian Osler (Bath) Francis (1841–1915). His mother (born Marian Osler) was the daughter of Edward Osler (1798–1863), who was the brother of William Osler's father, Featherstone Lake Osler (1805–1895). Thus, Bill Francis was William Osler's first cousin once-removed.

Marian Francis Kelen, the author of these reminiscences, was born on 10 January 1922, several days after her parents arrived in Oxford. Marian Grace Francis. Her given names derived from her paternal grandmother (born Marian Osler) and Lady Osler (born Grace Revere), who was her godmother. Her god-father was Dr. T. Archibald Malloch (1887–1953), who joined the Osler household in December 1919, served as one of William Osler's physicians during the last month of his life, and later assisted W.W. Francis catalogue William Osler's enormous collection of rare books, the *Bibliotheca Osleriana*.

In 1985 Frederick B. Wagner, Jr., (1916–2004) brought out *The Twilight Years of Lady Osler: Letters of a Doctor's Wife*, based largely on Lady Osler's letter to T. Archibald Malloch. She expresses great affection for Archie Malloch but is ambivalent about Bill and Hilda Francis and their daughter, Marian ("Maisie"). Wagner generalizes: "Lady Osler experienced increasing irritation, frustration, and intolerance of the entire Francis family." Hilda Francis took "refuge with the baby," and it was "a great blow to Lady Osler's ego and possibly a source of guilt feelings that Mrs. Francis could not find happiness in residence at The Open Arms." We must remember that Lady Osler was lonely and probably depressed after the loss of her husband and son.

Marian Francis Kelen's reminiscences of 13 Norham Gardens, and also of her father, are published here for the first time. Most of the photographs reproduced here are likewise published here for the first time. These reminiscences and photographs present a more optimistic view of life at 13 Norham Gardens, and a different view of W.W. Francis, than those presented in Wagner's monograph on *The Twilight Years of Lady Osler*. They demonstrate that Francis was energetic, enjoyed his family, and had a great sense of fun, as evidenced also by the tributes from his friends published in 1956 by the Osler Society of McGill University.

Although Lady Osler sometimes considered her a "brat," Marian Grace ("Maisie") Francis went on to a happy and productive life. Her parents returned to Montreal when she was nearly seven, and by 1945 she had received her B.Sc. and M.D.C.M. degrees from McGill. In 1946 she married Andrew (Andy) Kelen (1918–2006), a fellow medical student at McGill whom she met on a ski trail.

Susan Kelen adds:

> Andy Kelen graduated from McGill Medical School in 1945 in an expedited wartime programme. After the war, he completed an M. Sc. in neurology at the Montreal Neurological Institute and then took the family to Rochester, Minnesota, for a fellowship in internal medicine at the Mayo Clinic. The couple left Canada with three children and returned with four. He then settled the family in Ormstown, Quebec, to work in a small group practice which at its height had ten physicians including my mother.

The Ormstown Medical Centre was considered novel and was modelled after the Mayo Clinic. They shared their clinical files and patients and support staff. Their building was directly attached to the 75-bed community hospital. The Medical Centre included an X-ray department and laboratory which the hospital did not have. The Centre shared these facilities with the hospital. Canadian Medicare began offering health coverage to all citizens starting in 1968 as it does to this day. Ormstown is a small town only 34 miles from Montreal so my parents went frequently to rounds at the Montreal Neurological Institute or to see their own parents.

Andy worked as an internist and in family practice for 38 years. My mother worked in Family Practice at the same clinic for 18 years having a taken off the previous 18 years to raise the family. At work, she was sometimes known as "Mrs. Dr. Kelen" to differentiate her from my father. My parents were best friends and did everything together. They enjoyed outdoor activities and modelled community involvement to their children all their lives. My father was a founder of the local children's music festival and the Driver's Education programme and my mother was involved with environmental groups.

Andrew Kelen and Marian Francis Kelen had five children: Michael (born 1948) became a Federal Court judge; Charlotte ("Sari," born 1949) a teacher; Steve (born 1951) a social worker; Susan (born 1952) a psychologist; and Wendy (born 1956) a MA nurse specializing in diabetes education.

In December 2020, I had the privilege of orchestrating a teleconference (Zoom conference) between all five of Marian's children and Dr. Joseph Hanaway, co-author of the two-volume *McGill Medicine* (1996 and 2006) and also of *The General: A History of the Montreal General Hospital* (2016). Dr. Hanaway exclaimed afterwards, "What a great Canadian family!"

—Charles S. Bryan

Second Lieutenant Edward Revere Osler: His Service, Wounding, and Medical Care—A Reassessment

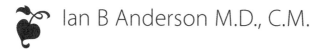 Ian B Anderson M.D., C.M.

William Osler met Dr. and Mrs. Samuel W. Gross soon after his move from Montreal to Philadelphia in 1884 and was a frequent guest at their home on Walnut Street.[1, i: 239] Samuel Gross died unexpectedly in April 1889, shortly before Osler left Philadelphia for Baltimore. Osler found something unique and enduring in Grace Revere Gross and, although little is known of their courtship, they married in May 1892.[1, i: 306] A son, whom they named Paul Revere Osler, was born the following February but died within a week. A second son arrived 28 December 1895 in Baltimore. William wrote: "Mrs. Osler had a small boy last week—both are doing splendidly. We are of course delighted, and he looks a strong and durable specimen."[1, i: 426] He was a much anticipated and loved baby; William and Grace were 46 and 42 years old, respectively, and they had feared they would not have children. Revere, as they called him, was close to his mother and shared her interest in art. His father tried unsuccessfully to interest him in natural science including microscopy but was devoted to him and followed his development closely (Figure 1). In 1905 the family moved to Oxford, where Revere went to a local school before going to Winchester, one of the famous English public schools (boarding schools). Revere was an average student who needed guidance and tutoring. His interests leaned toward inner-directed activities: sketching, photography, woodworking, and, especially, fishing. His parents arranged vacations around good fishing spots, and William utilized *The Compleat Angler* by Izaac

Presented in part at the forty-ninth annual meeting of the American Osler Society, Montreal, Quebec, Canada, on 13 May 2019.

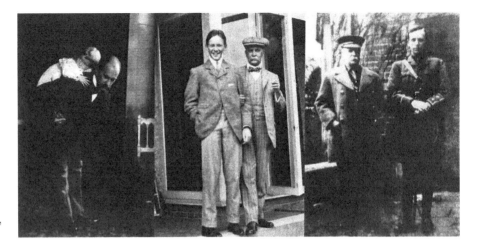

Figure 1.   William Osler and his son, Edward Revere Osler, in the nursery at 1 West Franklin Street, Baltimore, circa 1898; on vacation in Wales in 1911; and in their Army uniforms, circa 1916–1917.
Credit: Osler Library of the History of Medicine, McGill University.

Walton (1593–1683) to encourage an interest in books, which eventually took.[2] Revere grew up a happy, gentle, and artistic young man with numerous interests, including a budding interest in architecture. But his story came to epitomize the tragedy that was the Great War, now known as World War I.

Revere joins the Army

On leaving Winchester, Revere needed some seasoning (and tutoring) before the next step—Oxford. He passed the entrance examinations on his second try and in October 1914 entered Christ Church. It was a fateful time to be 18 years old. The war consumed all thought and life. Sir William wrote of wounded Germans, Belgians, and refugee Belgian professors as early as September 1914.[1, ii: 435,439] By the end of the First Battle of Ypres in December 1914, the British had suffered over 80,000 casualties, at least 16,200 of them fatal. Revere joined the Oxford Training Corps and his mother rather defensively wrote: "Revere's heart is not in drill or in the war. . . . A great question must be decided about him soon, and of course he will do his duty when the time comes."[1, ii: 453–454] "Too immature" was the assessment of his instructors. He left Oxford in January 1915 and considered enlisting as a soldier in the Public Schools Battalion. By now the first Canadian contingent had arrived in Salisbury Plain and Sir William had been in continuous communication with them even before they sailed from Quebec. The commanding officer of the McGill Hospital, Colonel Herbert Stanley Birkett (1864–1942), offered to take Revere as an orderly officer. The unit eventually arrived and initially set up in England. They deployed to Dannes-Camiers, France, on 19 June 1915, where they stayed for a year until moving to Boulogne for the remainder of the war.[3] While there was no "safe billet" in France, Revere no doubt felt frustration at being away from the action just as his parents feared the same, writing on 7 February 1916: "Revere is with the McGill Unit but he will exchange to the artillery & take his chances with his chums."[1, ii: 515] While still an entirely volunteer army, the British had introduced a massive recruitment of the Kitchener-inspired "Pals Battalions"—600,000 soldiers in 1915.[4, p.217] By the summer of 1916, having suffered a million casualties, and soon to suffer another million, the British government would be in crisis mode over manpower and conscription. A bill "making all men between the ages of eighteen and forty-one subject to compulsory enlistment" received Royal Assent 25 May 1916.[5] Nevertheless, the idea of "those who joined together would serve together" brought in millions of volunteers but did not see the "awful warning" of the impact of the huge casualties on the small towns, associations, and businesses that supplied the Pals battalions the cannon fodder.[4, p. 218] Revere originally tried to transfer to a Field Ambulance Unit but unable, after several months, was able to obtain a commission in the Royal Field Artillery.[1, ii: 530]

The Royal Field Artillery

Now Second Lieutenant Osler, Revere apparently found himself in the artillery, becoming by all accounts a model soldier through the hard work of a subaltern. His father wrote: "You never saw such a burly looking fellow—so grown & filled out, with hands like a navie & a face weather-beaten like leather."[1, ii: 568] But the field artillery was dangerous—the entire front was dangerous back to about 15 miles—the range of heavy artillery.[6] The field artillery was doubly so as they were exposed to snipers, machine guns and all the artillery. Three-quarters of all casualties on both sides were from artillery.[7] The Osler clan had already lost two soldiers who had enlisted in the Canadian army at the start of the war. Both were cousins of Revere. Major Ralph Featherstone Osler was wounded in the abdomen at Mount Sorrel 13 June 1916 and died of wounds 16 June 1916. Major Campbell Gwyn was killed 9 April 1917 in the assault on Vimy Ridge. Both Ralph Osler and Campbell Gwyn were mortally wounded during Canadian assaults on German-held high-ground—costly but successful assaults that are still celebrated a century later.

The Third Battle of Ypres had officially started 31 July 1917 and went through numerous phases—the actual Battles of Passchendaele lasted from 12 October to 10 November 1917. Typical of the generalship of the day, the 31 July assault came after a two-week artillery "softening up" and it was an unusually wet summer.[8, pp. 304–308,555] On 29 August 1917, while on a work party with the battery commander, Revere and 18 other soldiers were preparing the area to move the 18-pounder guns forward. A German shell landed in their midst killing eight

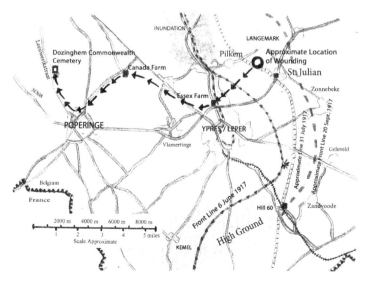

Figure 2. Map of the Ypres Salient, circa 1917, showing the possible evacuation route of Revere Osler to Essex Farm and then to Canada Farm (large arrows). Most of the land east of Poperinge was devoid of vegetation, and much of it consisted of churned mud up to nine feet deep, resulting from one of the wettest summers in decades. Some of the buildings in Ypres/Leper remained intact, but most structures east of Poperinge had been reduced to rubble. All the roads had vanished. The high ground was vital to both armies. Hill 60 was thus named because it was 60 meters above sea level.

outright. Revere had fragments in the thighs, abdomen, and chest. Dragged into a shell hole or firing pit until safe, a man-carry of 3000 yards brought him to Essex Farm (famous as the site where John McCrae wrote "In Flanders Field" two years before). Remember that the entire area was churned mud and barren of trees and vegetation from three continuous years of shelling. It would take at least four to six soldiers to manhandle a stretcher this distance and take hours.[9] Revere was then sent on to Canada Farm Advanced Dressing Station by narrow railway, and road ambulance to Number 47 Casualty Clearing Station (CCS) at Dozinghem (Figure 2).[10] He was awake but critically injured and in shock. Within minutes at least one telegram went out to a nearby CCS requesting "Major Cushing come immediately." Within one to two hours, five leading American surgeons—Harvey Cushing, George Crile, William Darrach, George Brewer, and Arthur Eisenbrey—arrived. It is not clear how the other surgeons were summoned, but telegraph was the usual and most efficient means of military communication. Revere recognized those around him. Crile organized a blood transfusion and Brewer and Darrach took him to the operating room for a laparotomy.[10] There is nothing recorded about the thoughts of the regular medical staff to this invasion, but they had sent for them in the first place and there were other American medical personnel embedded in this CCS.

Surgery was a forlorn hope. According to Cushing the procedure started just after midnight. Crile administered another blood transfusion during the procedure. The operative findings included two large rents in the colon and several mesenteric vessels. No clear description is made of the important issue of the chest injury,[10] but Crile mentions much blood in the chest.[11] "Obviously all was lost" He deteriorated and died around 07:00 according to Cushing. He was promptly buried in the trench prepared for the day's dead. Alder branches helped keep the body out of the muck and water. He was wrapped in an army blanket and covered with a British Union Jack, a brief burial service read and back to work. The war continued and the American surgeons had full working days ahead of them. Cushing was at Number 46 CCS, Crile and Eisenbrey at Number 17 CCS, and Brewer at Number 4 CCS, all treating British battle casualties.[12]

Effect on Sir William and Lady Osler

Sir William received a telegram the afternoon of 30 August from Cushing; it had been sent the previous evening and delayed: "Revere dangerously wounded, comfortable, and conscious, condition not hopeless."[1, ii: 577] He felt deep down that more and worse news would quickly follow as it did that evening of Revere's death. Lady Osler later spoke of "the months of dread—of the telephone, the messenger boy, the postman. Whenever she saw the telegraph boy at a distance he would quickly shake his head—'not for you this time.'"[10, p. 296] Sir William on the surface carried on: "He began that very night to shield others—his wife, his friends, the medical officers whose efforts to save his boy had been futile" The letters and telegrams came from mainly American friends—"The English in these days sorrowed in silence for one another. It was too common a story." Friends and colleagues remarked that on the surface, Sir William continued as before "in his gay old way" but when alone "we all knew his heart was broken" and "alone with me—he sobbed like a child."[1, ii: 578,580]

Revere's death likely accelerated Sir William's aging and death. Cushing reported Sir William contracting "the flugrip"[1, ii: 620] in October 1918 at the height of the great pandemic but recovered. He caught a cold in early October 1919, and this quickly evolved into pneumonia. While he carried on an active correspondence and continued revisions of his textbook, he knew from long experience and deep analysis of his condition that it could only end one way. His mind was active to the end planning the distribution of his library. He died at home amongst friends and family at 16:30 on 29 December 1919.[1, ii: 684]

The effort by American surgeons, and especially Harvey Cushing, to save Revere was one of the Oslers' few consolations, and a comfort to Lady Osler during her long widowhood She wrote: No one in the world could have done as much and no one had been fonder of him."[13]

American surgeons and support for France and Britain in the war

In the lead-up to America entering the war, less than half the population favored hostilities. Large numbers of German and Irish Americans opposed involvement and President Wilson tried to avoid war.[14] Nevertheless, the reintroduction of unrestricted submarine warfare and the infamous Zimmerman Telegram propelled the United States to war even though woefully unprepared. The US regular army ultimately swelled to the largest in Europe but as a fighting force, even by spring 1918, they still had only 318,000 troops in France, and these needed further training.[15]

As early as August 1914, the US Ambassador to France helped form the American military hospital and motor ambulance at the pre-existing American Hospital at Neuilly-sur-Seine. These were set up as university-based units that rotated. George Crile and the Cleveland Lakeside Unit served during January–March 1915 and were succeeded by the Harvard Unit with Harvey Cushing during April–June.[12] Before war was declared, the American Red Cross with many experienced doctors had been "contingency planning" for some time. Experienced surgeons including Crile, Cushing, Brewer, William Mayo, and

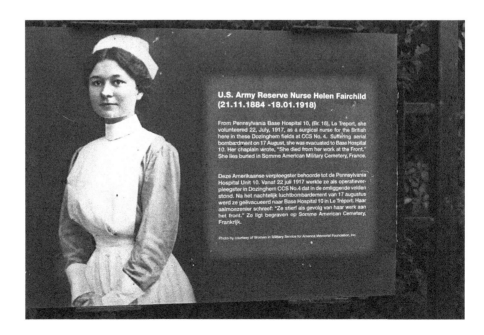

Figure 3. Poster at Dozinghem Cemetery commemorating U.S. Army Reserve nurse Helen Fairchild (see text). *Credit:* Author photograph.

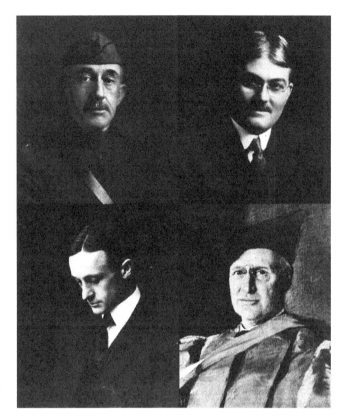

Figure 4. The all-star cast of U.S. Army surgeons who attended Revere Osler included (clockwise from upper left) George Brewer, George Crile, William Darrach, and Harvey Cushing. Not shown is Arthur Eisenbrey. *Credits:* National Library of Medicine.

John Finney formed the Committee on Standardization of Medical and Surgical Supplies and Equipment, which went a long way to preparing at least the United States Army Medical Corps for the coming deluge.[12] With hostilities, the War Department assumed control and surgical teams were sent to France in the summer of 1917. United States Base Hospitals were set up in Rouen, France (with Crile as clinical director), Boulogne, France (with Cushing as clinical director), and other locations. Nevertheless, these were associated with British units and initially attached to the British Expeditionary Force.[12] However, American medical personnel were soon working further forward in British Casualty Clearing Stations where there were threats from many sources. The German air force deliberately bombed medical units including Dozinghem. US Army Reserve Nurse Helen Fairchild had volunteered to work at No. 47 CCS and was seriously injured on 17 August 1917. She died of wounds 18 January 1918 (Figure 3).

Blood transfusion medicine: The advances to 1917

War has always been a motivating force for revolutionary advances in medicine and the influence of World War I on advances in transfusion medicine is one example.[16] Karl Landsteiner (1868–1943) had discovered the basics to determine blood group incompatibility in 1901.[17] Research and innovation quickly followed, centered in New York. Blood grouping techniques were refined by Moss and Ottenberg; Carel and Crile developed direct transfusion procedures by vein-to-vein anastomosis; Lindeman, Kimpton, Brown, and Unger worked on indirect transfusion techniques.[16–18] The Canadian Lawrence Bruce Robertson trained in New York including work in Lindeman's laboratory. The year 1914 found him working back in Toronto but quickly volunteered for the army. He was working in France by fall 1914. He carried out early transfusions and worked to convince British surgeons the importance of blood transfusions.[19] His techniques were risky (no cross matching) and labour intensive with syringe transfer without anticoagulant. Blood transfusions, while not routine in 1917, were recognized as having a place but was the exception not the rule. Blood transfusion in 1917 was truly labour intensive. It was still the era of real pioneers. The discovery of citrate as a safe anticoagulant permitted donated blood to be held longer.[20] L.B. Robertson's name was often confused with that of the American Oswald Hope ("O.H.") Robertson (1886–1966), who arrived in France in May 1917, had also worked in Lindeman's laboratory, and had learned valuable lessons in blood storage and better indirect techniques such as the transfusion bottle. O.H. Robertson helped convince British and American senior commanders of the importance and safety of blood transfusion. He established "blood depots" while serving with the U.S. Army Medical Corps, and therefore receives credit for the idea of blood banks. These developments, however, came too late to save Revere Osler.[16]

Crile gave Revere Osler two separate blood transfusions.[10] These donations were from men with less serious injuries who volunteered. While the blood would have been whole blood donations—the best type, with fresh young red cells and a full quota of clotting agents and platelets—they would have been single units. Two units would have been too little, too late in this grave situation.

The influence of the name Osler on the surgical care of Revere

The five American surgeons who attended Revere were all leaders and respected experts in their fields:

- George Washington Crile (1864–1953), a pioneer in blood transfusion who later co-founded the Cleveland Clinic.
- William R. Darrach (1876–1948), a leading New York surgeon who specialized in orthopedics and later orthopedic surgeon who later became dean of the Faculty of Medicine of Columbia University.
- George Emerson Brewer (1861–1939), a New York surgeon specializing in urology who founded the Society of Clinical Surgery and served as president of the American Surgical Association and other organizations.
- Arthur Bradley Eisenbrey (1880–1933), a Cleveland surgeon whose research at the Bellevue Hospital in New York and at the Carnegie Laboratory included studies of shock and inflammation.
- Harvey Williams Cushing (1869–1939), often considered the father of neurosurgery as we now know it, who was a close friend of the Oslers and later received the Pulitzer Prize for *The Life of Sir William Osler.*

Cushing's diary records the moment "when came this shocking message: 'Sir Wm. Osler's son seriously wounded at 47 C.S.S. Can Major Cushing come immediately?'"[10]

Cushing arrived at around 22:30—six hours after wounding, two hours after Revere's arrival at No 47 CCS and recognized immediately the grave situation—yet Revere must have been conscious on and off and recognized his father's

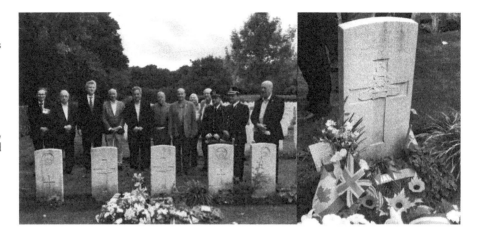

Figure 5. Participants at a remembrance ceremony on 30 August 2018 included civic leaders, Menin Gate buglers, Friends of Flanders Field Museum, diplomats, teachers, and Osler family members. Revere Osler's gravesite is shown on the right. *Credit:* Author photographs.

old friend. It would have depended on how busy the CCS was and how many urgent surgical cases were waiting. Stable cases were sent by rail to other base hospitals or even to England by rail ferry.[21] William Heneage Ogilvie (1887–1971), then a junior surgeon but later chief of British army surgery during the Second World War, stated that abdominal wounds during World War I carried a 60 percent mortality.[22]

Had he not been an Osler, the American surgeons would not have been summoned (they were busy at their own units) and he would not have received a blood transfusion. With three systems injured (chest, abdomen, and extremities) multiple procedures would have been needed. He was far too shocked for transfer. Whether he would have been operated on or treated expectantly is speculative, but he did not survive despite heroic attempts to save his life.

It is difficult to compare outcomes for combat casualties during World War I (second-generation warfare) with those of recent fourth-generation ("asymmetric") warfare. We can state with reasonable certainty, however, that, in current asymmetric-combat theaters, Revere would be evacuated by helicopter promptly and taken to a forward surgical team or a Role Three Medical Unit. He would receive banked red cells and a chest drain and then undergo laparotomy to control bleeding and repair the injury to his colon. His potential for survival would be high.[23-26]

A remembrance of Revere during 2018

The site of Number 47 Casualty Clearing Station (CCS) is now Dozinghem Commonwealth War Cemetery a short drive north of Poperinge where graves are in order of their death—3,427 graves from World War I along with several dozen from the World War II era (mainly aircrew)—all meticulously maintained by the Commonwealth War Graves Commission. Visits by friends and descendants are quite common. Many people including members of the Osler family commemorated the centenary of Revere's death. A note written by Susan Kelen, granddaughter of W.W. Francis, the first Osler Librarian at McGill, was left at the grave. This was seen by local historians and stimulated interest. This led to the remembrance in 2018. The note identified who Revere was and gave him personality as a fisherman—and the location of his fishing gear if he needed it in the next world (Figure 6).

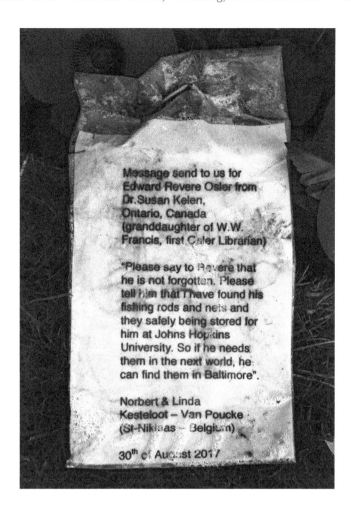

Figure 6. Note by Susan Kelen left at Revere's gravesite in 2018.
Credit: Author photograph.

Following this, on 30 August 2018 representatives of Osler family descendants, Friends of the Flanders Fields Museum, the City of Ypres/Leper, buglers from the Menin Gate honour guard, the Canadian Embassy, friends, guides, and teachers assembled to honour the memory of the only child of Sir William and Grace Osler who died of wounds 101 years before. "I think that my note took Revere from being one of 3,000 young men buried in Dozinghem Cemetery to a person with interests and personality and with friends who were still interested in him."[27] Edward Revere Osler, American, Canadian, and British citizen, lies in Flanders Fields, Section IV, Row F, Plot 21.

Reflections

Second Lieutenant Osler, like most of his generation, wanted to make a real contribution in the war and bravely suffered a significant wound. His best friend, Jack Slessor (later, Sir John Cotesworth Slessor [1897–1979], Marshal of the Royal Force) opined that Revere would have been a great man had he lived.[28] Revere died a cold, painful, lingering death but he was not alone—he was comforted and cared for by friends. He rests in Flanders Fields with friends now—there are several soldiers from the field artillery buried in the same row who died the same or next day. Their grave markers are the same as the hundreds of thousands that mark the graves in Commonwealth War Cemeteries around the world. That August 1917, the British offensive in the Ypres salient cost them 68,000 casualties, 3400 of them officers—including Second Lieutenant Edward Revere Osler.[8, p. 308]

> They shall not grow old, as we that are left grow old:
> Age shall not weary them, nor the years condemn.
> At the going down of the sun and in the morning
> We will remember them.

> —"For the Fallen," by Robert Laurence Binyon (1869–1843)

References

1. Cushing H. *The Life of Sir William Osler.* Oxford: Clarendon Press; 1925, i: 239.
2. Harrell GT, The Oslers' son—Revere. *Bulletin of the History of Medicine* 1980; 54(4): 561–571.
3. MacPhail A. *History of the Canadian Forces 1914–1919: Medical Services.* Ottawa: Department of National Defence; 1925: 215.
4. Keegan J. *The Face of Battle.* London: Jonathan Cape; 1976: 217.
5. Gilbert M. *Winston S. Churchill. Volume III. The Challenge of War, 1914–1916.* Boston: Houghton Mifflin Company; 1971: 755–758.
6. Ogilvie WH. *Forward Surgery in Modern War.* London: Butterworth London; 1944.
7. Nicholson GWL. *Seventy Years of Service.* Ottawa: Borealis Press; 1977: 87.
8. Nicholson GWL. *Canadian Expeditionary Force 1914–1919. Official History of the Canadian Army in the First World War.* Montreal: McGill–Queen's University Press; 2015.
9. https://commons.wikimedia.org/wiki/File:Cyril_Henry_Barraud-The_Stretcher-bearer_Party_(CWM_19710261-0019).jpeg, accessed 17 November 2020.
10. Cushing H. *From a Surgeons Journal,* 1915–1918. Boston: Little, Brown and Company; 1936: 197–198.
11. Crile G, ed. *George Crile, an Autobiography.* New York: Lippincott; 1947; volume 2: 308–309.
12. Nathoo N, Lautzenheiser FK, Barnett GH. Historical vignette: George W. Crile, Ohio's first neurosurgeon, and his relationship with Harvey Cushing. *Journal of Neurosurgery* 2005; 103(2): 378–386.
13. Muirhead A. *Grace Revere Osler: A Brief Memoir.* Oxford: Oxford University Press; 1931: 6
14. Tooze A. *The Deluge: The Great War, America, and the Remaking of the Global Order,* 1916–1931. New York: Viking; 2014: 66.
15. Keegan J. *The First World War.* Toronto: Vintage Canada Random House; 2000: 372.
16. Stansbury LG, Hess JR. Blood transfusion in World War I: The roles of Lawrence Bruce Robertson and Oswald Hope Robertson in the "most important medical advance of the war." *Transfusion Medicine Reviews* 2009; 23(3): 232–236.
17. Pinkerton PH. Canadian surgeons, blood transfusions in the Great War, and founding of Royal College. *Annals of the Royal College of Physicians and Surgeons of Canada* 2002; 35(6): 369–373.

18. Unger LJ. A new method of syringe transfusion. *Journal of the American Medical Association* 1915; 64(7): 582–584.

19. Robertson LB. The transfusions of whole blood: A suggestion for its more frequent employment in war surgery. *British Medical Journal* 1916; 2(2897): 38–40.

20. Mollison PL. The introduction of citrate as an anticoagulant for transfusion and of glucose as a red cell preservative, *British Journal of Haematology* 2000; 108(1): 13–18.

21. Anderson IB. Advanced Surgical Centres: past, present, and future. *Annals of the Royal College of Physicians and Surgeons of Canada*; 1998: 31(7): 341–347.

22. Ogilvie WH. Surgery goes to war. In Ogilvie WH. *Surgery, Orthodox and Heterodox.* Oxford: Blackwell; 1948: 224.

23. Barnett RW. *Asymmetrical Warfare: Today's Challenge to U.S. Military Power.* Dulles, Virginia: Brassey's; 2003: 9–23.

24. Hirshberg A, Mattox KL. Top Knife: The Art and Craft of Trauma Surgery. Shrewsbury: tfm Publishing; 2005: 1–17.

25. Holcomb JB, Hess JR. Early massive trauma transfusion: state of the art. *Journal of Trauma* 2006; 60(6 Supplement): S1–S2.

26. Roberts DJ, Ball CG, Feliciano DV, et al, History of the innovation of damage control for management of trauma patients: 1902–2016. *Annals of Surgery* 2017; 265(5): 1034–1044.

27. Wuyts F. In *Flanders Fields Belgium—A Tourist's Map of West Flanders Military Heritage.* Brussels: National Geografisch Instituut; 2009.

28. Dewey N. Revere Osler and Jack Slessor. *Osler Library Newsletter* 1981, No. 37(June): 1.

Maude Abbott and the History of the Eponym "Tetralogy of Fallot"

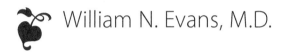 William N. Evans, M.D.

Maude Elizabeth Abbott (1869–1940), the famed early-twentieth-century Canadian clinician and cardiac pathologist, founded the discipline devoted to the understanding and care of those born with cardiovascular malformations. Abbott's lifetime commitment to the study of congenital heart disease was directly influenced by her mentorship and collaboration with William Osler. Of Osler, Abbott evocatively said, "his keen interest in my work and broad human sympathy pierced the veil of my youthful shyness with a personal stimulus that aroused my intellect to its most passionate endeavor."[1,2] Then, shortly following Osler's death in 1919, Abbott conceived, organized, and strenuously labored over the 600 plus page "Sir William Osler Memorial Volume" published in 1926.[1,3] She followed up the memorial volume with countless presentations on William Osler's life and influence for various groups, both lay and medical, in Canada and the United States over the next decade and a half of her life, earning, in my opinion, the title *La Prima Dona* Oslerian.

The tetralogy of Fallot

Even though Abbott did not coin the eponym "tetralogy of Fallot," she nevertheless popularized the term, and by doing so, embedded it into the lexicon of

Presented at the forty-ninth annual meeting of the American Osler Society, Montreal, Canada, on 15 May 2019. Portions of this manuscript were published previously in *Pediatric Cardiology* (2008; 29[3]): 637–640) and *Cardiology in the Young* (2009; 19[2]: 119–128, and also 2020; 20[2]: 124–132) and are reproduced with permission.

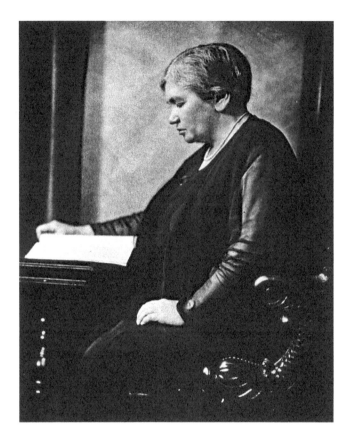

Figure 1.   Maude Elizabeth Seymour Abbott.
Credit: National Library of Medicine.

congenital heart disease.[4,5] World-wide, about 65,000 babies are born annually with tetralogy of Fallot. From the dawn of time until four years after Maude Abbott's death, mortality was 100 percent. In 1944 the first palliative surgery was introduced at the Johns Hopkins Hospital by pediatric cardiologist Helen B. Taussig (1898–1986), research-laboratory director Vivien Thomas (1910–1985), and cardiovascular surgeon Alfred Blalock (1899–1964).[6,7] Nevertheless, for long-term survival, the condition requires a definitive, complete surgical repair, introduced a decade later in the 1950s, by C. Walton Lillehei (1918–1999) at the University of Minnesota and John W. Kirklin (1917–2004) at the Mayo Clinic.[8,9] Currently, for those born into a society with advanced cardiovascular surgical services, survival into adulthood is nearly 99 percent. Nevertheless, even in the twenty-first century, many infants still die from this and other critical congenital cardiac malformations, as advanced cardiac surgical services often remain unavailable in parts of the developing world.

Although post-mortem anatomical descriptions of hearts malformed by the lesions comprising tetralogy of Fallot predated him by 200 years;[4] nonetheless, it was Étienne Louis Arthur Fallot (1850–1911) who detailed the condition's anatomical description in a lengthy multi-part article published in 1888 in the journal *Marseille Médical: Contribution à l'anatomie pathologique de la maladie bleue (cyanose cardiaque)*[10] Little is known about Étienne-Louis Arthur Fallot, as he insisted that no obituary be published upon his death. He was born in Sète, close to Marseille, on the southern coast of France.[4,11,12] He received his medical education at the Faculty of Medicine of the University of Marseille, graduating in 1876. Later he rose to professor of hygiene and legal medicine at the University of Marseille in 1888. Also, in Marseille, he was the chief of the clinic at the Hotel-Dieu,

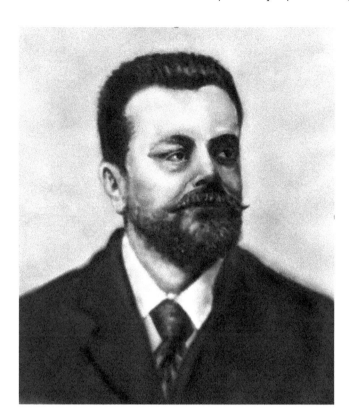

Figure 2. Étienne-Louis Arthur Fallot. *Credit:* Unknown artist/ Wikimedia Commons.

Chief of Service at Immaculate Conception Hospital, and he attended at the Ambroise-Paré Hospital. He assiduously insisted that anatomical-clinical correlations required verification by autopsy. The conclusions he drew in his landmark paper on *la maladie bleue* were arrived at by studying the clinical and pathological features in three individuals he cared for that died of the condition, coupled with descriptions from previously published papers by others in 50 more cases. Previous works included, among others, those by Danish anatomist and naturalist Niels Stensen (1638–1686) and the Dutch physician Edouard Sandifort (1742–1814). Fallot began his article by the translated quote, "One of the happy situations for the clinician to instruct himself, has come in a period of several years to our eyes in three cases of a rare and curious malady, on the pathologic anatomy of which, even in the expert medical public, there are serious errors and uncertainties: we had the possibility to observe during their life and at autopsy following their death, three subjects afflicted with the malady called cardiac cyanosis, and it would be, according to us, much more correct to designate this disease exclusively under the name of blue malady." He concluded his work by describing that the condition comprised four distinct anatomical findings similar in each patient: (1) pulmonary stenosis (PS), (2) a ventricular septal defect (VSD), (3) aorta rightward displaced overriding the ventricular septum, and (4) right ventricular hypertrophy (RVH). These pathological findings are displayed in figure 3[13] and further emphasized in figure 4 by a labeled photograph of a specimen from the Maude Abbott Medical Museum at McGill University in Montreal, Canada, a specimen currently on display. Although Fallot compiled the four anatomical components, his paper also clearly revealed he understood the tetralogy morphogenesis was related to a solitary intrauterine pathologic developmental process involving the right-ventricular infundibulum, resulting in the aorta being pulled rightward, opening the ventricular septum to create the VSD, and narrowing the pulmonary valve causing pulmonary stenosis and the resulting right ventricular hypertrophy.

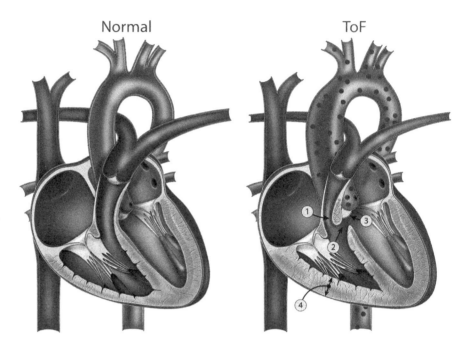

Figure 3. Normal heart and great vessels versus tetralogy of Fallot (ToF), demonstrating (1) pulmonic stenosis, (2) ventricular septal defect, (3) rightward-displaced aorta, overriding the ventricular septum, and (4) right ventricular hypertrophy.

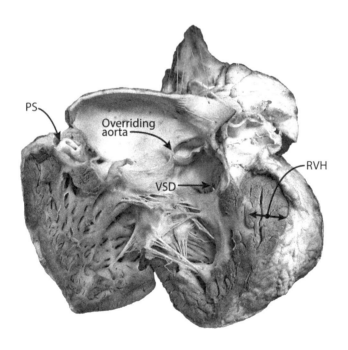

Figure 4. Heart and great vessels with tetralogy of Fallot in the Maude Abbott Medical Museum.
Credit: Maude Abbott Medical Museum, McGill University.

Evolution of the eponym

The term "*tetralogie de Fallot*" first appeared in print in the French medical literature, eight years after the publication of Fallot's report, in Pierre Marie's (1853–1940) *Leçons Clinique Médicale.*[14] This publication recapitulated lectures Marie gave at the Hotel-Dieu in Paris between 1894 and 1895. Pierre Marie was born in Paris and received his medical degree from the University of Paris in 1883. He was noted to be a brilliant student and became a protégé of the famed French neurologist and professor of anatomical pathology, Jean-Martin Charcot (1825–1893) of Charcot-Marie-Tooth disease and many other conditions Charcot first described.[15]

Pierre Marie's role in the history of the tetralogy of Fallot eponym leads to the following William Osler story detour, which eventually returns to the history of tetralogy of Fallot.

William Osler had affection and admiration for French medicine.[16] In May of 1903, the Osler family sailed for Europe. As part of this trip, Osler and his Johns Hopkins physician friend and traveling companion, Henry Barton Jacobs, and their wives spent time in Paris. Pierre Marie was one of their hosts. Years later, Marie wrote an account of a dinner held at his house, "after dinner I thought that both [Osler and Jacobs] may take some interest in seeing medals of Physicians and Surgeons of Paris; it was the custom that friends and students present a gift

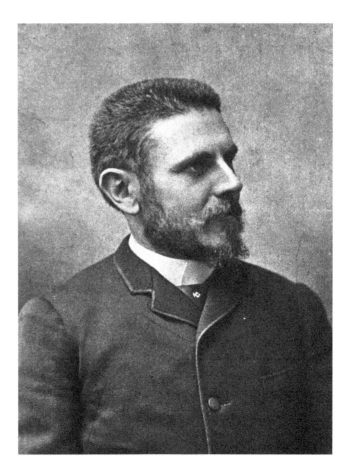

Figure 5.   Pierre Marie.
Credit: National Library of Medicine.

to their masters... Sir William and his friend had greatly admired the medals made by Vernon [the medalist Frédéric-Charles Victor de Vernon] ... [Jacobs] took me aside and asked me to enable him to have Vernon make, within days, the medal of Sir William... "[17,18] This casting was made by the Ferdinand Barbedienne Foundry in Paris and became known as the Vernon plaque. Five plaques were struck in bronze in the original size, 273 × 103 mm (about 10" × 4"), and were distributed to Grace Osler, Osler's mother (Ellen Pickton Osler), The Johns Hopkins Hospital, Henry Jacobs, and a friend. Twelve smaller versions, 108 × 75 millimeters (or about four × three inches) were also struck and distributed to Grace Osler, her sister (Susan Chapin), and to other close associates, such as Harvey Cushing. The ashes of William and Grace Osler and W.W. Francis (the first Osler librarian) lie behind a larger replica of the original Vernon plaque that was later cast by Limerick Company of Baltimore for the Osler Library at McGill University (Figure 6).[18]

Previously in 1902, Osler's friend Henry Barton Jacobs had married Mary Frick Garrett, the widow of Jacobs's patient, Robert Garrett. Members of the Garrett family were wealthy Baltimoreans and patrons of Johns Hopkins. Consequently, Mary Frick Jacobs was a doyen of Baltimore society. Mary's will stipulated that after her and Henry Jacobs's deaths, a portion of the estate would go to the Robert Garrett Fund (named for Mary's first husband) for Surgical Treatment of Children at Johns Hopkins. Subsequently, the Garrett Fund supported the critical research that led to the Blalock-Taussig-Thomas palliative shunt for tetralogy of Fallot.[19]

Returning to the history of the eponym, the story jumps to the Americas. Writing in the Spanish medical literature, the Buenos Aires physician Manuel A. Santas used the term *tetralogía de Fallot*, as if it were a common, in his 1905 *Estudio Semiológico de las Anomalías Congénitas del Corazón*.[20] Manuel Santas was a founder of Argentina's Pediatric Society and one of its enthusiastic supporters. He served as the organization's seventh president. Santas was professor of Semiology and later of Pediatrics at the Faculty of Medicine of the University of Buenos Aires.[4,21] In his

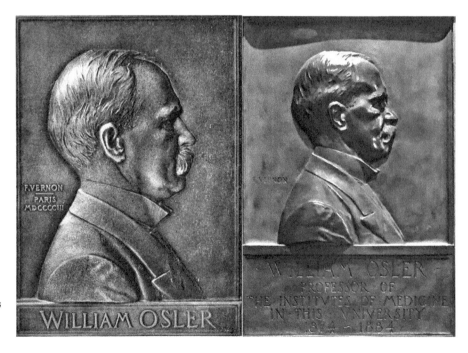

Figure 6. Original Vernon Plaque with relief of William Osler (left), and replica cast for the Osler Library of the History of Medicine (right). The original measures 10 inches by four inches; the replica is much larger, measuring 30 inches by 20 inches.

book Santas referenced an 1899 article on ventricular septal defects authored by another Argentinean physician, Horacio Piñero, who also employed the eponym's Spanish language version in his paper on ventricular septal defect.[22] From 1896 to 1899, Piñero had studied physiology and psychology in Europe. Additionally, Piñero cited Pierre Marie's Parisian lecture series in his 1899 ventricular septal defect article. Piñero likely wrote this article during his European studies. (As a footnote, Manuel Santas's son, Andrés Adolfo, was awarded a Rockefeller Foundation Fellowship in 1948 and spent time between 1948 and 1949 at Johns Hopkins in cardiac surgery with Alfred Blalock.[23])

Abbott's role in popularizing the eponym in English

Maude Abbott was likely among the first to employ the English-language "tetralogy of Fallot" in a 1924 article on classifying congenital heart defects.[24] In a previous 1923 article, she employed descriptive language rather than the eponym.[25] In fact, Abbott wrote two 1924 reviews on the classification of congenital heart malformations. In another 1924 article, distinct from the one above, she referred to the condition as "Fallod's tetralogy."[26] It is not clear if this was a typographical error in the printed work or a simple name variation with a hard-consonant ending. In Abbott's 1924 article, where she used the term tetralogy of Fallot, she also noted that the "French writers" had also used the term "tetralogy of Fallot" (Abbott placed quotes around the term). However, despite indicating that there were multiple French publications using the term, she only referenced Fallot's 1888 article, making no reference to Pierre Marie's use of *tetralogie de Fallot* in his *Leçons Clinique Médicale*. Nevertheless, Fallot had not audaciously referred to the condition as tetralogy of Fallot!

"Fallot" became common in English when its use spread from specialized pathology and cardiology literature to general pediatric textbooks. Tetralogy of Fallot is not listed in the 250-page index of Isaac Abt's 1926 eight-volume, 8300-page pediatric textbook.[27] However, in Griffith-Mitchell's 1933 *Diseases of Infants and Children* (forerunner of *Nelson's Textbook of Pediatrics*),[28] it is mentioned only once (on page 777). Maude Abbott was clearly responsible for the use of this eponym becoming standard in English after a quarter of a century, lagging behind the French and Spanish language medical literature. Interestingly, the eponym "tetralogy of Fallot" held true to its romance-language roots and has not become commonly Anglicized to "Fallot's tetralogy," instead it kept the "of" or "de" format.

In 1888, Etienne-Louis Arthur Fallot described hearts from cyanotic patients that had four abnormal cardiac anatomic characteristics. However, it took half a century for "tetralogy of Fallot" to become a commonly used eponym for the condition. During that time, Maude Abbott evolved into the world's congenital heart disease expert. Rather than creating an alternative shorthand noun from Stensen or Sandifort's name, she popularized the Fallot eponym as a permanent descriptor for the collective pathologic conditions of pulmonary artery stenosis, ventricular septal defect, a rightward-displaced aorta, and right ventricular hypertrophy. Maude Abbott's publications were many and culminated in her 1936 Atlas.[29] Paul Dudley White, a charter member of the American Osler Society and a pioneer in American cardiology, penned the preface to Abbott's atlas: "It was left to Maude Abbott, fired by a spark from Osler, to make the subject one of such general and widespread interest that we no longer regard it with either disdain or awe as a mystery for the autopsy table alone to discover and to solve. She has been the most important of the pioneers in establishing congenital heart disease as a living part of clinical medicine."

Abbott's lasting importance

Maude Abbott's contributions to the discipline of congenital heart disease spread across space and time, which moved others to study, to understand, and to develop methods for diagnosing and treating cardiac malformations. By 1945 the management of tetralogy of Fallot by Taussig, Blalock, and Thomas constituted the foundation of the care for other forms of congenital heart disease, following the world's first therapeutic, surgical procedure to relieve *la maladie bleue*, which opened the door for the modern era of congenital cardiovascular surgery.

References

1. MacDermot HE. *Maude Abbott: A Memoir.* Toronto: Macmillan; 1941.
2. Evans WN, Béland MJ. The paediatric cardiology Hall of Fame: Maude Elizabeth Abbott. *Cardiology in the Young* 2010; 20(2): 124–132.
3. [Abbott ME, ed.]. Bulletin No. IX of the *International Association of Medical Museums and Journal of Technical Methods. Sir William Osler Memorial Number. Appreciations and Reminiscences.* Montreal: Privately printed [Murray Printing Co., Limited, Toronto]; 1926.
4. Evans WN. "Tetralogy of Fallot" and Etienne-Louis Arthur Fallot. Pediatric Cardiology 2008; 29(3): 637–640.
5. Van Praagh R. Etienne-Louis Arthur Fallot and his tetralogy: a new translation of Fallot's summary and a modern reassessment of this anomaly. European Journal of Cardiothoracic Surgery1989; 3(5): 381–386.
6. Blalock A, Taussig HB. The surgical treatment of malformations of the heart in which there is pulmonary stenosis or pulmonary atresia. *Journal of the American Medical Association* 1945; 128(3): 189–202.
7. Evans WN. The Blalock-Taussig shunt: the social history of an eponym. *Cardiology in the Young* 2009;19(2): 119–128.
8. Lillehei CW, Cohen M, Warden HE, Varco RL. Complete anatomical correction of the tetralogy of Fallot defects: report of a successful surgical case. *AMA Archives of Surgery* 1956; 73(3): 526–531.
9. Ellis FH Jr, Kirklin JW, Clagett OT. Tetralogy of Fallot. *Surgical Clinics of North America* 1955; Mayo Clinic number: 1013–1021.
10. Fallot EA. *Contribution à l'anatomie pathologique de la maladie bleue (cyanose cardiaque) Marseilles Med* 1888; 25: 77–93,138–158, 207–223, 270–286, 341–354, 403–420.
11. Zampieri F, Thiene G. Fallot, Étienne-Louis Arthur (1850–1911). In van Krieken J, ed. *Encyclopedia of Pathology.* Springer, Cham; 2017 https://doi.org/10.1007/978-3-319-28845-1_4080-1.
12. Baille Y. Arthur Fallot (1850–1911) et la maladie bleue [Arthur Fallot (1850–1911) and blue disease]. *History of Science and Medicine* 2011; 45(1): 81–84.

13. Evans W, Acherman R, Luna C. *Simple & Easy Pediatric Cardiology: The Basics for Everyone Caring for Children*. Las Vegas: Children's Heart Center Nevada Press; 2013.
14. Marie P. *Leçons de clinique médicale. Hôtel-Dieu 1894–1895*. Paris: Masson; 1896.
15. Almeida GM, Germiniani FM, Teive HA. The seminal role played by Pierre Marie in neurology and internal medicine. *Arquivos de neuro-psiquiatria* 2015; 73(10): 887–889.
16. Coury C. Sir William Osler and French medicine. *Medical History* 1967;11(1): 1–14.
17. Cushing H. The master-word in medicine. Chapter 22 in Cushing H. *The Life of Sir William Osler*. Oxford: Clarendon Press; 1925: i: 600–625.
18. Golden RL. Medallic tributes to Sir William Osler and their historical associations. *Journal of the American Medical Association* 1979; 242(26): 2862–2867.
19. Bryan CS. Henry Barton Jacobs, William Osler's intimate friend. *Baylor University Medical Center Proceedings* 2017;30(1): 101–105.
20. Santas MA. *Estudio Semiológica de las Anomalías Congenitas del Corazón*. Buenos Aires: Agustín Etchepareborda; 1905.
21. Cien años de crecimiento—Sociedad Argentina de Pediatría. https://www.sap.org.ar/uploads/archivos/general/files_libro-100-anos-cap3_1530580473.pdf
22. Piñero HG. Dificultad del diagnóstico de la enfermedad de Roger, La tetralogía de Fallot fisiopatología y clínica de estas lesions congénitas del corazón. *Revista de la Sociedad Medica Argentina* 1899; 7: 155–200.
23. United States. Report to Congress on physician exchange visitor programs. Rockville: U.S. Dept. of Health & Human Services, Public Health Service, Health Resources and Services Administration, Bureau of Health Professions, Division of Medicine; 1983: 75.
24. Abbott ME, Dawson WT. The clinical classification of congenital cardiac disease. International Clinics 1924; 4: 156–188.
25. Abbott ME, Lewis DL, Beattie WW. Differential study of a case of pulmonary stenosis of inflammatory origin (ventricular septum closed) and two cases of (a) pulmonary stenosis and (b) pulmonary atresia of developmental origin with associated ventricular septal defect and death from paradoxical cerebral embolism. *American Journal of the Medical Sciences* 1923; 165: 636–659.
26. Abbott ME. The treatment of congenital heart disease. In: Blumer G, ed. *Billings-Forchheimer's Therapeusis of Internal Diseases*. New York: Appleton; 1924; 5: 344.
27. Abt IA. *Abt's Pediatrics*. Philadelphia & London: WB Saunders Company; 1923–1926.
28. Griffith JPC, Mitchell AG. *The Diseases of Infants and Children*. Philadelphia & London: WB Saunders Company; 1933: 777.
29. Abbott ME. *Atlas of Congenital Heart Disease*. New York: American Heart Association; 1936.

John M.T. Finney: Distinguished Surgeon and Oslerphile

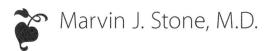 Marvin J. Stone, M.D.

John M.T. Finney (1863–1942) was born near Natchez, Mississippi in a plantation house in the midst of a Civil War battle. After the death of his mother when he was only a few months old, he lived in four different foster homes.[1] His fourth foster mother, "Aunt Lizzie," had a major impact on his life, enabling him to attend Princeton University and taking care of him later in Boston when he was a medical student. Finney was the only person to play varsity football at both Princeton and Harvard. He received his M.D. from Harvard and interned at Massachusetts General Hospital following which he moved to Baltimore to join the new Johns Hopkins Hospital and Medical School. Finney served 33 years under his chief of surgery, William Halsted. During this prolonged period, he received only one compliment from Halsted. Finney was a member of the "All-Star" surgical team (Figure 1).[2] He performed an appendectomy on Halsted's wife, Carolyn Hampton Halsted. Finney developed special interest and expertise in abdominal surgery, especially surgery of the stomach and duodenum. He was one of the pioneers in the operation of pyloroplasty. He saw a number of private patients particularly at the Union Protestant Hospital and developed a first-rate surgical program at that hospital. Later, he was able to admit private patients at Johns Hopkins. He had the appointment as Professor of Clinical Surgery at Johns Hopkins.

Finney had a long and close relationship with William Osler. The two met when the hospital first opened in 1889 and Finney referred to him as 'the Chief'. Finney was a lifelong admirer of Osler. In his autobiography, Finney describes Osler on rounds: "But in order to get a glimpse of the real "Chief," of the many sides of his character; his wonderful memory for cases, the inexhaustible storehouse of medical lore with which his mind was filled, his remarkable insight into

Presented in part at the forty-fifth annual Meeting of the American Osler Society, Baltimore, Maryland, on 28 April 2015.

This paper was previously published in *Baylor University Medical Center Proceedings* (2016; 29[1]: 91–93) and is reproduced with permission.

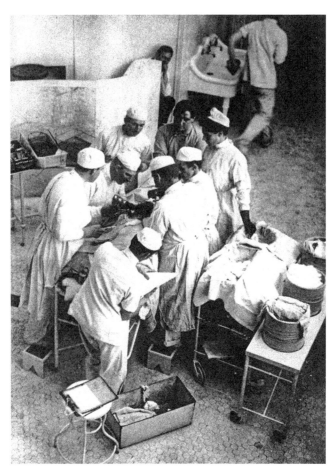

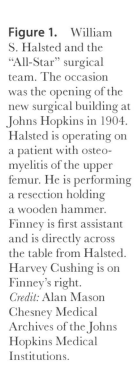

Figure 1. William S. Halsted and the "All-Star" surgical team. The occasion was the opening of the new surgical building at Johns Hopkins in 1904. Halsted is operating on a patient with osteomyelitis of the upper femur. He is performing a resection holding a wooden hammer. Finney is first assistant and is directly across the table from Halsted. Harvey Cushing is on Finney's right. *Credit:* Alan Mason Chesney Medical Archives of the Johns Hopkins Medical Institutions.

human nature, his intimate knowledge of disease and its protean manifestations; in order to feel the magic of his personality, one must watch him by the bedside of his patient, surrounded by his students, the ideal clinician and teacher. There he sits in characteristic pose in the midst of them, his exquisite hands palpating the patient or toying with a stethoscope, of thoughtful mien, his mind alert, never missing an opportunity to direct attention to some point of interest illustrated by the case or to point out to the students some way in which by study and research additions could be made to existing knowledge. Nor does he fail to take advantage of the opportunity to try in his own delightful way to stimulate in the minds of his students the desire for real accomplishment in their work."[1, p. 280]

Finney was a member of the first resident staff at John's Hopkins (Figure 2).[3,4] Finney recommended William S. Thayer, his medical school classmate at Harvard, to replace Henry Lafleur, Osler's first chief resident. Thayer stayed on in that capacity with Osler for seven years.

Harry Friedenwald, an ophthalmologist, and son of Aaron Friedenwald, also an ophthalmologist, contacted Osler in Canada when the elder Friedenwald became ill with an abdominal mass. Osler wrote a letter back to Friedenwald recommending surgical exploration by Finney saying ". . . you could not be in better hands." Moreover, Osler said, "Finney has been most successful . . . and his judgment is so good."

Figure 3 shows Osler's handwritten letter to Friedenwald. Osler said he would not be able to do anything other than urge surgical exploration because

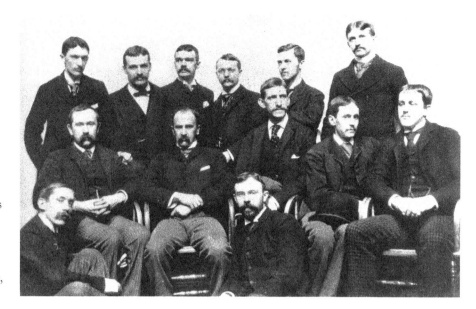

Figure 2. William Osler with the first resident staff at Hopkins 1889–1890. Finney is in the back row, second from left.
Credit: Osler Library of the History of Medicine, McGill University.

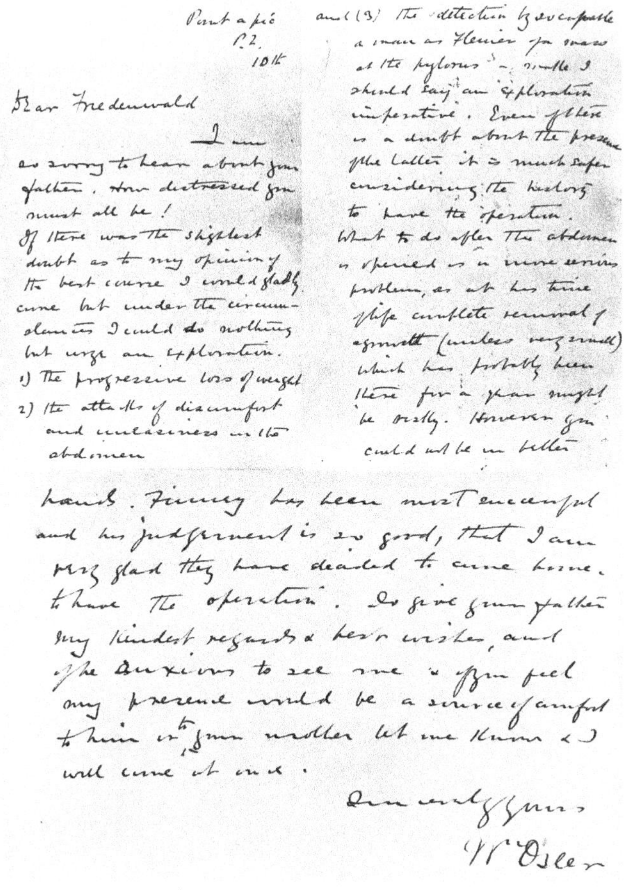

Figure 3. Osler's handwritten letter to Harry Friedenwald about his father. The elder Friedenwald died sixteen days after this letter was written.
Credit: Collection of Marvin J. Stone.

of the progressive loss of weight and the discomfort and uneasiness in the abdomen and a palpable abdominal mass. Later on, in the letter Osler concludes by saying, "Do give your father my kindest regards and best wishes, and if he is anxious to see me or if you feel my presence would be a source of comfort to him or to your mother let me know and I will come at once." The letter was signed, "Sincerely yours, Wm Osler." Not only was Finney an Oslerphile, but Osler was quite definitely a Finneyphile.

Finney had a number of offers during his career, one of which was to become the president of Princeton. After consideration he decided not to do that but did become a life trustee of the university. After Halsted's death Finney was offered the chair of surgery at Hopkins but declined feeling that he was too old and that the post should go to a younger person. At one point he was touted to run for candidate for Senator from Maryland, but he did not really pursue that.

Finney did accept a number of positions including being founder and first president of the American College of Surgeons (Figure 4).[5,6] He served on the editorial board of *Surgery Gynecology & Obstetrics* from 1913 until his death. Finney was also president of the American Surgical Association and the Society of Clinical Surgery. He was a member of the Board of Trustees at Lincoln University and received many honors and degrees throughout his career.

Finney served in the Armed Services during World War I. He achieved the rank of Brigadier General in the US Army Medical Corps, and he also served as Chief Surgical Consultant to the Allied Expeditionary Forces. He participated in studies for new methods of wound care. He was decorated by the United States, France, and Belgium, including receiving the Legion of Honor from France.

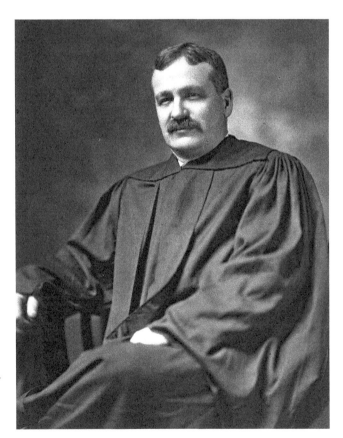

Figure 4. Finney at age fifty when he was elected first president of the American College of Surgeons.
Credit: American College of Surgeons.

Finney had a long career as mentor and counselor to students and young physicians in training. He gave many addresses to Princeton undergraduate students in an informal medical club atmosphere. These were collected in a small book called *The Physician*.[7] Twenty-one topics were published including chapters on experience, ethics, criticism of colleagues, altruism, humor, the grateful patient, causes of failure and other selected subjects.

At the conclusion of his autobiography Finney stated, "The true physician is supremely happy in his work. He could not be happy doing anything else. Once having caught the vision as it unfolds before his gaze, all else fades into insignificance."

John Finney was an outstanding clinician and a master surgeon who rose to international prominence during his long career at Johns Hopkins. His standards and ideals were of the highest caliber. Finney was an inspiration and role model for generations of students and physicians.

Summary

John Finney (1863–1942), the son of a clergyman, was born on a plantation near Natchez, Mississippi in the midst of a Civil War battle. An outstanding athlete, he was the only person to play varsity football for both Princeton and Harvard. After receiving his MD from Harvard, he interned at Massachusetts General Hospital and then went to Baltimore to become one of the first interns at the new Johns Hopkins Hospital. He met William Osler the day the hospital opened and became a lifelong admirer of "the Chief." Finney specialized in gastrointestinal surgery and was recognized for his expertise in the field. In a letter to a physician colleague whose father was seriously ill with an abdominal tumor, Osler recommended surgical exploration by Finney and wrote "you could not be in better hands . . . Finney has been most successful and his judgment is so good . . ." Finney served for 33 years under William Halsted at Hopkins and received only one compliment from him. After Halsted's death, Finney was offered the Chair of Surgery at Johns Hopkins but declined. He was a founder and first president of the American College of Surgeons. He also served as president of the American Surgical Association and the Society of Clinical Surgery. Finney became Chief Surgical Consultant for the Allied Expeditionary Forces in WWI. He was decorated by the United States, France, and Belgium. Finney was a master surgeon and a role model for generations of students and physicians.

References

1. Finney JMT. *A Surgeon's Life. The Autobiography of J.M.T. Finney*. New York: Putman; 1940.
2. Harvey AM, Brieger GH, Abrams SL, Fishbein JM, McKusick VA. *A Model of its Kind: A Pictorial History of Medicine at Johns Hopkins*. Baltimore: The Johns Hopkins University Press; 1989; volume 2: 81.
3. Harvey AM, Brieger GH, Abrams SL, McKusick VA. *A Model of its Kind: A Centennial History of Medicine at Johns Hopkins*. Baltimore: The Johns Hopkins University Press; 1989; volume 1: 39.

4. Bliss M: *William Osler A Life in Medicine.* New York: Oxford University Press; 1999: 213–214.
5. Finney JMT: Presidential Address: American College of Surgeons. First Convocation, November 13, 1913.
6. Cameron JI: John Miller Turpin Finney: The first president of the American College of Surgeons. *Journal of the American College of Surgeons* 2009; 208(3): 327–332.
7. Finney JMT. *The Physician.* New York: Scribner; 1923.

In Osler's Wake: The Legacy of Archibald Garrod

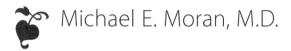 Michael E. Moran, M.D.

In 2020 the Royal Swedish Academy of Science awarded the Nobel Prize in Chemistry to Jennifer A. Doudna of the United States and Emmanuelle Charpentier, a French-born scientist working in Germany, "for the development of a method of genome editing" that involves a system known as CRISPR/Cas9 ("genetic scissors"). We are now close to fulfilling the dream of curing "inborn errors of metabolism," a term and concept introduced by Sir Archibald Edward Garrod (1857–1936) during his 1908 Croonian Lectures at the Royal College of Physicians, London. Garrod has been called "the physician father of biochemistry," "the father of clinical genetics," and, more recently, "the father of precision medicine." He gave the first demonstration that a disease of "chemical individuality" followed the laws of Mendelian inheritance. The disease in question was alkaptonuria. Garrod acknowledged the assistance of William Osler, and he later succeeded Osler as Regius professor of medicine at Oxford.[1–9]

Alkaptonuria is an autosomal-recessive deficiency of the enzyme homogentisate 1,2 dioxygenase, which is the only enzyme capable of breaking down homogentisic acid. It affects nearly all ethnic groups with an incidence of one in 250,000 to one in a million live births. Blackish discoloration of the urine on exposure to air (or after the addition of alkali) is the earliest and most characteristic feature of alkaptonuria. "Black urine" is a benign condition, but buildup of homogentisic acid in tissues—connective tissue (notably, cartilage) and elsewhere—results in ochronosis, manifested by arthritis and other complications.

Alkaptonuria was the first of four conditions hypothesized by Garrod to represent inborn errors of metabolism; the others are albinism, cystinuria, and pentosuria. All four have now been shown to reflect specific point mutations in the genome, the "one gene–one enzyme" paradigm.[10] In 1999 the Johns Hopkins

Presented in part at the forty-seventh annual meeting of the American Osler Society in Atlanta, Georgia, on 11 April 2017.

pediatrician and geneticist Barton Childs (1916–2010) wrote: "No one would deny that Osler was the hero of the medicine of the twentieth century. It is likely that Garrod will be the icon of the twenty-first."[11]

Garrod was not the only member of his family to achieve eminence in science. His father, Sir Alfred Baring Garrod (1819–1907) demonstrated the role of uric acid in gout, coined the term "rheumatoid arthritis," and suggested lithium as treatment for mental illness. His daughter, Dorothy Annie Elizabeth Garrod (1892–1968), became an iconic figure in archaeology. My purpose is to summarize the lives of these remarkable individuals.

Sir Alfred Baring Garrod

Alfred Garrod was born in Ipswich, the son of a tenant farmer who founded a firm of real estate agents and auctioneers.[11] Alfred aspired from childhood to be a doctor and to that end served as an apprentice at Ipswich Hospital. He later moved to University College, London, where, after qualifying as MB in 1842 and MD in 1843, he worked in the chemical department "occupied chiefly in the analysis of morbid fluids and other substances." He branched out into clinical medicine and reported in 1848 that uric acid was increased in patients with gout but not in patients with acute rheumatism or Bright's disease.

In 1855 Alfred Garrod brought out *The Essentials of Materia Medica, Therapeutics and Pharmacopœa*, which went through 13 editions, and in 1859 he brought out *The Nature and Treatment of Gout and Rheumatic Gout* (Figure 1). He coined the term "rheumatoid arthritis" after rejecting such previous concepts as "chronic rheumatism" described by William Heberden (1710–1801) and "rheumatic gout" described by Henry William Fuller (1820–1873). In 1863 Alfred resigned from University College Hospital after William Jenner (1815–1898), rather than he, was

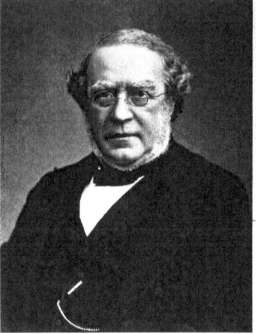

Figure 1. Alfred Baring Garrod and his treatise on *The Nature and Treatment of Gout and Rheumatic Gout* (1859). *Credit:* Wikimedia Commons.

made professor of the principles and practice of medicine. However, he went on to a highly successful career in private practice, was knighted, became physician extraordinary to Queen Victoria, and, with his wife, the former Elizabeth Ann Colchester from Ipswich, entertained prominent Victorian personalities at their home at 63 Harley Street.

Alfred and Elizabeth Garrod had six children, four boys and two girls. A boy and a girl died young, but three of the boys enjoyed successful careers: Alfred Henry Garrod (1846–1879) as a vertebrate zoologist, Henry Baring Garrod (1850–1912) as a classics scholar and educator, and "Archie," who was named after the Archibald Campbell Tait (1811–1882), Archbishop of Canterbury. Archie, despite an early interest in the taxonomy of butterflies, was thought by his father to be "unpromising."

Sir Archibald Edward Garrod

At age 15, Archie Garrod was sent to a boarding school, Marlborough College, where he initially did poorly because of disinterest in the classics. Intervention by his older brother Alfred and the kindly headmaster, Frederic William Farrar (1801–1903), saved him from expulsion and he went on to receive prizes in physics and geography. He then entered Christ Church, Oxford, where he fell under the influence of the biologist Ray Lankester (1847–1929) and the chemist A.G. Vernon Harcourt (1834–1919), both of whom coached him in scientific writing. During his last year at Oxford, he won the coveted Johnson Memorial Prize for his essay on "The Nebulae: A Fragment of Astronomical History."[13]

Garrod graduated from Oxford with first-class honors ("a First") in natural science. He moved back in with his parents in London and attended St. Bartholomew's Hospital Medical School ("St. Barts"), where he developed lifelong friendships and was mentored by the likes of Emmanuel Edward Klein (1844–1925), the "father of British bacteriology," William Selby Church (1837–1928), a prominent consulting physician, Samuel Jones Gee (1839–1911), who described celiac disease, and the chemist William James Russell (1830–1900). He became

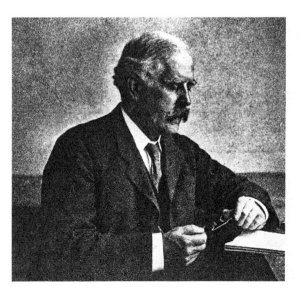

Figure 2. Archibald Edward Garrod in later life and his Croonian Lectures on *Inborn Errors of Metabolism* (delivered in 1908 and published in book form in 1909). *Credit:* Wellcome Collection CC BY.

interested in otolaryngology and, with Samuel Osborne Habershon (1825–1889), went to Vienna to work with Leopold von Schrötter (1837–1908) and Johann Schnitzler (1835–1893). This led to Garrod's his first book, *An Introduction to the Uses of the Laryngoscope* (1886),[14] which was well-received.

Returning to London, Garrod became house physician at St. Bart's for Dyce Duckworth (1840–1928), well-known as a physician, surgeon, dermatologist, and author of *A Treatise on Gout* (1889). A chance meeting with Sir Thomas Smith (1833–1909), a friend of Archie's father, led to an invitation to Stafford Place for tea where Garrod met Smith's daughter, Laura. The story goes that Archie proposed to Laura while rowing with a rose attached to the bow of the boat. Samuel Habershon was best man at their wedding on 27 May 1886. Duckworth counseled Garrod to become a clinician but to always pursue scientific interests, especially in chemistry. Archie dedicated his first major work, *A Treatise on Rheumatism and Rheumatoid Arthritis* (1890),[15] to his father. Over the next decade he studied rheumatic diseases with an interest on the possible impact of heredity.

In 1892 Garrod was appointed assistant physician to the Hospital for Sick Children in London (later known as the Great Ormond Street Hospital). Pediatrics was just coming into its own as a medical specialty. Building on his experience in chemistry, Garrod collaborated with Frederick Gowland Hopkins (1861–1947), the biochemist who later shared the Nobel Prize for discovery of vitamins. In 1897 a woman arrived with an infant whose diaper was stained brownish black. Garrod soon saw other patients with this condition—alkaptonuria—and on review of the literature realized that 40 such cases had been reported since 1822. After presenting five cases of his own in 1899 to the Royal Medical and Chirurgical Society of London,[16] he began to observe the disorder among first cousins. He sought out William Bateson (1861–1926),[17] the English biologist who popularized the ideas of Gregor Mendel and coined the term "genetics," and with Bateson's help began to suspect that transmission of alkaptonuria followed Mendelian principles. Bateson presented Garrod's findings to the Royal Society on 17 December 1901, a few weeks after Garrod updated his observations in *The Lancet*.[18]

Osler was among those who took note. He wrote Garrod requesting 100 copies of his recent article. He helped Garrod find additional cases. In 1902 Garrod wrote Bateson: "I am gradually getting in some further information about alkaptonuria and heredity.... Prof. Osler is kindly following up some American cases for me." Preserved in the Osler Library of the History of Medicine at McGill are seven letters from Osler to Garrod written between 23 January 1902 and 2 January 1903 and pertaining to cases of alkaptonuria in the practices of two of Osler's close friends: Henry V. Ogden, Jr. (1857–1931) of Milwaukee, Wisconsin, and Thomas B. Futcher (1871–1938) of Baltimore.[19] Futcher had reported the first case of alkaptonuria in the US in 1898,[20] and his experience included an entire family. Osler relayed the information to Garrod.

On 13 December 1902, Garrod's paper entitled "The Incidence of Alkaptonuria: A Study of Chemical Individuality" was published in *The Lancet*.[21] He now had data about heritability, some of it from Osler and his colleagues:

> Hitherto nothing has been recorded about the children of alkaptonuric parents, and the information supplied by Professor Osler and Dr. Ogden on this point has therefore a special interest. Whereas Professor Osler's case shows that the condition may be directly inherited from a parent Dr. Ogden's case demonstrates that none of the children of such a parent need share his peculiarity. As the matter now stands, of five children of two alkaptonuric fathers whose condition is known only one is himself

> alkaptonuric. It will be interesting to learn whether this low proportion is maintained when larger number of cases shall be available. That it will be so is rendered highly probable by the undoubted fact that a very small proportion of alkaptonurics are the offspring of parents either of whom exhibits the anomaly.

In today's terms, Garrod was describing an autosomal-recessive disorder due to a single gene mutation. Garrod went further:

> If it be, indeed, the case that in alkaptonuria and the other conditions mentioned [albinism and cystinuria] we are dealing with individualities of metabolism and not with the results of morbid processes the thought naturally presents itself that these are merely extreme examples of varia-tions of chemical behaviour which are probably everywhere present in minor degrees and that just as no two individuals of a species are abso-lutely identical in bodily structure neither are their chemical processes carried out on exactly the same lines.

In this now-classic paper, Garrod extended "my very special thanks . . . for invalu-able aid in collecting information" to Osler and the German physician-chemist Karl Hugo Huppert (1832–1904). He included Futcher and Ogden among the 18 additional persons who helped him.

In 1904 Osler reported in *The Lancet* two brothers with alkaptonuria and its long-term complication, ochronosis. Among his observations was the occur-rence of bilateral pigmentation in the sclera midway between the cornea and the outer and inner canthi at the insertion of the recti muscles—a finding sometimes known as "Osler's sign."[22,23] He had seen the first brother, a 57-year-old US politician with presumed diabetes, in 1895, at which time "I was impressed by a remarkable appearance of the sclerotic which showed small V shaped areas of pigmentation near the cornea. . . ." Futcher, then a resident, later determined that the patient did not have diabetes but rather had alkaptonuria and reported the case.[20] Six years later Futcher's patient was admitted to the Johns Hopkins Hos-pital under Osler's care. The pigmented appearance of the "sclerotics" [sclerae] had "extended considerably," and Osler learned that the patient's brother also had "pigmented sclerotics and ears." Osler induced the brother to come to the laboratory where alkaptonuria was confirmed. Osler pointed out that both broth-ers had ochronotic osteoarthropathy and pointed out the clinical significance of cartilaginous pigmentation in cases of alkaptonuria.[23]

Osler and Garrod enhanced their friendship after Osler moved to Oxford in 1905 to become Regius professor of medicine. In 1907 Osler invited Garrod to become an editor of the new *Quarterly Journal of Medicine.* In 1908 Garrod delivered the Croonian Lectures on inborn errors of metabolism, published the next year in book form (Figure 2) and now considered a landmark in the history of genet-ics and biochemistry.[24,25] That same year, Osler and Garrod helped Edgar Reid, a physician in Swansea, Wales, bring out a case report of ochronosis associated with alkaptonuria.[26]

Garrod's career as a laboratory scientist effectively ended with the Croonian Lectures but he continued to be clinically active, wrote essays on the importance of basic science and especially biochemistry to medicine,[27–29] and co-edited a text-book of pediatrics.[30] During the Great War he served in the Army Medical Service in Malta as director of the war hospitals there. After succeeding Osler as Regius professor of medicine at Oxford, he wrote glowingly about his predecessor noting, however, that "Osler was very human, and his weakness added to his attraction."[31]

Archie and Laura Garrod had three sons and a daughter. All three sons enlisted in the British armed forces. Lieutenant Thomas Martin Garrod of the Loyal North Lancaster Regiment died from war injuries on 10 May 1915 at the age of 20, and Lieutenant Alfred Noel Garrod of the Royal Army Medical Corps died of wounds on 25 January 1916 at the age of 28. The youngest son, Basil Raheer Garrod of the Royal Air Force, died on 9 February 1919 of influenza during the occupation of Germany. There remained only the daughter, Dorothy Annie Elizabeth Garrod. Dorothy studied classics and history at Newnham College, Cambridge, where she converted to Catholicism during her first year. Graduating from Newnham College, she served in France during the war with the Catholic Women's League. After she was demobilized in 1919, she joined her father in Malta.

Dorothy Garrod

In Malta, Dorothy Garrod became intrigued by the relics of ancient civilizations. By one account, her father "in his wisdom distracted her mind towards interest in the antiquities,"[32] and with his encouragement she studied at Oxford under the anthropologist and archaeologist Robert Ranulph Marrett (1866–1943). She graduated in 1921 with distinction and decided to focus on the archaeology of the Paleolithic Age. To that end she spent two years studying with Henri Édouard

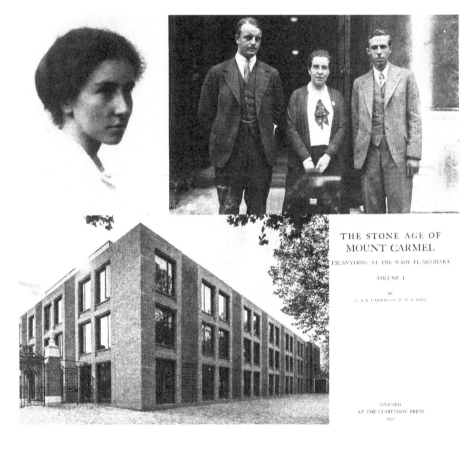

Figure 3.   Dorothy Garrod. *Clockwise from upper left:* As a young woman; with two colleagues after defending her views on historic Palestine at the International Congress on Prehistoric and Prothistoric Sciences at King's College, London; her treatise on *The Stone Age of Mount Carmel: Excavations at the Wadi El-Mughara* (1937, with D.M.A. Bate); and the Dorothy Garrod Building, Newnham College, Cambridge, dedicated in 2019. *Credits:* Archive PL/Alamy Stock Photo; Smith Archive/Alamy Stock Photo; Robert Evans/Alamy Stock Photo.

THE STONE AGE OF
MOUNT CARMEL

EXCAVATIONS AT THE WADY EL-MUGHARA

VOLUME I

BY
D. A. E. GARROD and D. M. A. BATE

OXFORD
AT THE CLARENDON PRESS
1937

Prosper Breuil (1877–1961), commonly known as Abbé Breuil, who was a Jesuit priest, archaeologist, anthropologist, ethnologist, geologist, and authority on cave art.

Breuil and Garrod were among the first to think globally about human prehistory. Breuil encouraged her to excavate on Gibraltar, and it was there that Dorothy discovered five skull fragments of a male child—maxillary, mandibular, temporal, parietal, and cranial—that when pieced together were concluded to be the second Neanderthal skull ever found. She named it "Abel" but it is commonly known as "Gibraltar 2" or the "Devil's Tower Child." In 1926 she brought out *The Upper Palæolithic of Britain*,[33] for which she was received a B.Sc. degree from Oxford. In 1928 she led an expedition to South Kurdistan and in 1929 she was appointed to supervise excavations in Palestine in a project jointly sponsored by the British School of Archaeology in Jerusalem and the American School of Prehistoric Research. Working with the Welch paleontologist and archeologist Dorothea Minola Alice Bate (1878–1951), also known as Dorothy Bate, she demonstrated sequential occupation of a series of caves by Lower Paleolithic, Middle Paleolithic, and Epipaleolithic cultures. Additionally, she coined the term "Natufian culture" to designate a late Epipaleolithic culture of the Levant that supported a sedentary or semi-sedentary population prior to the introduction of agriculture. In 1937 Garrod and Bate brought out the first volume of *The Stone Age of Mount Carmel*, summarizing much of this research.[34]

These accomplishments did not go unnoticed by the larger academic community. In 1939 Dorothy Garrod was elected Disney Professor of Archæology at Cambridge, becoming the first woman to hold a chair at either Cambridge or Oxford. This appointment was hailed as "an immense step towards complete equality between men and women at the University," but it was not until 1948 that women became full faculty members with voting privileges at Cambridge. In the meantime, Garrod served in the Women's Auxiliary Air Force during the Second World War as a section officer in a photographic interpretation unit. (Garrod is credited as being the first to use aerial photography in archaeological excavations.) She retired from Cambridge in 1952 and moved to France where she continued to excavate.

Dorothy Garrod is recognized not only as a major figure in British archeology and the study of human evolution but also as a quiet champion for gender equality in science and academia.[35,36] In 2019 the multipurpose Dorothy Garrod Building was dedicated to her memory at the University of Cambridge (Figure 3).

References

1. Bearn AG. *Archibald Garrod and the Individuality of Man*. Oxford: Clarendon Press; 1993.
2. Bearn AG, Miller ED. Archibald Garrod and the development of the concept of inborn errors of metabolism. *Bulletin of the History of Medicine* 1979; 53(3): 315–328.
3. Dronamraju K. Profiles in genetics: Archibald E. Garrod (1857–1938). *American Journal of Human Genetics* 1992; 51(1): 216–219.
4. Childs B. Sir Archibald Garrod's conception of chemical individuality: a modern appreciation. *New England Journal of Medicine* 1970; 282(2): 71–77.
5. McKusick VA. Osler as a medical geneticist. *The Johns Hopkins Medical Journal* 1976; 139(4): 163–174.

6. Perlman RA, Govindaraju DR. Archibald E. Garrod: the father of precision medicine. *Genetics in Medicine* 2016; 18(11): 1088–1089.

7. Piro A, Tagarelli A, Tagarelli G, Lagonia P, Quattrone A. Archibald Edward Garrod: the physician father of biochemistry. *Metabolism, Clinical and Experimental* 2009; 58(4): 427–437.

8. Prasad C, Galbraith PA. Sir Archibald Garrod and alkaptonuria—'story of metabolic genetics'. *Clinical Genetics* 2005; 68(3): 199–120.

9. Scriver CR. Garrod's Croonian Lectures (1908) and the charter 'Inborn Errors of Metabolism.' *Journal of Inherited Metabolic Diseases* 2008; 31(5): 580–598.

10. Pierce SB, Spurrell CH, Mandell JB, Lee MK, Zeligson S, et al. Garrod's fourth inborn error of metabolism solved by the identification of mutations causing pentosuria. *Proceedings of the National Academy of Sciences of the United States of America* 2011; 108(45): 18313–18317.

11. Childs B. *Genetic Medicine: A Logic of Disease.* Baltimore: The Johns Hopkins University Press; 1999: 16.

12. Storey GD. Alfred Baring Garrod (1819–1907). *Rheumatology* 2001; 40(10): 1189–1190.

13. Garrod AE. *The Nebulae: A Fragment of Astronomical History.* London: Parker & Co.; 1882.

14. Garrod AE. *An Introduction to the Use of the Laryngoscope.* London: Longmans, Green & Company; 1886.

15. Garrod AE. *A Treatise of Rheumatism and Rheumatoid Arthritis.* London: Charles Griffin & Co., Ltd.; 1890.

16. Garrod AE. A contribution to the study of alkaptonuria. *Medico-Chirurgical Transactions* 1899; 82: 367–394.

17. Keynes M, Cox TM. William Bateson, the rediscoverer of Mendel. *Journal of the Royal Society of Medicine* 2008; 101(3): 104.

18. Garrod AE. About alkaptonuria. *Lancet* 1901; 158(4083): 1484–1486.

19. William Osler to Archibald E. Garrod, 23 January 1902, 20 February 1902, 8 April 1902, 19 August 1902, 4 October 1902, 26 November 1902, and 2 January 1903. Osler Letter Index, CUS417/98.7, CUS417/98.8, CUS417/98.9, CUS417/98.10, CUS417/98.11, CUS417/98.12, and CUS417/98.13, Osler Library of the History of Medicine McGill University.

20. Futcher TB. Alkaptonuria. *New York Medical Journal* 1898; 67: 69–74.

21. Garrod AE. The incidence of alkaptonuria: a study of chemical individuality. *Lancet* 1902; 160(4137): 1616–1620.

22. Toodayan N. Osler's sign (ochronisis; alkaptonuria). In Bryan CS, ed. *Sir William Osler: An Encyclopedia.* Novato, California: Norman Publishing/HistoryofScience.Com; 2020: 601–602.

23. Osler W. Ochronosis: The pigmentation of cartilages, sclerotic, and skin in alkaptonuria. *Lancet* 1904; 163(4192): 10–11.

24. Garrod AE. The Croonian Lectures on inborn errors of metabolism. *Lancet* 1908; 172(4427): 1–7; 172(4428): 73–79; 172(4429):142–148; 172(4430); 214–220.

25. Garrod AE. *Inborn Errors of Metabolism.* London: Henry Frowde and Hodder & Stoughton; 1909.

26. Reid E, Osler W, Garrod AE. On ochronosis: report of a case: the clinical features; the urine. *Quarterly Journal of Medicine* 1908; 1(o.s.)(2): 199–208.

27. Garrod AE. Where chemistry and medicine meet. *British Medical Journal* 1911; 1(2633): 1413–1418.

28. Garrod AE. The Harveian Oration: The debt of science to medicine. *British Medical Journal* 1924; 2(3330): 747–752.

29. Garrod AE. The place of biochemistry in medicine. *British Medical Journal* 1928; 1(3521): 1099–1101.

30. Garrod AE, Batten FE, Thursfield H, eds. *Diseases of Children by Various Authors.* London: Edward Arnold; 1913.

31. Moran ME. Garrod, Sir Archibald Edward, Reminiscences of William Osler. In Bryan CS, ed. *Sir William Osler: An Encyclopedia.* Novato, California: Norman Publishing/HistoryofScience.Com; 2020: 291.

32. Weinstein-Evron M. *Archaeology in the Archives: Unveiling the Natufian Culture of Mount Carmel.* Boston: Brill; 2009: 1.

33. Garrod DAE. *The Upper Palæolithic Age in Britain.* Oxford: Oxford University Press; 1926.

34. Garrod DAE, Bate DMA. *The Stone Age of Mount Carmel. Excavations at the Wady el-Mughara. Report of the Joint Expedition of the British School of Archæology in Jerusalem and the American School of Prehistoric Research, 1929–1934.* Volume 1, Oxford: Clarendon Press; 1937.

35. Davies W, Charles R, eds. *Dorothy Garrod and the Progress of the Palæolithic.* Oxford, United Kingdom: Oxbow Books; 1999.

36. Bar-Yosef O, Callander J. Dorothy Annie Elizabeth Garrod (1892–1968). In Cohen GM, Joukowsy MS, eds. *Breaking Ground: Pioneering Women Archaeologists.* Ann Arbor: University of Michigan; 2005.

Henry Ware Cattell and Walt Whitman's Brain

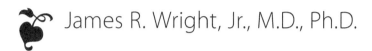 James R. Wright, Jr., M.D., Ph.D.

Henry Ware Cattell (1862–1936) (Figure 1) was a prominent pathologist and medical editor in late-nineteenth and early-twentieth-century America. Strangely, his name is unknown to most medical historians but is more widely known by aficionados of Walt Whitman's poetry. There is currently no single adequate biographical source on Cattell and so this summary was pieced together from newspaper articles, obituaries, and alumni records in his file at the University Archives at the University of Pennsylvania (hereafter, Penn).[1] Here, I will provide a detailed biographical sketch of Cattell, address his sibling rivalry with his more famous brother, James McKeen Cattell (1860–1944), briefly discuss the fad of nineteenth century intellectuals embracing the pseudo-science of phrenology and their participation in anatomical "brain clubs," and, finally, address the mystery of what happened to Walt Whitman's brain after his autopsy on 27 March 1892.

Cattell's family background

Henry Ware Cattell's life course and career were facilitated by being born into a well-educated and influential family. His Quaker ancestors arrived in America in 1648 and settled in New Jersey in about 1732. His family and ancestors included merchants, bankers, academics, religious leaders, and politicians, including an uncle who was a long-serving US senator from New Jersey.[1] His father, Reverend William C. Cattell, was a Presbyterian scholar and the seventh president of Lafayette College in Easton, Pennsylvania. After serving as associate principal

Presented in part in at the forty-ninth annual meeting of the American Osler Society, Montreal, Quebec, Canada, on 13 May 2019. This paper was previously published in *Clinical Anatomy* (2018; 31[7]: 988–986) and is reproduced with permission.

at a preparatory school in Princeton, New Jersey, he taught Latin and Greek at Lafayette College for five years before resigning to become pastor at a Presbyterian church in Harrisburg, Pennsylvania. During the Civil War, Lafayette College suffered a financial crisis due to severely reduced student enrollment and was nearing bankruptcy when its Board of Trustees approached William to become college president, which he accepted. William was tasked with fund-raising and was successful in this endeavor, saving the College. He continued another 20 years as president of Lafayette. After retirement, he served as secretary of the Board of Ministerial Relief of the Presbyterian Church, raising over three million dollars for widows and orphans. In 1859, William married Elizabeth "Lizzie" McKeen (1835–1917), the daughter of James McKeen, a member of the Lafayette College Board of Trustees who left her a substantial inheritance when he died. They had two children, James McKeen Cattell and Henry Ware Cattell, and the Cattells often used their wealth and influence to help further their sons' careers. William remained on the Lafayette College Board of Trustees until his death in 1898.[2]

Henry's older brother, James McKeen Cattell (1860–1944), was born in Easton, received his A.B. from Lafayette College in 1880, and studied in Leipzig, Paris, Geneva, and Gottingen for two years before receiving his A.M. from Lafayette College in 1882. After two years as a philosophy fellow at Johns Hopkins University (1883–1884) he returned to Leipzig to complete his Ph.D., which he received in 1886. He then became an assistant under Wilhelm Wundt (1832–1920), who is widely regarded as the father of experimental psychology, at the University of Leipzig. Upon returning home, he was appointed the first professor of psychology in America, working at the University of Pennsylvania (Penn) from 1888 to 1891. He finished his academic career at Columbia University where he was professor of experimental psychology, anthropology, and philosophy (1891–1917). He served as the editor-in-chief for *Popular Science Monthly* (1900–1915) and co-editor of the *Psychological Review* (1894–1903) and also *The American Naturalist* (1907–1944). He bought the journal *Science*, which had fallen on hard financial times, in 1894 for $500. J. McKeen Cattell arranged for *Science* to become the official journal of the American Association for the Advancement of Science (AAAS) in 1900, but he retained ownership until his death in 1944, when the journal's ownership was transferred to the AAAS.[3-5] He published at least 75 papers in *Science* between 1893 and 1942. He also originated, edited, and published *American Men of Science* directory (1906–1938). James McKeen Cattell's distinguished 50-year career was colored by arrogance, self righteousness, and an often-antagonistic approach to others.[6,7] J. McKeen's extreme success combined with certain aspects of his personality may have made life difficult for Henry, who desperately wanted to follow in his family's highly accomplished footsteps.

Henry Ware Cattell

Henry Ware Cattell was born in Harrisburg, Pennsylvania, on 7 October 1862. He attended a prestigious preparatory boarding school, the Hill School, in Pottstown, Pennsylvania. and then went to Lafayette College, from which he received his A.B. in 1883. Following in his brother's footsteps, he moved to Leipzig and attended medical school there for one year (1883–1884), but he actually received his M.D. degree from Penn, where William Osler (1849–1919) was one of his teachers, on 2 May 1887. He received a "prize for best collection of anomalies in the dissecting room,"[1] which may have helped him decide to become a

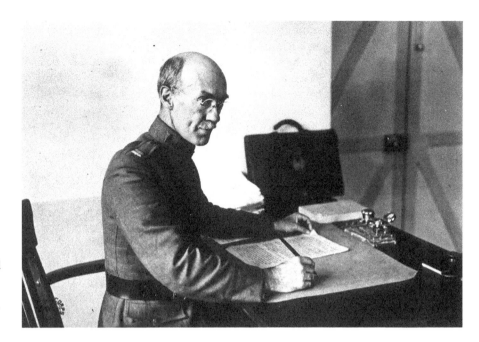

Figure 1. Captain Henry Ware Cattell in military uniform seated at desk during World War I, 1918.
Credit: National Library of Medicine.

pathologist. Henry also spent time studying abroad in 1886 (receiving an A.M. from Lafayette), 1890, and 1895.

Henry Cattell's early career was as a laboratory physician and pathologist. He began his academic career as an assistant demonstrator of chemistry at Penn (1887–1892). This was probably awkward as his brother, who was only two years his elder, was at Penn as the first professor of psychology in the United States. Next, at the same time that his brother relocated to a prestigious position at Columbia University, Henry became demonstrator of morbid anatomy (1892–1897) at Penn. During the 1890s, he was also an assistant pathologist at Blockley Hospital, an almshouse that played an important role in Philadelphia's status as the leading American city for medical education in the nineteenth century; it was later renamed Philadelphia General Hospital.[8] Cattell was eventually appointed its pathologist by the Board of Charities and Correction at Blockley, succeeding Juan (or John) John Guitéras (1852–1925) when he resigned. Cattell held this position from 1898 to 1900.[8] Cattell also worked as a forensic pathologist. From 1896 to 1898 he was senior coroner's physician of Philadelphia; he continued to serve as an expert witness in murder trials until at least the late 1920s, and, according to obituaries in several Philadelphia newspapers, "was one of the City's first 'Crime Scientists.'" Next, he served as director of Ayer Chemical Laboratory at the prestigious Pennsylvania Hospital (n.b., this was the first hospital in the U.S., founded in 1751 by Benjamin Franklin and Dr. Thomas Bond) from 1899–1901. He also worked as a pathologist at Presbyterian Hospital, many small Philadelphia hospitals, and at the Institution for Feeble-Minded Children at Elwyn, Pennsylvania.[1]

In 1892 an incident abruptly changed Cattell's life and reduced his commitment to pathology as a career. He had been serving as the pathologist/prosector for the American Anthropometric Society (AAS, see below) at the time the poet Walt Whitman died. Cattell, as pathologist for Penn's Wistar Institute, performed Whitman's autopsy on 27 March 1892; Whitman's brain was removed and was to join those of other prominent American intellectuals who had donated their brains to the Society's "Brain Club." As discussed in detail below, something went horribly wrong (apparently, he discretely told a few AAS colleagues that an assistant had dropped the brain and destroyed it, but otherwise he kept the matter a secret). Full of self-doubt, Cattell was anguished about his inadequacies as a pathologist and was extremely worried about how all of this would affect his career when discovered. While continuing to practice hospital-based pathology, he began to transition into an author and editor. Not surprisingly, there is no mention of any of this in his Penn file, which Cattell appears to have updated regularly.

In 1894 Cattell self-published his first book, *Notes on the Demonstration of Morbid Anatomy (Including Autopsies) Delivered in the Medical Department of the University of Pennsylvania before the third-year class*, using his International Medical Magazine Company.[9] In addition to explaining how to perform an autopsy, his book provides insights on how to obtain autopsy consent and permission to retain organs: "You should be sure you have the right to make the post-mortem before you begin. The nearest relative, or the one who is going to pay the expenses of the funeral, should give consent in writing."[9, p. 90] As will be seen later, Cattell did not always follow these basic rules. In 1896–1897, he translated Ernst Ziegler's *Text-Book of Special Pathological Anatomy* from German to English.

In 1903 Cattell published his own mainstream pathology textbook entitled *Post-Mortem Pathology*, which was followed by subsequent editions in 1905 and 1906. This book provides a detailed description of contemporary autopsy technique and is historically important as it provides the only detailed description, including some illustrations, of how to perform Howard A. Kelly's covert "arm's length" autopsy technique, in which the entire body can be eviscerated (except for brain removal) through the vagina in women or the anus or a small incision in the "crack" behind the scrotum in men.[10] This method allowed the covert collection of pathological teaching specimens without any telltale external incisions that could be noticed by family members. In addition to outlining autopsy consent regulations, his book provides unique insights into local autopsy-consent "practice" in Philadelphia in the 1880s which allowed William Osler and other Philadelphia pathologists to get away with performing autopsies at Blockley Hospital without legal consent.[11] Related to "practice," Cattell is a little more flippant in how he describes autopsy consent noting that "there should be a law permitting post-mortem examinations of the bodies of all persons dying in charitable institutions" as exists in Germany. He also notes that such a law does not exist, but, although it was not strictly legal, "this custom prevailed . . . with practically no opposition, until lawsuits, arising out of this custom, caused it to be discontinued." His book also gives practical advice for obtaining consent to retain organs as teaching specimens: "When portions of the body are desired for future study or for preservation, permission to remove them should be obtained from someone connected with the household, though not necessarily from the nearest relative." He further added that "it is, of course, unnecessary to tell how much is to be taken away!"[12, pp. 5–6] Clearly, these questionable and highly paternalistic approaches to autopsy consent, although morally reprehensible now, permitted the outstanding clinico-pathological correlations that helped make Blockley an excellent teaching environment.

While not stopping pathology practice entirely, Cattell began to recast himself as a medical editor in the late 1890s (once again following in his brother's footsteps). In 1894–1897, Cattell served as editor of *International Medical Magazine* and from 1894–1896 served as a co-editor of *International Clinics: A Quarterly of Clinical Lectures*. Beginning in 1900 he served intermittently as editor of *International*

Clinics: A Quarterly of Clinical Lectures (1900–1903, 1910–1916, and 1922–1932), which published papers by important clinicians including William Osler, who was a "collaborating editor" for 17 years[13]; according to one obituary, he published 78 volumes of this book between 1900 and 1932. From roughly 1905–1911, Cattell was editor of *Medical Notes and Queries*, an independent medical journal which he used to cause trouble for Penn administration (see below). Cattell also edited the *Lippincott's Medical Dictionary* in 1910 and 1913, and published a limited-edition book entitled *Tait McKenzie's Medical Portraits* in 1925.[14] McKenzie was a famous Canadian physician, athlete, soldier, painter, sculptor, and educator who resided in Philadelphia and was Penn's first professor of physical education.[15]

Cattell served as a Major during World War I and was initially in charge of pathology at the Army Medical Museum in Washington, D.C.[16] He was sent to France, where he served as a pathologist at Base Hospital No. 17 during 1918–1919 and was also in charge of all post-mortem records for the American Expeditionary Forces (AEF). Details on the AEF autopsy service can be found elsewhere.[17]

Cattell was outspoken throughout his life and, as the son of a minister, projected strong moral convictions related to certain vices. For instance, he was opposed the sale of cigarettes to minors, long before this was known to have public-health implications. One of his last public appearances was testifying at House and Senate committee hearings, where he spoke about the intoxicating effects of alcohol.[1]

The Cattell brothers' outspoken views on municipal and university administration

Henry Ware Cattell had a series of battles with the city of Philadelphia and Charles C. Harrison (1844–1929), Penn's Provost. In 1905, he found out that Penn was planning to build a veterinary hospital in West Philadelphia adjacent to his property; he wrote Provost Harrison and city health officials, and, when this proved ineffective, filed a formal complaint. Next, he precipitated newspaper coverage suggesting that, since animals with infectious diseases would be treated there, it would be impossible to achieve adequate isolation in such a built-up portion of the city.[1]

In 1908 he participated in a grassroots attempt to reform municipal politics by joining with the upstart City Party and agreeing to run for coroner. A local paper called him the "first serious City Party candidate." Shortly after this, Cattell wrote an editorial to a Philadelphia daily newspaper, the *Public Ledger*, suggesting that land occupied by the city's commercial museums had been sold to Penn for about 25 percent of the market value, and then personally offered to buy city land for twice that price. This caused some turmoil as both the buyer and seller had been on public record that the sale was at market price.[1]

Cattell's new perception that city land could be obtained so inexpensively soon led him to suggest a total reorganization of medical training in Philadelphia. In an editorial in the May 1910 issue of his *Medical Notes and Queries*, Cattell proposed that "the time is now propitious for placing the University of Pennsylvania under absolute State control, and for the reunion of the Medico-Chirurgical College and the Jefferson Medical School." He further suggested that if Penn were under state control, "everybody knows that the present gang (of administrators) will soon be out of power, then the institution may hope for some larger measure of independence." Cattell noted that the numbers of medical students enrolled at the Medico-Chirurgical College and Jefferson Medical College exceeded those enrolled at Penn. Cattell considered these to be "practical teaching schools," unlike Penn, which was becoming increasingly focused on becoming a scientific institution turning out "laboratory workers and ultra-scientists." He envisaged a full merger "with sufficient endowment to erect on the new boulevard a group of buildings commensurate with the combined prestige of both institutions." He considered all of this as necessary to "continue Philadelphia as one of the great medical centers of the world." His editorial received extensive press coverage and resulted in the press contacting the deans of all three medical schools for comments.[1] Cattell proved to be right about a merger but he picked the wrong partner; the Medico-Chirurgical College merged into the University of Pennsylvania in 1916.[18]

In late 1910 Cattell again used his *Medical Notes and Queries*, this time to publically accuse Penn of selling professorships, which generated considerable newspaper coverage in Philadelphia[1] as well as the *New York Times*.[19] Cattell's assault on Penn included a fake "advertisement" that he had created "For sale. Professorship vacancies in the University of Pennsylvania. Prices ranging from $100,000 to $1,000,000," which Cattell believed should be placed in newspapers around the country. This new issue was addressed in two successive editions of the *Medical Notes and Queries* (November and December) as well as the extensive press coverage he was able to generate. While Cattell was initially vague and refused to supply names, it soon became clear that Cattell was referring to the appointments of Barton Cooke Hirst as professor of obstetrics in 1889 and J. William White as the John Rhea Barton Professor of Surgery in 1900. In no instance was there alleged to be direct payment by a candidate, but Cattell believed that decisions were made based upon which candidate would most financially benefit Penn. For instance, White and two others were trustees under the will of Edmund A.W. Hunter, who died in 1895, conditionally leaving an extremely valuable estate to Penn. The final decision as to the disposition of the estate was solely under the control of the trustees, and they could, at their discretion, substitute another medical school for Penn.[1] Cattell may have been right about White's appointment, but Jefferson Medical College (JMC) seemed to be taking the same approach. When JMC anatomy professor William Pancoast retired in 1886, there were two strong candidates to replace him, W.W. Keen, a world-renowned surgeon, and William S. Forbes. Forbes, like White, was in a position to designate whether the large estate of one of his former patients would be donated to JMC and Forbes beat out Keen, who appeared to be the much stronger candidate.[20] If Cattell was aware of this, he simply ignored that Penn was not unique and that JMC was also guilty.

Once again, as in all the above-mentioned stories, Cattell suggests that Charles C. Harrison should resign. However, this time, the allegations were addressed by provost-elect Edgar F. Smith, Harrison's replacement. Smith said the charges were "absolutely without foundation." Cattell's response still focused on Harrison: "If Charles C. Harrison has the real interests of the University of Pennsylvania at heart, he will resign from the board of trustees … and not handicap his successor by his policies, which have shown themselves to be so detrimental to education at the University of Pennsylvania and to civic reform in the city of Philadelphia."[1]

In criticizing administrators, Henry Cattell was preceded by his brother, J. McKeen Cattell, who beginning in 1902 criticized the tight control exerted by

American university administrators. McKeen Cattell used his journals, *Science* and *Popular Science Monthly*, for this purpose.[21,22] McKeen Cattell also featured "professor protest literature" by other authors in these journals. In 1913, he ratcheted it up a few notches by bundling many of these protest papers together and then editing a book, *University Control*.[23] McKeen Cattell thus used his publishing empire to spearhead a revolt among American university professors against their universities. This resulted in the formation of the American Association of University Professors in 1915.[24] This revolt may no doubt have factored into the decision by the Columbia University administration to fire McKeen Cattell in 1915, despite his prominence in academia, although the ostensible reason was his public opposition to conscription when the US entered World War I. While Cattell and others claimed he was a martyr for academic freedom, the story was much more complex.[6] J. McKeen Cattell, who according to his biographer never had a moment of self-doubt during his life, "fought back first by supporting a Socialist candidate for NYC Mayor and then by a long series of *ad hominem* attacks on [the president of Columbia University]" (Michael M. Sokal, personal communication, 15 July 2018).

It seems likely that knowledge of his famous brother's actions influenced Henry Ware Cattell in his attacks on Penn administration and that this is where he got the idea to publish critical papers in his journal, *Medical Notes and Queries*. Like his brother, he pushed for the need for Penn faculty member unionization in some of his press coverage in Philadelphia news papers. However, it seems unlikely that Henry discussed his ideas with James as they were not close and did not correspond. The primary route through which the brothers received information about each other was via letters from their mother (Michael M. Sokal, personal communication, 8 July 2018). She died in 1917, closing this avenue of indirect communication between brothers.

Henry Ware Cattell's later life

Three years before his death, Henry Cattell retired and moved to Burlington, New Jersey. Cattell, perhaps, in part, because he was not close to his famous brother, was extremely proud of his career-long association with his even more famous former teacher Sir William Osler, who died in 1919. Cattell was enamoured with Osler's skills as an editor, and he contributed his reminiscences about Osler in Maude Abbott's *Sir William Osler Memorial Number*. His contribution, "Osler, the Medical Editor," is not one of Cattell's strongest literary efforts. Ironically, using his own sometimes highly pretentious text, Cattell describes how Osler's writings were not pretentious. Cattell reminded his readers that Osler was the chief editorial writer for the *Medical News* while he was in Philadelphia. Cattell stated that "editors, like poets, are born, not made. And Osler was a born medical editor of the best type. . . ."[13] It is ironic that Cattell, considering his dubious history with Walt Whitman's brain (see below), chose poets as his comparator. Cattell frequently gave lectures about Osler and, according to one of his obituaries, had been working at the Surgeon General's Office in Washington, D.C. writing a book about Osler until shortly before his death.[1] Cattell also had a fondness for Osler's famous successor as physician-in-chief at Johns Hopkins, Lewellys F. Barker M.D. (1867–1943). The last book Cattell edited was a limited edition 534-page *Festschrift* in honor of Barker's sixty-fourth birthday in 1932.[25]

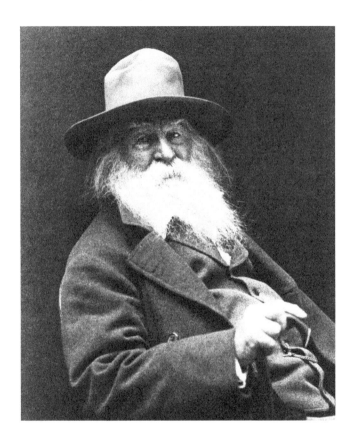

Figure 2.   Walt Whitman (photograph by George C. Cox, 1887).
Credit: US Library of Congress.

Cattell appears to have grown more contentious with age. In his declining years, he was involved in several public altercations with friends that, because of his prominence, resulted in local newspaper coverage. In 1931 he accused a friend, Major Joshua F. Bullitt (1856–1933), a prominent Philadelphia attorney, of slapping him during an argument and had him arrested.[1] According to newspaper coverage in 1933, Cattell sought a court order to prevent his friend of 50 years, "Dr. Daniel Longacker" (*sic*), from selling the hospital grounds of the Burlington County Hospital at sheriff's sale over a $3,000 debt. Cattell owned both the hospital and the grounds, but his friend held a mortgage on the land. This was eventually settled out of court.[1] Ironically, Cattell's friend had also been involved in the Walt Whitman scandal, as at the time of his death, Dr. Longaker (1858–1949) was Whitman's friend and personal physician, having replaced Silas Weir Mitchell (1829–1914) and William Osler. He was likely also a member of the Anthropometric Society in Philadelphia which, along with Cattell, played a role in the loss of Whitman's brain (see below).[26] Longaker attended Whitman's fateful autopsy,[27] which is discussed further below.

Cattell, who was single, died of heart disease at Mount Alto Veterans Hospital in Washington, D.C.; his brother arranged for his obituary to appear in *Science* a mere five days later on March 13, 1936.[28] A brief obituary appeared in the *Journal of the American Medical Association*.[29]

Phrenology, Walt Whitman, and Whitman's brain

The concept of phrenology (literally, science of the mind) was invented by Franz Joseph Gall (1758–1828) in Vienna during the last decade of the eighteenth century and was further developed by his sometime colleague Johann Cristoph (Gaspar) Spurzheim (1776–1832) in the first few decades of the nineteenth century. Phrenologists believed that palpable bumps on the skull reflected the degree of development of 27 different underlying areas ("organs") of the brain and that these bumps correlated with the degree of function of these 27 specific organs, which were believed to control 27 specific personality traits. Therefore, phrenologists believed that one could determine a person's psychological strengths and weaknesses by palpating his/her skull. While this pseudo-science was mostly discredited by the mid-nineteenth century, it had wide public appeal and a large impact on the medicine, science, and culture in the nineteenth century.[30–33] Writers, poets, and other intellectuals readily embraced the concept that their brain anatomy was somehow demonstrably better. While phrenology was no longer considered viable science by the second half of the nineteenth century, it gave birth to legitimate scientific interest in whether the brains of geniuses were structurally different than those of people of normal intelligence. Initially, it was simply assumed that the gifted would have heavier brains than the less gifted, but this did not prove to be uniformly true and so the relationship must be more complex requiring further study. Therefore, it was in vogue in some intellectual circles in the late-nineteenth century to donate one's brain to science for study after death. This brain donation society trend began in France in 1876 with the Société Mutuelle d' Autopsie (Society of Mutual Autopsy) and was soon replicated in Philadelphia in 1889 by the American Anthropometric Society (AAS), started by a small but prominent "who's who" group of former and current Philadelphia medical professors, including the Penn provost William Pepper (1843–1898), Penn anatomy professor Joseph Leidy (1823–1891), JMC neurology professor Francis X. Dercum (1856–1931), Penn physiology professor Harrison Allen (1841–1897), JMC anatomy professor Edward Anthony Spitzka (1876–1922), Penn professor of comparative anatomy and zoology Andrew Jackson Parker (1855–1892), Silas Weir Mitchell, and William Osler.[26,34,35] At one point there were reportedly 300 AAS members, but only a few went public and so it mostly functioned as a secret society.

Early in his career, Walt Whitman (Figure 2), like many of his colleagues, was a staunch believer in phrenology and he had his bumps charted at the Phrenological Museum of Orsen Fowler (1809–1887) and Horatio Wells (1820–1875) in 1849. Whitman's belief in phrenology was reflected in some lines and verses of his early poetry; however, in later editions, he had re-written these portions as he no longer believed in phrenology. Whitman cited the physician and poet Oliver Wendell Holmes (1809–1894) for his change of mind, quoting Holmes: "you might as easily tell how much money is in a safe feeling the knob on the door as tell how much brain a man has by feeling bumps on his head."[26] This change of beliefs is important when considering the likelihood that Whitman had actually personally agreed to donate his brain to the AAS shortly before his death, as several AAS physicians involved in his autopsy claimed. It should be noted that there was no documentation in writing to support this contention and Whitman's brother was staunchly opposed to him having an autopsy or brain removal. However, Whitman's personal physician Daniel Longaker stated that he had witnessed Whitman's verbal consent to an autopsy and this was corroborated by Harrison Allen.[26] As noted above, autopsy consent and organ retention abuse was not uncommon in late-nineteenth century Philadelphia[11]; it may have happened here!

When members of the Society died, the autopsies were initially performed by other Society members, primarily Allen and Dercum. However, since Allen and Dercum were busy as fee-for-service clinicians, scientists, and medical educators, they needed someone to assist with the autopsies and preserve the brains. The Society hired Henry Ware Cattell as it "prosector" in 1892. The prosector, not always a physician, was the person wielding the knife for the supervising physician. Whitman's autopsy was performed at Whitman's Mickle Street house. According to the autopsy report, Dercum removed the brain himself and then entrusted it to Cattell for transport, fixation, and storage.[26] Cattell performed the remainder of the autopsy, which concluded that Whitman died of pleurisy of the left lung, consumption of the right lung, general miliary tuberculosis, and parenchymatous nephritis, under Dercum's supervision.

Whitman's brain was removed, carried to Penn in a specialized transport sack impervious to fluid, weighed, and then fixed, likely in a glass jar containing Müller's fluid and absorbent cotton (n.b., formalin was not yet in use as a fixative). The process for brain fixation that Cattell used is likely as described in his autopsy textbook; proper fixation would have taken several months with fixative changes at regular intervals, initially daily, then every other day for three successive weeks, twice a week for the next three weeks, and then once a week for the next three weeks.[9] Had the brain been dropped after the fixation process was well underway, it would not have been destroyed. Therefore, Cattell's apparent story that the brain had been dropped by a bumbling assistant before it was fixed was credible, but this was only known by a few AAS insiders for the next 15 years.

In a 1907 Edward Spitzka, AAS member and professor of anatomy at JMC, published a 133-page-long paper entitled "A study of the brains of six eminent scientists and scholars belonging to the American Anthropometric Society, together with a description of the skull of Professor E. D. Cope" in the *Transactions of the American Philosophical Society*. While the science in the paper was not well-received, one sentence was memorable and he likely regretted its inclusion: "The brain of Walt Whitman, together with the jar in which it had been placed, was said to have been dropped on the floor by a careless assistant. Unfortunately, not even the pieces were saved."[36] Immediately, the most important revelation in what he believed to be a monumental scientific achievement was that Walt Whitman's brain had been dropped and destroyed. There was extensive coverage of this tidbit and little notice of Spitzka's science.

This indelicate but intriguing story is now believed to have influenced the filming of the movie *Frankenstein* (1931). When Mary Shelley wrote her novel in 1818, it was not generally known that the mind was centered in the brain and the technology to remove and preserve brains did not yet exist. Removing brains, placing them in fixative, and creating museum collections was not commonplace until the late-nineteenth century. Brian Burrell, in his meticulously researched paper "The strange fate of Whitman's brain," published in 2003 in the *Walt Whitman Quarterly Review*, not only attempts to ferret out what happened to Whitman's brain, but also builds a compelling case that the story of dropping the glass container holding Whitman's brain inspired the scene in the 1931 classic film in which the hunchback assistant Fritz drops the container labelled "normal brain" and is forced to provide Dr. Frankenstein a brain labelled "abnormal," that had been removed from a murder.[26]

What really happened to Walt Whitman's brain?

After Spitzka's article, it was widely reported that the brain had been dropped by Cattell's assistant and had been destroyed. However, before Spitzka's article, Cattell apparently tried to pre-empt future blame and added to the confusion using a story about the AAS that appeared in the *New York Herald* on 4 September 1898. In this story, Cattell had only removed, weighed, and examined Walt Whitman's brain, and then returned it to the body because the family objected to him taking it away. However, this version seems implausible as, had Cattell not taken the brain back to Penn, there would have been no way to accurately weigh it in Whitman's home. Burrell[26] likens this story as "the obfuscations of a guilty man" and notes the statements are inconsistent with Cattell's handwritten autopsy report which indicated that the brain was removed, fixed, and stored by the AAS. In general, none of the diverse stories offered over the years were internally consistent. Most people believed until recently that someone dropped the brain, and it had been destroyed. What could not be understood is why the fragments had been discarded as there still would have been some value in examining these. Less clear was whether it was an assistant or Cattell who destroyed Walt Whitman's brain. As Burrell noted, this statement was imprecise and could have two interpretations, since literally Cattell was serving as an assistant in the autopsy.

In December 2012, Henry Ware Cattell's recently discovered diary was sold on EBay to a private collector and this diary tells a radically different story; it documents that Cattell placed the brain in a jar of fixative but apparently forgot to cover it, and, when he later discovered this, the brain was "spoiled." Diary entries document, starting about October 14, 1892 (i.e., six and a half months after the autopsy), Cattell's sudden feelings of inadequacy, musings about his forgetfulness, concerns for his future career when his secret is found out, suicidal thoughts, and guilt about his continuing financial success, which was fully contingent on continuing to dodge culpability for the destruction of Walt Whitman's brain. It also appears that he had fired an assistant named Edwards (possibly the one he blamed), and that he was now being blackmailed by him.[36] On 15 May 1893, Cattell wrote:

> I am a fool, a damnable fool, with no conscious memory, or fitness for any learned position. I left Walt Whitman's brain spoil by not having the jar properly covered. Discovered it in the morning. This ruins me . . . How I ever got in such financial straits [I] do [not] know. When I broke with Edwards I should have told him to go to thunder. Borrowed over $500 more from P & M (Pa and Ma, his parents). They are too good & kind. I would have killed my self before this a dozen times over if it had not been for them.[36]

Clearly, Cattell had left Whitman's brain uncovered in a jar of fixative for possibly as much as six and a half months. The fixative was not regularly changed and had evaporated; Walt Whitman's brain had simply decomposed.

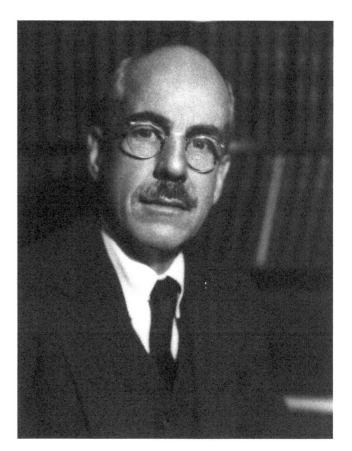

Figure 3. James McKeen Cattell (1860–1944), Henry Cattell's older brother, was the first professor of psychology in the U.S. and was hailed at the time of his death by the *New York Times* as "the dean of American Science."
Credit: National Library of Medicine.

In hindsight, negligence in maintaining Whitman's brain should have been suspected, and likely Spitzka knew this was the actual case when he published his paper, hence his less than definitive wording of the sentence that started the scandal ("was said to have been dropped on the floor by a careless assistant"). Spitzka was aware that several of the other elite brains under the care of the AAS had been destroyed through poor attention to fixation and/or long-term specimen maintenance while on Cattell's watch (1892–1897). Ironically, one of these was the brain of J. William White,[26] the surgeon Cattell later accused of having bought his professorship at Penn.

When Cattell stepped down as demonstrator of anatomy at Penn to devote more time to editing, he also ceased to be the prosector for the AAS.

Conclusion

Henry Ware Cattell did not achieve the level of success of either his father or his older brother. His anguish about his career is expressed sporadically throughout his diary.[36] The Reverend William C. Cattell papers are held by the Presbyterian Historical Society in Philadelphia and the James McKeen Cattell papers are held by the Library of Congress. It is telling that in stark contrast, Henry Ware Cattell's diary was held by an unknown person who sold it on EBay. If the brothers had sibling rivalries, there is no question the elder brother won!

Henry Ware and James McKeen Cattell (Figure 3) were apparently not close in life and little correspondence between them exists amongst J. McKeen's papers (Michael M. Sakol, personal communication, 8 July 2018). Perhaps, J. McKeen showed a tinge of regret for the estrangement when he arranged for Henry Ware Cattell's obituary to appear in his *Science*, a journal he edited, less than a week after Henry's death: it states: "Dr. Cattell was unmarried; his only near relative was his brother, Dr. J. McKeen Cattell."[28] For Henry, being snubbed by his brother likely made him cherish his longstanding relationship with Sir William Osler even more; however, a reality check suggests that this relationship may have been mostly one-sided. While Cattell wrote often and fondly about Osler, it does not appear that, even though Osler remained close to many of his former students and corresponded with them regularly, that Cattell was amongst this cohort, as the Osler Library of the History of Medicine at McGill, which is the repository for Osler's papers, does not have any record of correspondence with Cattell. It does, however, hold two more reprints of papers Cattell wrote about Osler.[37,38]

Unfortunately, because of a momentary lapse in concentration, Henry Ware Cattell's career will always be linked to Walt Whitman's brain—and now, even more strangely, with EBay. Ironically, this provides one more connection with Cattell's old teacher Sir William Osler. Osler, who died in Oxford in 1919, was a member of the AAS, and he insisted shortly before his death that his brain be sent to the Wistar Institute; like Whitman, he had an autopsy performed in his home; Osler's brain, after appropriate fixation, was hand-carried by a friend to Philadelphia, thus beginning the first of many afterlife adventures[34,35,39]; however, none of these scholarly papers describe its most recent travels. Osler biographer Michael Bliss recently wrote in an autobiography: "I . . . won an auction on eBay to buy a (microscope) slide of William Osler's brain tissue. . . . I paid about $1,400 for my little bit of Osler's brain."[40]

There is no record of whether Henry Ware Cattell was himself ever a member of the AAS. If he was, by the time he died, Spitzka was already dead and the AAS was no longer collecting the brains of intellectuals.

Acknowledgments

I thank the staff of the University of Pennsylvania Archives for access to the Henry Ware Cattell files; Lily Szczygiel of the Osler Library of the History of Medicine, McGill University; and Kristin Rodgers, collections curator of the Ohio State University Health Sciences Library Medical Heritage Center. I also thank Michael M. Sokal, PhD, for helpful insights on James McKeen Cattall. Finally, I thank Charlotte Monroe, the University of Calgary Interlibrary Loan service, and Thomas Kryton for digitally enhancing the figures.

References

1. Cattell, Henry Ware, 1887 MD file. University Archives, University of Pennsylvania, Philadelphia.

2. Cattell WC. *Memoir of William C. Cattell, D.D., LL.D. 1827–1898*. Philadelphia: JB Lippincott Co.; 1899: 1–104. https://archive.org/details/memoirofwilliamc00phil, Accessed 22 November 2020.

3. Pillsbury WB. Biographical memoir of James McKeen Cattell, 1860–1944. *National Academy of Sciences of the United States of America Biographical Memoirs*. 1947; 25: First Memoir. http://www.nasonline.org/publications/biographical-memoirs/memoir-pdfs/cattell-james-m.pdf. Accessed 22 November 2020.

4. Sokal MM. The unpublished autobiography of James McKeen Cattell. *American Psychologist* 1971; 26(7): 626–635.

5. Sokal MM. Science and James McKeen Cattell, 1894 to 1945. *Science* 1980; 209(4452):43–52.

6. Sokal MM. James McKeen Cattell, Nicholas Murray Butler, and academic freedom at Columbia University, 1902–1923. *History of Psychology* 2009; 12(2): 87–122.

7. Sokal MM. 2016. Launching a career in psychology with achievement and arrogance: James McKeen Cattell at the Johns Hopkins University, 1882–1883. *Journal of the History of the Behavioral Sciences* 2016; 52(1): 5–19.

8. Croskey JW. History of Blockley: a history of the Philadelphia General Hospital from its inception, 1731–1928. Philadelphia: F.A. Davis Company; 1929: 1–765.

9. Cattell HW. *Notes on the Demonstration of Morbid Anatomy (Including Autopsies) delivered in the Medical Department of the University of Pennsylvania before the third-year class*. Philadelphia: International Medical Magazine Company; 1894: 1–376.

10. Wright JR Jr. Sins of our fathers: Two of "The Four Doctors" and their roles in the development of techniques to permit covert autopsies. *Archives of Pathology and Laboratory Medicine* 2009; 133(12): 1969–1974.

11. Wright JR Jr. Why did Osler not perform autopsies at Johns Hopkins? *Archives of Pathology and Laboratory Medicine* 2008; 132(11): 1710 (letter).

12. Cattell HW. *Post-Mortem Pathology: A Manual of Technic of Post-Mortem Examination and the Interpretations to be Drawn Therefrom: A Practical Treatise for Students and Practitioners*. Philadelphia: J.B. Lippincott Company; 1906: 5–6.

13. Cattell HW. Osler, the Medical Editor. In [Abbott ME, ed.]. Bulletin No. IX of the *International Association of Medical Museums and Journal of Technical Methods. Sir William Osler Memorial Number. Appreciations and Reminiscences*. Montreal: Privately printed [Murray Printing Co., Limited, Toronto); 1926: 91–93.

14. Cattell HW. *Tait McKenzie's Medical Portraits*. Philadelphia: J.B. Lippincott Company; 1925.

15. R. Tait (Robert Tait) McKenzie Papers 1880–1940. University Archives, University of Pennsylvania, Philadelphia. https://www.archives.Penn.edu/faids/upt/upt50/mckenzie_rt.html. Accessed 22 November 2020.

16. Henry RS. *The Armed Forces Institute of Pathology: Its First Century, 1862–1962*. Washington, D.C.: Office of the Surgeon General Department of Army; 1964: 1–422.

17. Wright JR Jr, Baskin LB. Pathology and laboratory medical support for the American Expeditionary Forces by the US Army Medical Corps during World War i. Archives of Pathology and Laboratory Medicine 2015; 139(9): 1161–1172.

18. Medico-Chirurgical College and Hospital of Philadelphia Records 1881–1955 (bulk 1881–1922). https://www.archives.Penn.edu/faids/upc/upc50_3.html. Accessed 22 November 2020.

19. Charges University barter; Dr. Cattell says Pennsylvania professorships are rated even at $1,000,000. *The New York Times*, 8 December 1910.

20. Wright JR Jr. The Pennsylvania Anatomy Act of 1883: Weighing the roles of Professor William Smith Forbes and Senator William James McKnight. *Journal of the History of Medicine and Allied Sciences* 2016; 71(4): 422–446.

21. Cattell JM. Concerning the American University. *Popular Science Monthly* 1902; 61: 170–182.

22. Cattell JM. University control. *Science* 1906; 23(586): 475–477.

23. Cattell JM. *University Control*. New York City, New York: Science Press; 1913: 1–501.

24. Veblen T. *The Higher Learning in America: A Memorandum on the Conduct of Universities by Business Men*. Annotated edition, Baltimore: The Johns Hopkins Press; 2015: 1–240.

25. Cattell HW. *The Lewellys F. Barker M.D., LL.D., Festschrift in Honor of Sixty-Fourth Birthday on September 16th, 1931*. Philadelphia: J.B. Lippincott Company; 1932.

26. Burrell B. The strange fate of Whitman's brain. *Walt Whitman Quarterly Review* 2003; 20(Winter): 107–133.

27. Singley CJ. Longaker, Dr. Daniel (1858–1949). In: LeMaster LR, Kummings DD, eds. *Walt Whitman: An Encyclopedia*. New York: Garland Publishing; 1998. https://whitmanarchive.org/criticism/current/encyclopedia/en'try_238.html.Accessed 22 November 2020.

28. [Cattell JM]. Obituary: Henry Ware Cattell. *Science* 1936; 83(2150): 252.

29. Unsigned. Henry Ware Cattell (obituary). *Journal of the American Medical Association* 1936; 106(14): 1218–1219.

30. Stern MB. Emerson and phrenology. *Studies in the American Renaissance* 1983; n.v. (31 December): 213–228.

31. Greenblatt SH. 1995. Phrenology in the science and culture of the 19th century. *Neurosurgery* 1995; 37(4): 790–804 (discussion, 804–805).

32. Hagner M. Skulls, brains, and memorial culture: on cerebral biographies of scientists in the nineteenth century. *Science in Context* 2003; 16 (1–2): 195–218.

33. Boshears R, Whitaker H. Phrenology and physiognomy in Victorian literature. *Progress in Brain Research* 2013; 205: 87–112.

34. Rodin AE, Key JD. Osler's brain and related mental matters. *Southern Medical Journal* 1990; 83(2) 207–212.:

35. Feindel W. Osler's brain again. *Osler Library Newsletter* 1990; No. 64; page numbers 1–3. https://www.mcgill.ca/library/files/library/No64June1990.pdf. Accessed 26 November 2020.Spitzka, EA. 1907. A study of the brains of six eminent scientists and scholars belonging to the American Anthropometric Society, together with a description of the skull of Professor E. D. Cope. *Transactions of the American Philosophical Society* 1907; 21(new series) (4): 175–308.

36. Gosline SL. "I am a fool": Dr. Henry Cattell's private confession about what happened to Whitman's brain. Walt Whitman Quarterly Review 2014; 31(4): 158–162.

37. Cattell HW. "Omnes Viae Medicinae Propriae ad Oslerem docunt." *Medical Notes and Queries* 1926; 8(1): 1–6.

38. Cattell HW. Some personal reminiscences about Sir William Osler, Bart., Canada, the United States of America, Great Britain, and of the world. *International Clinics* 1930; 3(Series 40): 291–297.

39. Robb-Smith AHT. The examination of Sir William Osler's brain. *Osler Library Newsletter* 1989; No. 60: page number. 1 ; https://www.mcgill.ca/library/files/library/No60February1989.pdf Accessed 26 November 2020

40. Bliss M. *Writing History: A Professor's Life*. Toronto: Dundurn Press; 2011: 1–432.

Rudyard Kipling's Medical Addresses and his Relationship with Sir William Osler

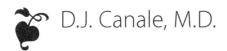 D.J. Canale, M.D.

During his career Rudyard Kipling (1865–1936) became one of the most widely read writers in his era of prose and poetry in England and soon afterwards in North America. Although he wrote both prose and poetry on a number of subjects, some readers have suggested that he has received less credit than he deserves in the literature of medical history.[1] E.P. Scarlett explains: "Because of the close relation which existed between Kipling and the medical profession no one outside the ranks of the profession has written with more understanding of the work of the physician."[2] He had reason to be familiar with medicine and doctors and wrote numerous stories and poems with medical themes. He had closely witnessed malaria, cholera, and typhoid epidemics in India and later while serving as a correspondent in South Africa during the Boer War. He estimated that 4,000 Boers were killed, with the English losing six-times as many due to preventable disease.[3] On returning to England after seven years in India Kipling himself suffered recurrent bouts of malaria and dysentery. In later years he suffered from recurrent bouts of duodenal ulcer.

This essay focuses on three addresses Kipling made to the medical profession: to the students at the Medical School of the Middlesex Hospital,[4] to the Royal College of Surgeons,[5] and to the Royal Society of Medicine.[6] Typically,

Presented at the forty-eighth annual meeting of the American Osler Society, Pittsburgh, Pennsylvania, on 14 May 2018.

This paper was previously published in the *Journal of Medical Biography* (2019; 27[4]: 204–212) and is reproduced with permission.

lay persons invited to address medical organizations will talk on whatever profession or activity in which they currently are involved. Kipling's addresses, on the other hand, focused on doctors and medical subjects from his view as a layman. While his writings, in both prose and poetry, touched on many medical subjects, I discovered that he gave only three published medical addresses which I obtained over the years and which became the subject of this paper.

Prologue

As a prologue to our story, it is important to briefly mention the high points of Kipling's life. He was born on 30 December 1865 in Bombay, India where his father was Professor of Architectural Sculpture at the newly founded School of Art in Bombay. Kipling's parents as did Rudyard himself considered themselves "Anglo-Indians" a term denoting people of British origin living in India.[7] His younger sister Alice, known as Trix, was born two and a half years later in 1868. In 1871 six-year-old Rudyard and three-year-old Trix were taken to Southsea, Portsmouth, to board with an older couple, and be educated in England as was common with Britishers living in India. Rudyard would later describe his stay as miserable; he felt he had become the black sheep of the new family in the "House of Desolution.[3, p. 19; 7, p. 20] At age twelve he resumed his education at the United Services College at Westward Ho, Devon.[7, p. 23] It was here that Kipling first began to write. Upon seeing Kipling's aptitude for writing the headmaster gave him the run of his library. At 13, Rudyard knew he belonged to a "different world from the other boys at his school or rather he belonged to two worlds. theirs and the world of literary London."[7, p. 28]

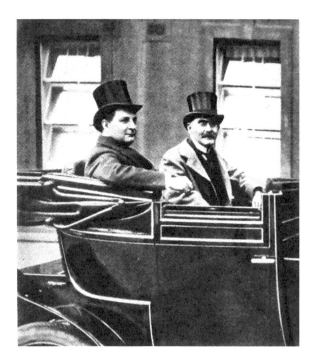

Figure 1.   Sir John Bland-Sutton and Rudyard Kipling on the way to Middlesex Hospital to deliver Kipling's address on "Doctors," 1 October 1908.

He finished his schooling in 1882. He did not have the grades nor did his family have the resources for him to further his education at Oxford. It was decided he would return to India. He was only 16 years old when he joined his family in Lahore, Punjab. His father Lockwood had arranged for him to become assistant editor of a small local newspaper, *The Civil and Military Gazette.* Later he was given a higher position on the *Pioneer* at Allahabad. Much of his writings during this time were based on his travels throughout northern India. He left India after seven years and returned to London in 1889.

Kipling married an American, Caroline "Carrie" Balestier (1862–1939), in London in 1892. They honeymooned in America and soon settled on the Balestier estate in Brattleboro, Vermont where they built a house they named "Naulakha" in which they lived for four years. Carrie's brother suffered financial loses which resulted in serious conflict between him Carrie and Rudyard. Differences were not reconciled and the Kiplings left Brattleboro in 1896 and returned to England where they settled in East Sussex.[7, p. 239] In September 1902 they purchased "Batemans," a seventeenth-century Jacobean stone house in a lonely valley in Burwash, East Sussex.

Kipling's success and fame continued to grow. The Nobel Prize had been established in 1901, and Kipling, awarded the Nobel Prize for Literature in 1907, became the first English honored recipient. He turned down the honor of becoming Poet Laureate and refused a knighthood. The Kiplings lived in Burwash until he died. Kipling suffered for years from duodenal ulcers. While in London he suffered a severe gastrointestinal hemorrhage and underwent surgery for a perforated duodenal ulcer by Sir Alfred Webb-Johnson (1880–1958). He died one-week later, on 17 January 1936, at age 70.[8]

Address Delivered to the medical students of the Middlesex Hospital, London

Kipling's first address to the medical profession was titled "Doctors" and was delivered to the students at the Medical School of the Middlesex Hospital on 1 October 1908.[4] The address called the attention of an unreflecting generation to certain aspects of a doctor's life which are persistently ignored. He opened by stating there are two classes of mankind in the world, doctors, and patients, with the average patient looking upon the average doctor very much as the non-combatant looks upon the troops fighting on his behalf. The fight is against death, which is always bound to win in the long term. We look to the physician whose business is to make the best terms with death and to see how his attacks can best be delayed or diverted. He noted that in due time the students, will be drafted into the permanently mobilized army which is always under fire against death.

Kipling told the students they would have no working hours that anybody is bound to Respect: "Have you ever heard of any bill for an eight-hour day for doctors?" With becoming a doctor, he said, come privileges of access in emergences to areas denied to ordinary persons and the power of quarantine. He told the students they would be exposed to the contempt of the gifted amateur—the gentleman who thinks he knows by intuition everything it has taken the doctor years to learn and those with undisciplined emotions who would limit and hamper medical research. (The surgeon Stephen Paget [1855–1926] invited Kipling to become vice-president of the Research Defence Society in 1908 to defend the use of animals in scientific experiments.[9]) In closing, Kipling noted that medicine's high ideals and lofty ethics bring tremendous privilege, yet the profession is marked by the highest death rate for its practitioners of any profession in the world. His wish for the students was what all men desire, enough work to do and the strength enough to it.

The Spectator on 10 October 1908 reported that "The public no less than the profession should return thanks to Mr. Kipling. He has done what only a man of literary genius can do, he has heightened and deepened an almost universal sentiment by its strong and gracious expression."[10] Further, writes Victor Bonney, "No writer has depicted the technical and spiritual aspects of medicine so understandingly as Kipling and therein medical men are indebted to him forever."[11] This address illustrates Kipling's remarkable awareness of the challenges a young physician can expect to encounter.

Address delivered to The Royal College of Surgeons, England

Kipling's second address to the medical profession was at the Annual Dinner of the Royal College of Surgeons, London, 14 February 1923.[5] This date is the anniversary of the birthday of England's great surgeon-naturalist John Hunter (1728–1793). Hunter is acknowledged to be the founder of experimental and surgical pathology. Kipling's friend and personal surgeon, Sir John Bland-Sutton (1855–1936) gave an oration in the afternoon and Sir Anthony A. Bowlby (1855–1929) delivered the Annual Hunterian Oration. Kipling's tribute to the medical profession was delivered at the annual dinner. Kipling's address was printed in full in the *Times* newspaper edition on 22 February 1923 and by Lieutenant Colonel Fielding Garrison (1870–1935) in *The Military Surgeon*, August 1923.[12] (Of interest is that my copy of his address was the limited first U.S. edition printed for copyright purposes. Earlier Kipling had begun to copyright his works in the U.S. to prevent the pirating of his work by American publishers.)

Kipling introduced himself as a "dealer in words," and said, "words are, of course, the most powerful drug used by mankind."[5, p. 3] He then cited an ancient legend wherein man's divinity was stolen by the wisest of the Gods, Brahma who hid it inside man himself, where man would never dream of looking for it. The ancient practitioners, medicine-men, and the astrologer-physician searched for man's eternal woes, but their search was in vain.

Later when the embargoes on the healing art were lifted and the physician was permitted to look openly into the bodies of mankind, the surgeon, as he had become known, found more wonders beneath the knife than ever before. Man's boldest dream was that one would find the ultimate secret of his being where Brahma had hidden it. Kipling noted that the surgeon's calling should exact the utmost that man can give, and that the surgeon should be prepared to dismiss every preconceived idea and accept those new discoveries. Furthermore, such "virtue is not reached or maintained except by a life's labor, a single-minded devotion."[5, p. 6] He acknowledged the gratitude of the layman, however: "the true reward is the dearly-prized, because purchasable or non-purchasable, acknowledgment of one's fellow craftsmen."[5, p. 7] Kipling notes the importance of anatomy which ushered in scientific surgery. This was primarily the work of the great Flemish anatomist Andreas Vesalius (1514–1564) and the publication of his *De Fabrica Human Corporis* (1543) in which human anatomy was first accurately described.

Address delivered to the members of The Royal Society of Medicine

Kipling's third address to the medical profession, "Healing by the Stars," was delivered to members of the Royal Society of Medicine on 15 November 1928.[6] Here, Kipling described himself as a "storyteller"[6, p. 3] and recounts a true story which occurred nearly 300 years before. The story is about Nicholas Culpeper (1616–1654), an astrologer-physician practicing in Spitalfields who was called in for a second opinion for a friend's maidservant in whom the local practitioner had diagnosed as plague, or the Black Death, as it was called in England. Culpeper consulted a horoscope and inquired of the heavens what the malady was. The face of the heavens indicated it was not plague but just smallpox and the girl recovered. Though such a theory might be preposterous, Culpeper believed that to understand the mystery of healing one must look as high as the stars. Kipling noted that in addition to a horoscope, Culpeper "used a pharmacopoeia and therapeutics that would have made a West African witch doctor jealous."

Kipling then mused about what Culpeper's reaction to the state of medicine would be if he returned to earth at the present time. Culpepper would be shown tissues that had been subjected to the influence of radium; but he, putting more emphasis on theory than research, would submit that tissue changes were more related to happenings in the heavens than to new discoveries in medicine. He would note that the significant medical revelations over the past few years have made men specialize more narrowly. One might ask what it matters if just a fraction of an idea helps advance medicine in the modern era. Is that not analogous to reaching to the heavens for answers where new advances in medicine surpass the wildest dreams of the ancient practitioners?

Sir William Osler

Kipling's address "Healing by the Stars," introduces one to his relationship with Sir William Osler (1849–1919). Osler mentioned Kipling in his address "The Master-Word in Medicine" to undergraduates at the University of Toronto in 1903. Osler borrowed the language for the title from Mowgli's "master word" in Kipling's *Jungle Book*.[13]

Kipling and Osler first met in Oxford in June of 1907 at Lord (George) Cruzon's (1859–1925) first Encaenia ceremony in which Kipling was awarded an Honorary D.Litt. The Kiplings stayed with the Oslers at 13 Norham Gardens in Oxford and both families got along well with Lady (Grace Revere) Osler (1854–1928) being especially charmed by Carrie. On 19 July 1907, William Osler wrote to his friend Mrs. Mabel Brewster: "I sent you a paper with an account of the Encaenia and the reception to Mark Twain (1835–1910) and Kiplings. The latter stopped with us—such a jolly fellow, so full of fun with an extraordinary interest in everything. Mrs K is very bright and we fell in love with them both. . . ."[14]

In 1910 Kipling sent Osler a copy of his just-published book, *Rewards and Fairies*.[15] Inscribed on the title page was, "Excellent herbs had our fathers of old." There was also a note of October 3rd. "Dear Osler, Here with my book of Tales. I wouldn't bother you with it except for ick Culpeper and [René] Laennec [1781–1826] for whom I feel you are in a way responsible. Yours very sincerely, Rudyard Kipling.[16]

Osler likely introduced Kipling to Nicholas Culpeper and René Laennec in Oxford in 1907, and both appeared in the children's stories of *Rewards and Fairies.* It was from Osler that Kipling acquired an interest in the history of medicine.[7, p. 421] After publishing this book, Kipling said the book "would need to be read by children before people realized it was meant for grown-ups."[7, p. 269] This collection of short stories contained two medical stories. "Marklake Witches" was based on René Theophile Laennec with his little wooden trumpets and his diagnosis of tuberculosis. Laennec, who became a famous physician and whose description of tuberculosis Osler felt to be "perhaps the most masterly chapter in clinical medicine."[17] "A Doctor of Medicine" deals with the "physician-astrologer" Nicholas Culpeper. In this children's story Dan and Una (modeled after Kipling's children John and Elsie) are introduced to Nicholas Culpeper by Puck the fairy. Culpeper tells of his being faced with an outbreak of the plague in Sussex. One evening Culpeper notes the death of three rats described as creatures of the moon; under the influence of Mars the rats die. By consulting divine astrology Culpeper concludes that rats are the source of the plague and urges the villagers to "take a bat and kill a rat."[13, p. 269] Osler likely drew Kipling's attention to the 1908 India Plague Commission report that concluded for the first time that Bubonic plague in man is entirely dependent on the disease in the rat.[18] Culpeper could not have known anything about the connection between rats and plague.[19] Culpeper on the other hand was said to be a charlatan who mixed astrology with medicine in sufficient proportion to suit the popular taste. Engle, however, did not consider Culpeper a quack and noted that Kipling "had long been interested in Culpeper.[20]

The late Alex Sakula, a fellow Oslerian, wrote a splendid paper on the correspondence between Kipling and Osler.[16] They greatly admired each other but were together only four times—not surprising since both were at the height of their careers and remarkably busy. Both lost their only sons during the great war; John Kipling (1897–1915) died on 25 September 1915 during the Battle of Loos and Revere Osler died on 28 August 1917 during the Third Battle of Ypres. The last time Kipling and Osler were together was on 1 April 1919, in London. Osler was elected to "The Club" (Dr. Johnson's Club) the most famous of dining clubs of the world. Osler noted "Kipling was present and in very good form." Osler died later that year in December.[14, ii: 639]

A fourth address by Kipling to a medical audience took place on December 15, 1927, and was given to the Fountain Club, a dining club associated with St. Bartholomew's Hospital. This address is cited in "Uncollected Speeches" edited by Thomas Pinney (b. 1932). This unpublished address is recorded in part in the Minute Book of the Fountain Club. Kipling spoke of the barber surgeons and the physician apothecaries but described the physicist as the "accoucheur of new ideas" who would, in due course, short circuit both the physician and surgeon. Whether indeed the physicist deserves such praise, one cannot help noticing the remarkable contributions of the physicist to the development of the CT and MRI scans, PET scans and proton beam radiation, cardiac ultrasound, and robotic surgery, to cite a few examples.[21]

Summary

Rudyard Kipling was one of the most widely read writers of prose and poetry during his lifetime. His wide travels—he was born in India and lived in England and The United States and made frequent visits to South Africa—led to many encounters with physicians and medicine. His unique addresses to the medical profession reveal his knowledge of medical subjects. His three major medical addresses concern medical subjects in contrast to most laymen addressing physicians, who typically speak about their own areas of expertise.

Acknowledgment

The author is grateful to Margaret Seicshnaydre for her valuable assistance and contributions to this manuscript.

References

1. Beatty WE. Some medical Aspects of Rudyard Kipling. *The Practitioner* 1975; 215: 532–542.
2. Scarlett EP. The medical jackdaw: Kipling and the doctors. *Group Practice* 1962;11: 634–638.
3. Kipling R. *Something of Myself.* London: Macmillan and Co.; 1937: 165.
4. Kipling R. *Doctors. An Address Delivered to the Students of the Medical School of the Middlesex Hospital, 1st. October, 1908.* London: Macmillan and Co.; 1908.
5. Kipling R. *Address at the Annual Dinner of the Royal College of Surgeons London, February 14, 1923.* Garden City, New Jersey: Doubleday, Page & Co.; 1923.
6. Kipling R. *Healing by the Stars. Address to the Members of the Royal Society of Medicine November 15, 1928.* Garden City, New Jersey: Doubleday, Doran & Co.; 1928.
7. Carrington C. *Rudyard Kipling: His Life and Work.* London: Macmillan & Co.; 1955: 14.
8. Ricketts H. *Rudyard Kipling: A Life.* New York: Carrol & Graf; 1999: 388.
9. Sheehan G. Some of Kipling's medical acquaintances. *Kipling Journal*, Reader's Guide, June 23, 2004.
10. *The Spectator*, 10 October 1908, 534.
11. Bonney V. Kipling and Doctors. *Kipling Journal* 1937; 42(June): 48–56.
12. Garrison FH. Kipling on John Hunter. *Military Surgeon* 1923; 36(August): 141–143.
13. Kipling R. *The Jungle Book.* London: Macmillan and Co.; 1902: 48.
14. Cushing H. *The Life of Sir William Osler.* Oxford: The Clarendon Press;1925; ii: 97.
15. Kipling R. *Rewards and Fairies.* London: Macmillan and Co.; 1910.
16. Sakula A. Rudyard Kipling, Sir William Osler, and the History of Medicine. *Kipling Journal* 1983; 57(226) (June): 10–24.

17. Osler W. *The Evolution of Modern Medicine.* New Haven: Yale University Press; 1922: 204.

18. Osler W. *The Principles and Practice of Medicine.* Seventh edition, London: D. Appleton and Co.; 1909: 240.

19. Horton, Dr. A Doctor of Medicine. *Kipling Journal* 1956; 23(120) (December): 10–12.

20. Engle G. Excellent herbs had our fathers of old. *Kipling Journal* 2003; 77(306) (June): 34–49.

21. Pinney T, ed. *Rudyard Kipling's Uncollected Speeches: A Second Book of Words. With a Checklist of His Speeches.* Greensboro, North Carolina: ELT Press; 2008.

Friendship, Philanthropy, and Fish Sauce: Sir William Osler and Charles W. Dyson Perrins

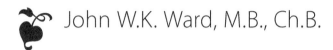 John W.K. Ward, M.B., Ch.B.

J. Brett Langstaff (1889–1985), in an article entitled "Youthful Recollections," highlighted the hospitality he received at 13 Norham Gardens, Oxford, even after he had moved to London to head the Magdalen College Mission.[1] The last paragraph of Langstaff's article deals with a 1919 visit to the Osler residence:

> On one of my last visits to that house, so hospitable as to be known as "The Open Arms," I was sitting alone with Lady Osler when a long-distance call took her to a nearby telephone. It was a professional emergency for Sir William from Scotland, and so poor was the connection that Lady Osler could not distinguish the name of the person calling. After a struggle Lady Osler asked to have the name spelled out. Then I heard her exclaim, "I have it now. It's Perrins, as in fish sauce!" When she returned from the phone she was flushed with confusion because it really was the Mr. Perrins who had made a fortune selling Lee (*sic*) and Perrins Sauce. Later I learned that Sir William's immediate response to this call, despite the weather and his own unfitness at the time, brought on the bronchopneumonia from which he died four days after Christmas 1919.

The purpose of this article is to elaborate on "Perrins, as in fish sauce," who was clearly Charles William Dyson Perrins (1864–1958) (Figure 1), to explore his relationship with Osler, which led to Osler's last consultation, and to describe briefly how this consultation had fatal consequences for Osler.

Presented at the forty-seventh meeting of the American Osler Society, Atlanta, Georgia, on 12 April 2017.

Dyson Perrins

Perrins was born in May 1864, the youngest and only son among five children born to James Dyson Perrins (1823–1887) and his wife and cousin, Frances Sarah Perrins (1827–1918). He was the grandson of William Perrins, a manufacturing chemist who in 1823 had entered a partnership with another chemist, John Wheeley Lea.[2,3] Their business was essentially a pharmacy and several shops until the development of the Worcestershire sauce. Multiple stories exist about the origin of the sauce. One such is that an alleged governor of Bengal, freshly back from India asked the partners to create a facsimile of his favourite sauce but never returned for the result. However, no such person has been found despite extensive research to fit this description.[4] In the early nineteenth century chemists were known to experiment by trial and error using ingredients by trying things in combination. It is possible Lea and Perrins discovered the original which in 1835 tasted unpleasant. Serendipitously, they discovered that age and storage improved the sauce's flavour. In 1837 they began selling it locally, and its fame quickly spread throughout Britain and the Empire and then to the Americas. By the 1860s they had sold all the chemist shops, moved to new premises and concentrated on Lea & Perrins Sauce, a source of great wealth.

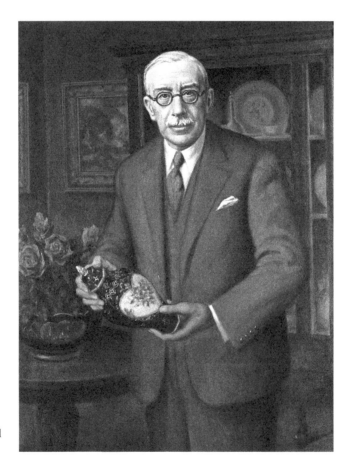

Figure 1.   *Charles William Dyson Perrins*, by Ernest Waldron West (1904–1994).
Credit: Museum of Royal Worcester.

Dyson's parents, James and Frances, had enormous influence on him, particularly on the importance of public service and philanthropy. They were generous with time and money in civic and business life and donated widely to academic, hospital and church charities.

At the age of fourteen Dyson became a boarder at Charterhouse, a public school with a strong Christian tradition. His school reports show he was stronger at mathematics than the classics. He entered Queen's College, Oxford, in 1882 to read law but left two years later without a degree, possibly because the course was not to his liking. He joined the British Army in the Highland Light Infantry and in 1889 became a captain. He developed a love of Scotland where he met and married his wife, Catherine Gregory (c.1865–1922). The wedding was a huge affair at St Giles' Cathedral in Edinburgh and the couple were to be blessed with five children.

Dyson bought the Ardross Estate in Ross-shire, complete with castle, as a holiday retreat and then bought neighboring properties so that in all he owned 42,000 acres in Scotland, with extensive grouse moors and deer forests. He developed these for the local people and provided much additional employment at a time of agricultural depression, in addition to giving sports facilities, a railway, a golf club, a bowling club and a centre in Alness with a library, reading room and billiard room.

Dyson's father died suddenly in 1887 and he had become a wealthy man. However, he didn't become a partner in Lea and Perrins till 1894 when he was thirty, two years after Wheeley Lea had retired. He had, however, moved to the family home, Davenham, in Great Malvern, and in 1891 been admitted to the board of Governors of Worcester Porcelain, a position no doubt stimulated by his hobby of collecting old Worcester ware. In 1898 he loaned the company £20,000 and in 1902 became chairman. In 1897 he became a justice of the peace and was elected mayor of Worcester. He became high sheriff of Worcestershire in 1899, and in 1903 gave financial support for a new Malvern library.

In 1904 Lea and Perrins was given the royal warrant by Edward VII, and in 1905 Dyson gave Malvern a new hospital. His multiple gifts and bequests during a long life—he died aged 93 in 1958 and was survived by his second wife, Frieda, whom he married in 1923, one year after Catherine died of a stroke—were too numerous to recount here. The Royal Worcester Museum remains a tangible testimony to his generosity.

In 2006 I presented a paper to the Osler Club of London entitled "William Osler and the Palace in Pall Mall."[5] This paper highlighted Osler's membership of the Royal Automobile Club (RAC) and his use of it for entertaining, especially during the XVIIth International Medical Congress of 1913. Osler was elected in September 1908, having been proposed by Harry Edwin Bruce Bruce-Porter (1869–1948) and seconded by Lord Montague of Beaulieu (1866–1929).[6] Dyson Perrins was also a member of this club. He was elected on 5 February 1908 and remained a member till his death in 1958. RAC archives do not have records of his proposers. Thus, Osler and Perrins possibly met through the Royal Automobile Club, but more likely through each of their memberships of both the Bibliographical Society and the Roxburghe Club.

The Bibliographical Society was founded in 1892 to promote and encourage study and research in historical, analytical and textual bibliography. Both Osler and Perrins were elected in 1906 and almost certainly attended the same meetings. In 1906 the club was dwindling in activities and numbers but Alfred W. Pollard (1859–1944), the secretary at that time was later to write that Osler was to provide inspiration for its flourishing. Osler was to become its president from 1913 till his death. Perrins, with characteristic modesty, steadfastly refused nomination as president but accepted the vice-presidency from 1925.[7]

The Roxburghe Club, a prestigious group with limited membership, is dedicated to printing unpublished documents and reprinting rare texts, among them unknown or neglected works of English literature and history.[8] The club was founded on 16 June 1812 when a group of book collectors and bibliophiles dined on the eve of the sale of the greatest private library of the age, that of John Ker, Third Duke of Roxburghe (1740–1804). The diners resolved to perpetuate the occasion by dining each year on 17 June, the anniversary of the sale. The early members reprinted fifteenth- and sixteenth-century pamphlets, usually in verse form, and gave the reprints to each other. As the club grew, the annual subscription was put towards publishing club books. The book collection is currently held in the Society of Antiquaries in London.

Perrins had a long appreciation of early medieval illuminated manuscripts and woodcuts, and most of his vast collection was assembled between 1900 and 1920. He once explained that he bought books with pictures so that he and Catherine, whose health was poor, could look at them together in the evenings. Elected to the Roxburghe Club in 1908 as member no. 178, Perrins chose as his presentation volume a 1495 edition of *Epistoli et Evangeli et Lectioni vulgari in Lingua Toscani*, which reproduced more than 500 Florentine woodcuts. Other books produced by the club, based on items Perrins owned, included the *Topographical Study of Rome* (1581) by Etienne de Perac.

In 1914 Osler was elected to the Roxburghe Club as member no. 192, but he apparently never produced a volume for the club members, probably because of the Great War. Items relating to the club in the *Bibliotheca Osleriana* include the 1812 sale catalogue, books of club regulations, membership lists, Perrins's presentation volume, and other club books.[9] Some of the club books contain papers relating to allied subjects, such as Osler's manuscript account of a dinner on 3 June 1919 on which he commented: "This was the first dinner since the War. We toasted Yates Thompson on the success of his sale held today, 30 items, £52,000!" This sale took place at Sotheby's and it was here that Perrins bought the *Winchester Binding*, a manuscript in original condition produced around 1150, which in 1947 he gave to Winchester Cathedral to accompany its twelfth-century *Winchester Bible*.

Osler's interest in rare books, especially those relating to science and medicine, is well known. In August 1913 Osler was chairman of the Section of Medicine at the XVIIth London International Medical Congress and entertained the officers and presenters of his section to dinner in the Great Gallery of the Royal Automobile Club. Despite his heavy workload and entertaining he also presented a paper to the History of Medicine Section in the Royal Society of Medicine. That paper entitled "The Earliest Medical Books to 1470" formed the basis of *Incunabula Medica, 1467–80*,[10] published in 1923 by the Bibliographical Society with a preface by Osler's dear friend, the bibliographer and scholar of English literature, Professor A.W. Pollard, whose own father had been a physician.[11]

Osler and Perrins were united by their love of books and their willingness to share their libraries, Osler with his latch-keyers and Perrins with friends and academics. Harvey Cushing tells us that opposite the entry for 13 June 1915 Osler wrote in his account book: "Perrins Library." This entry is explained by Pollard's introduction to *Incunabula Medica*. Osler had planned a brief bookman's holiday and asked two friends to accompany him. They left Oxford in Osler's car and that evening they reached Gloucester. After Sunday service the next day they visited the Cathedral library. The afternoon brought the small party to Malvern, and in Davenham they had a wonderful time with Dyson Perrins' illuminated manuscripts.[12]

Books were not the only bond between Osler and Perrins; there was also their common interest in the welfare of Oxford University. In 1912 William Henry Perkin, Jr., FRS (1860–1929), hitherto professor of organic chemistry at Manchester, was appointed Wayneflete professor of chemistry at Oxford with a fellowship at Magdalen College, which Waynflete had founded. Perkin had demanded a new laboratory before accepting his chair. Unfortunately, the Chancellor's Endowment Fund could only provide £15,000, a sum insufficient to allow a start to building. Then as now, fund-raising was an important facet of university life. A lunch was held at Magdalen hosted by Sir Herbert Warren (1853–1930), the college president, with Perkin in attendance and Dyson Perrins as a guest. Perrins heard of the problems with the new laboratory and promptly pledged £5,000 for equipment and £20,000 as a permanent endowment to make the laboratory function, independent of student fee income or of being a financial burden to the university. It was typical of Dyson's dry humour that on leaving Magdalen he was heard to comment, "This is the most expensive lunch I have ever had!" In the McGill Library is this letter from William Osler to Warren:

Dear Warren,

Congratulations on the Perrins Gift which we owe to you. It is splendid. Perrins wrote so enthusiastically about it and he was delighted with Perkin. I hope the news came in time to be announced today.

Sincerely yours,

W. Osler[13]

This letter raises the possibility that it was Osler who suggested Perrins as a possible benefactor to Perkin and Warren. Osler knew Perkin's father, who had founded the aniline dye industry, must have known Perkin, and was a friend of Warren, who was among those who encouraged Osler to move from Baltimore to Oxford. The Magdalen College archives do not yield an answer, but the current archivist, Robin Darwall-Smith, suggests a scenario. He observes that by 1915 Warren was one of the most eminent figures in Oxford. Warren had been vice-chancellor (1906–1910), was currently professor of poetry, was one of the foremost lion hunters and networkers of his age, and, moreover, the Prince of Wales had recently been a student at Magdalen. With Perkin, a fellow at Magdalen, and others pondering what to do about chemical facilities, and thoughts of Perrins as a possible benefactor, Warren invited Perrins to lunch along with the Wayneflete professor of chemistry. Once in Warren's charming clutches, there would be no escape for Perrins! The new laboratory was completed in 1916. In a speech of thanks to Perrins by Warren he gave some insight into Perrins's character: "Mr Perrins had not sought in any way to glorify himself. He gave them an endowment, and the proposal to attach his name to this fund was not Mr. Perrins' aim but that of the Hebdomadal Council."

Perrins received an honorary degree of Doctor of Civil Law from Oxford as testimony to his munificence. The number and sums involved in Perrins' long life beyond Osler's death in 1919 are beyond the remit of this paper but they were huge, local and general, cultural, educational, and health related.

Epilogue

Brett Langstaff's recollection of the telephone from "Perrins, as in fish sauce" provides a crucial detail to the events leading to Osler's death, as recounted by Osler biographers Harvey Cushing and Michael Bliss.

According to Harvey Cushing, the Oslers had returned to Oxford from a holiday on the Isle of Jersey on 12 September 1919 and were looking forward to a quiet time before the distractions of term time.[14] However a note in Osler's account book tells how this plan was interrupted: "Left here the night of Sept. 22nd to see Mrs. M. in Glasgow with Drs. [Robert Barclay] Ness, [Agnes Wallace] Cameron and [William Buchanan] Armstrong. Went on to Edinburgh, stayed with Lovell Gulland. Saw Harvey Littlejohn and others."

According to Bliss, the Jersey holiday had invigorated Sir William and over the six weeks there he had regained all of the 21 pounds he had lost during the war years. Back home he responded to a request for a consultation in Glasgow and, on 23 September 1919, accompanied by the three doctors, he saw Mrs. Fulton Martin, who had "one of those remarkable Erythema cases (all sorts of skin lesions and for three months on and off consolidation of both lower lobes)."[15] It is unknown what Osler said or prescribed. His bill for the consultation was £525, probably based on the common British travel fee for consulting of a guinea (21 shillings) a mile. This large bill was paid.

From Glasgow, Osler went to Edinburgh to see old friends and talk with medical people about future research grants that he would have a hand in doling out, having agreed to serve on the first government grants committee. While in Edinburgh he stayed with Dr. G. Lovell Gulland (1862–1941). Sir William returned to Oxford on 28 September. Lady Osler, in a letter to her sister on the following day, indicates the difficulties and tiring nature of his journey home due to a railroad strike, necessitating a long trip in an "old and slow" automobile. He took to his bed with a cold, which led to pneumonia, which led to lung abscess and empyema, from which he died on 29 December 1919.

Some residual questions remain about Osler's final consultation. Why was Perrins involved in calling Osler rather than a Glasgow doctor or a member of the Martin family? Why did Sir William respond so promptly and keenly? Bliss has suggested that Osler was keen to recoup the costs of his Jersey holiday but the more likely reason is his close relationship with Perrins.

Osler never begrudged Perrins for setting in motion the events that led to his fatal illness. On 26 November 1919, he wrote to Sue Chapin, his sister-in-law: "Complete change of pelvic crockery—the Crown Derby replaced by Worcester on account of my affection for Mr. Perrins, the President of the Co. These little acts of kindness cost nothing and are appreciated in this hard world."[16] The reference refers to the financial difficulties of the Royal Worcester China Company after the Great War, and how Perrins saved the company out of his own pocket. Thus, Osler appreciated Perrins to the end for his friendship and munificence.

Acknowledgments

I thank for archival assistance Lily Szczygiel of the Osler Library of the History of Medicine, McGill University, Robin Darwall-Smith, former archivist of Magdalen College, University of Oxford, and Trevor Dunmore, librarian of the Royal Automobile Club, London. I also thank my wife, Ruth Ward, for her unfailing support and suggestions.

References

1. Langstaff JB. Youthful Reminiscences, *Journal of the American Medical Association* 1969; 210(12): 2233–2235.
2. Rogers D. In *Oxford Dictionary of National Biography* (online): 2005.
3. Handley J. *The Quiet Hero.* Malvern: Aspect Design; 2010: 7.
4. Keogh B. *The Secret Sauce: A History of Lea and Perrins.* Leaper Books; 1997.
5. Ward J. William Osler and the Palace in Pall Mall. Osler Club of London archives; 2006.
6. Royal Automobile Club Year Book. 1909; RAC archives, London.
7. Pollard G. Obituary Notice of C.W. Perrins, *The Library* (Journal of the Bibliographic Society): volumes s5–XIII. Issue 2, June 1958, 129.
8. Timms J. *Clubs and Club Life in London.* London: Chatto and Windus; 1886: 159–165.
9. Osler W. *Bibliotheca Osleriana.* Oxford: Clarendon Press; 1929: Entries 4634, 4635, 4731, 6144, 7319–7333.
10. Osler W. *Incunabula Medica: A Study of the Earliest Printed Medical Books: 1467–1480.* Bibliographical Society, Oxford. Oxford University Press; 1923.
11. Greg W, revised by Woodhuysen H. *Oxford Dictionary of National Biography* (online): 2004.
12. Pollard AW. *Incunabula Medica.* Bibliographical Society, Oxford. Oxford University Press; 1923: Preface, vii.
13. William Osler to Herbert Warren, undated. Osler Letter Index, CUS417/34.50. Osler Library of the History of Medicine, McGill University.
14. Cushing H. *The Life of Sir William Osler.* Oxford: Clarendon Press; 1925: ii: 668.
15. Bliss M. *William Osler: A Life in Medicine.* Oxford: Oxford University Press; 1999: 467.
16. William Osler to Susan Chapin, 26 November 1919. Osler Letter Index, CUS417/130.94, Osler Library of the History of Medicine, McGill University.

SECTION IV

 Influences and the Osler Diaspora

Diabetes Mellitus and Pernicious Anemia: Interrelated Therapeutic Triumphs Discovered Shortly after William Osler's Death

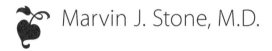 Marvin J. Stone, M.D.

Two monumental breakthroughs in medicine—the discovery of insulin for treatment of diabetes mellitus and the treatment of pernicious anemia with liver extract—took place within seven years of Sir William Osler's death. The purpose of this paper is to briefly review Osler's relationship to some of the protagonists in these exceptional events.

Diabetes mellitus and the discovery of insulin

Sir William Osler, who is sometimes considered the father of modern medicine, died in Oxford on 29 December 1919 at the age of 70. Less than one year later, Frederick Banting (1891–1941), a young surgeon, began research to find effective treatment for diabetes mellitus (DM) at the University of Toronto. J.J.R. Macleod (1876–1935) (director of physiology) granted Banting space, funding, and supplies for his research although Banting had never done any previous research.[1,2]

Presented at the forty-ninth annual Meeting of the American Osler Society, Montreal, Canada, on 14 May 2019. This paper is dedicated to the memory of Michael Bliss. It was previously published in *Baylor University Medical Center Proceedings* 2020;33(4):689–692 and is reproduced with permission.

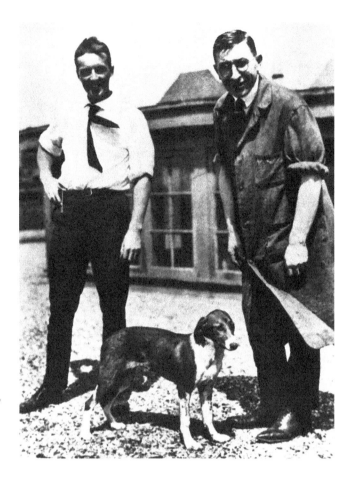

Figure 1. Charles Best, Frederick Banting, and an experimental subject.
Credit: Wikimedia Commons:

Charles Best (1899–1948), a medical student, joined the project soon after it began. Banting and Best's involvement in the DM research at Toronto was determined by the outcome of a coin flip.[3]

In 1921, Banting and Best isolated what came to be known as insulin from canine pancreatic extract (Figure 1). Banting injected pancreatic extract in himself for the first time in November 1921. No obvious reaction occurred, and no blood or other tests were performed. Biochemist J.B. Collip (1892–1965) improved the purification procedure. The first American patient was treated with purified pancreatic extract in May 1922 and showed remarkable improvement in blood sugar and diabetic control.[1,3] Similar results were obtained in other patients. In 1923, the Nobel Prize in Physiology or Medicine was awarded to Banting and Macleod for the epoch-making discovery of insulin (Figure 2). The omission of Best and Collip generated controversy throughout the scientific world. In addition, some felt that Macleod did not deserve the award. The prize money was shared with Best (from Banting) and Collip (from Macleod).

Pernicious anemia

George Richards Minot (1885–1950) (Figure 3), was born in Boston and lived there most of his life. As a young hematologist, he had an almost obsessive interest in the effect of diet on anemia. Early on, James Homer Wright, pathologist at the

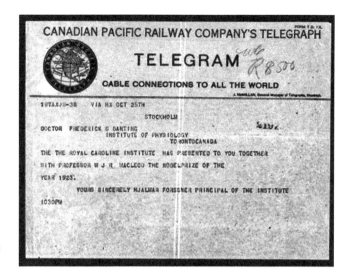

CANADIAN PACIFIC RAILWAY COMPANY'S TELEGRAPH

TELEGRAM

CABLE CONNECTIONS TO ALL THE WORLD

Figure 2. Telegram announcing the 1923 Nobel Prize in Physiology or Medicine to Banting and Macleod.
Credit: Reference 3, page 35.

Massachusetts General Hospital, taught Minot the significance of the reticulocyte count in the peripheral blood as an index of enhanced bone marrow response.[4-6]

In October 1921, Minot became ill and lost 12 pounds. He diagnosed his own case of severe diabetes.[7] He was unable to work and was seen by the prominent diabetologist, Elliott Joslin. In January 1923, Joslin obtained enough insulin from the Toronto group to treat Minot. He improved dramatically and was able to return to work.[7,8]

In 1926, Minot and William P. Murphy (1892–1987) presented their work on treatment of pernicious anemia (PA) with liver to the Association of American Physicians.[9] Later that year their exciting findings were published in the *Journal of the American Medical Association* (*JAMA*).[9,10] They abolished the anemia in 45 PA patients by feeding them one-half pound of "lightly cooked" beef liver

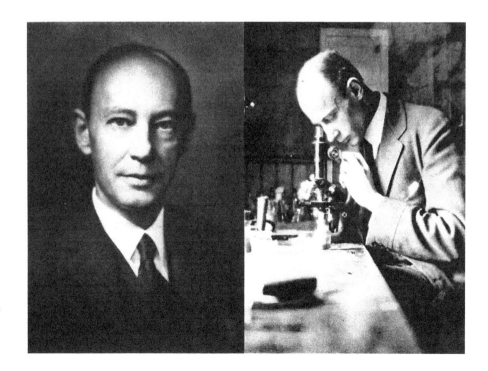

Figure 3. George Richards Minot.
Credit: Scott Podolsky and Stephanie Krauss, Countway Library of Medicine, Harvard University.

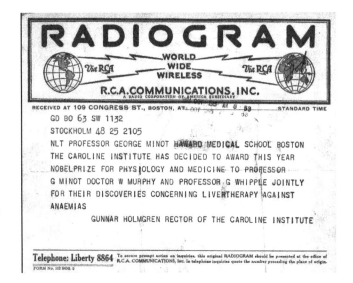

Figure 4. Telegram announcing the 1934 Nobel Prize in Physiology or Medicine to Minot, Murphy, and Whipple.
Credit: www.bonhams .com.

daily. Minot and Murphy overcame the objections of physicians who urged blood transfusion for severely anemic patients because Minot demonstrated the early rise in reticulocyte count shortly after liver therapy was begun and well before the rise in hemoglobin values.[4-6] In 1934, Minot, Murphy, and George H. Whipple (1878–1976) shared the Nobel Prize in Physiology or Medicine (Figure 4) for "liver treatment of anemia."[5,7] The identification and characterization of intrinsic factor and cobalamin (Vitamin B_{12}) completed the remarkable PA story.[5,6,11]

In deciding whether to attend the Nobel ceremony in 1934, Minot contacted Banting inquiring about the quality of insulin available in Sweden. Banting assured Minot that Swedish insulin was of excellent quality. Minot took insulin the rest of his life; without it, he would not have been able to discover the successful treatment for PA.[7]

Osler's studies on pernicious anemia

In Minot and Murphy's landmark 1926 *JAMA* article, Osler was cited, but only to the extent that some patients improved with "change in air" and better diet.[10] No mention was made of Osler's previous scientific contributions nearly 50 years before.

In 1877, William Gardner and Osler described a patient who was almost certainly the first with the clinical, hematologic, and pathologic features to leave no doubt he had Addisonian pernicious anemia.[12,13]

The case was that of a 52-year-old Englishman who complained of weakness and dyspnea on exertion, numbness of the fingers and the hands (difficulty buttoning his clothes), and a throbbing sensation in his temples. He died of progressive symptoms three months later. In the peripheral blood Osler described macroovalocytes that measured up to 14x9μ and large nucleated red cells with abnormal chromatin. At autopsy, pallor of the skin and organs as well as a peculiar lemon tint to the skin and a thin gastric membrane were described. The bone marrow disclosed intense hyperplasia and was filled with large nucleated red cells having homogeneous stroma and finely granulated nuclei. This was the first clear description of the megaloblast so named by Paul Ehrlich three years later.

Osler rejected William Pepper's idea that PA was a form of pseudo-leukemia but hypothesized instead that it was a reversion of the bone marrow to an embryonic state, though why he did not know. Osler remarked it was "A disease . . . concerning the pathology of which we still have a good deal to learn, and concerning the successful treatment of which we as yet know nothing."

In 1886, Frederick Henry and Osler reported a 42-year-old male with the clinical features of PA and atrophy of the stomach confirming the previous findings of Austin Flint and Samuel Fenwick.[12,14] Physical examination showed the skin to have a peculiar yellowish pallor, which by now Osler stated was almost pathognomonic of PA, along with pale mucous membranes. The red blood cell count was 790,000 per cu mm with some red cells four times normal size. The patient died six months later. The last red blood cell count was 315,000 per cu mm. Autopsy showed the gray pallor of the skin and all organs, and bone marrow hyperplasia. The stomach showed a grossly thin mucous membrane in the fundus but was otherwise unremarkable except for pallor and small nodular projections. A prominent feature of the gastric atrophy in this patient was round cell infiltration in all the layers of the stomach that we now know to be lymphocytes that evoke cell-mediated autoimmune attack on the gastric parietal cells.[11]

PA was almost always fatal. By 1881, Osler reported, "all of the Montreal cases have died." The duration of the disease was said to be three to twelve months with unusual cases lasting three to five years. It soon became evident that there was a classic triad consisting of sore tongue, jaundice (lemon yellow), and numbness and tingling of the fingers and toes. Later, other features such as premature graying, blue eyes, and vitiligo were identified.[11]

Osler and Banting

Frederick Banting's father, William, was baptized in Bond Head by Featherstone Osler on the same day in 1849 that he christened his own son, William.[15]

Frederick Banting never met William Osler. In 1923, Lady Osler invited the newly honored Frederick Banting to the Osler home at Oxford, 13 Norham Gardens—famous as the "Open Arms."[2] Banting slept in Osler's bed and remarked the next day:

> To have been in the same house, slept in the same bed, bathed in the same tub, shaved by the same mirror, talked on the same veranda, viewed the same books and pictures as Sir William Osler fills one with an inspiration that puts sleep to flight. Above me is the picture of his sainted father and mother. How proud they were of him! Lady Osler is charming. He had wonderful surroundings, friends, books, and a beautiful home—because he was the kind of man to whom all things were beautiful and to whom all people were good. He gave to others and it came back to him.[2]

The successful treatment of DM with insulin and PA with liver advanced scientific medicine in seven years far beyond anything that preceded it. Michael Bliss wrote "Osler would have been transported into ecstasy at the announcement in 1922 of the isolation of the internal secretion of the pancreas and its almost miraculous effect in bringing starved, dying children back to life and health. He would have been especially thrilled that the near resurrection happened in Canada at the University of Toronto."[1,3,15]

It is just as likely that Osler would have been euphoric four years later over the monumental breakthrough in the treatment of PA, even though his own significant scientific contributions a half-century before were largely neglected.[11,12]

Summary

William Osler died on December 29, 1919 at the age of 70. Less than one year later, Frederick Banting began a research project at the University of Toronto to find a treatment for diabetes mellitus. J.J.R. Macleod, director of physiology, gave him space, funding, and supplies. Charles Best, an undergraduate medical student, joined Banting. In 1921, Banting and Best isolated and purified insulin from pancreatic extracts of dogs. J.B. Collip, a biochemist, helped in the purification process. The first American patient was treated with Toronto insulin in May 1922. Banting and Macleod were awarded the Nobel Prize in 1923 "for the discovery of insulin." George Richards Minot, a young hematologist in Boston, had an obsessive interest in the effect of diet on anemia. In October 1921, Minot developed weight loss and was diagnosed with severe diabetes mellitus. By January 1923, the pioneering diabetologist Elliott Joslin began to treat Minot with insulin. Minot's condition improved and he returned to work. In 1926, Minot and W.P. Murphy amazed the medical world when they eradicated the anemia in 45 pernicious anemia patients by feeding them a half-pound of beef liver daily. Minot shared the 1934 Nobel Prize with Murphy and G.H. Whipple "for their discoveries concerning liver therapy in cases of anemia." Minot remained on insulin the rest of his life. Osler described the clinical findings and blood picture of pernicious anemia nearly a half century before Minot, but his observations were largely ignored. Osler had an intriguing connection to Banting. Had he lived Osler would have been ecstatic over these two monumental therapeutic breakthroughs.

Acknowledgments

Supported in part by the Edward and Ruth Wilkof Foundation. I thank Kathleen Shannon Stone and Cynthia Orticio for assistance with manuscript preparation.

References

1. Bliss M. *The Discovery of Insulin*. Toronto: McClelland and Stewart; 1982.
2. Bliss M. *Banting. A Biography*. Toronto: McClelland and Stewart 1984.
3. Bliss M. The Discovery of Insulin at the University of Toronto, 75th Anniversary exhibition and catalogue, 1996, pages 13–38.
4. Castle WB. The contributions of George Richards Minot to experimental medicine. *New England Journal of Medicine* 1952; 247: 585–592.
5. Castle WB. The Conquest of Pernicious Anemia. In *Blood, Pure and Eloquent*, Wintrobe MM, ed. New York: McGraw-Hill; 1980; chapter 10: 282–317.
6. Karnad AB. *Intrinsic Factors*. Boston: Harvard/Countway Library; 1997: 49–50.

7. Rackenann FM. *The Inquisitive Physician. The Life and Times of George Richards Minot MD.* Cambridge, Massachusetts: Harvard University Press; 1956.

8. Barnett DM. Elliott P Joslin MD: A Centennial Portrait. Joslin Diabetes Center, 1999.

9. Minot GR and Murphy WP. Observations on patients with pernicious anemia partaking of a special diet. A. Clinical Aspects. Transactions of the Association of American Physicians 1926; 41: 72–75.

10. Minot GR and Murphy WP. Treatment of pernicious anemia by a special diet. *Journal of the American Medical Association* 1926; 87: 470–476.

11. Chanarin I. A history of pernicious anemia. *British Journal of Haematology* 2000; 111: 407–415.

12. Stone MJ. William Osler's legacy and his contributions to haematology. *British Journal of Haematology* 2003; 123: 3–18.

13. Gardner W and Osler W. A case of progressive pernicious anemia. *Canada Medical and Surgical Journal* 1877; 5: 385–404.

14. Henry FP and Osler W. Atrophy of the stomach, with the clinical features of progressive pernicious anemia. *American Journal of the Medical Sciences* 1886; 91: 498–511.

15. Bliss M. *William Osler A Life in Medicine.* New York: Oxford University Press; 1999: 478–479.

Osler and his Australian Connections

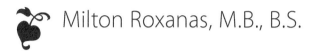 Milton Roxanas, M.B., B.S.

Osler's connections with Australia were relatively few during his Montreal (1870–1884), Philadelphia (1884–1889), and early Baltimore periods (1889–1896). However, in 1897, addressing the British Medical Association in Montreal[1] on "British Medicine in Greater Britain," Osler took the opportunity to describe the influence of British medicine on its colonies and predicted that a future meeting might be held in Australia.[2] He described the Australian population as more homogenous and was surprised "with the monotonous similarity of the diseases in the antipodes to those of Great Britain and of this continent." He noted the frequency of "parasitic infections and snake-bites" which were unusual in the northern hemisphere. He also commented that the medical profession in Australia was not as regulated as elsewhere because of the "absence of the military element" and was disappointed at the extent to which Australian physicians were adversarial toward each other, which he surmised from his reading.[2] Osler reported that "in the large Australian cities, differences and dissensions seem lamentably common," which he attributed to the three- or four-yearly reappointments in hospitals that involved soliciting votes.[1] Osler was scathing about the situation in Melbourne, where the election of hospital appointments was in the hands of "subscribers" and "election tickets were put in hotels and bars and even in stations and in cabs."[2]

In July 1900, Osler travelled to London to attend the Royal College of Surgeons centenary celebrations at the hall of Lincoln's Inn. Four chairs away sat Henry Simpson Newland (1873–1969), from Adelaide, who mentioned his interest in neurosurgery to Osler who then advised him to go to Baltimore and work with Harvey Cushing, which he did. Also in 1900 in the Osler and Thomas McCrae monograph on *Cancer of the Stomach*, the first chapter states "Our col-

Presented in part at the forty-fourth annual meeting of the American Osler Society, Philadelphia, Pennsylvania, on 2 May 2011. Portions of this manuscript were previously published in the *Medical Journal of Australia* (2010; 193[11–12]: 686–689, 690–693) and are used with permission.

leagues in Australia have demonstrated . . . the mortality figures (for cancer of the stomach) . . . show an increase at about the same rate as in England." They cite two references each from Australia and New Zealand.[2]

During Osler's 1907 address to students at St. Mary's Hospital in London, halfway through his lecture he deviated to verbally attack St. Mary's bacteriologist and immunologist, Sir Almroth Wright (1861–1947) who was cynical of clinical methods and clinicians.[3] The nature of Osler's attack on Wright is not recorded, but it is known that Osler and Wright had previously been on good terms despite Wright being very argumentative. Wright's contributions to medicine were outstanding and included discovering the role of calcium in coagulation, developing a typhoid vaccine, helping to found immunology as we now know it, and mentoring Alexander Fleming, who discovered penicillin.[4] He was appointed demonstrator in physiology at the University of Sydney in 1889.

Osler was travelling in Rome in April 1909 when he was asked to see a seriously ill Australian with severe purpura. He theorised that the capillaries allowed blood to leak out and postulated an anaphylactic reaction. Osler published an article about this patient, who died 15 minutes after Osler first saw him.[5]

In February 1911, Osler was invited by his brother Sir Edmund Boyd Osler to visit Egypt and the Nile Valley. As usual, Osler was able to make a good mix of vacation, history and medicine. He enjoyed visits to the Sphinx, various tombs, the Egyptian museum and was impressed by the beauty of the mosques. He took time to visit Kasr El Aini Hospital where he met Dr. Frank Cole Madden (1873–1929) who was born in Melbourne. Madden had a distinguish career as superintendent of the Hospital for Sick Children, Great Ormond Street, London, and was then surgeon, teacher and Dean of Faculty of Medicine at the University of Cairo. He was awarded the Order of the British Empire for his services in World War I but committed suicide, in April 1929, disheartened as a result of politics between university, Egyptian and British governments.[6]

Osler spoke about *The Evolution of Modern Medicine* in the Silliman Lectures at Yale University in April 1913. Demonstrating he was sufficiently knowledgeable about traditional Aboriginal "witchdoctors" with the power to heal or kill, he included them in how medicine and religion grew out of a mixture of magic, saying "among native Australians today it is still deliberately cultivated."[7]

Leslie Cowlishaw (1877–1943) was from Sydney, appointed officer-in-charge of invaliding in England in 1916, and an established collector of medical books when he met Osler. The two struck up a close relationship and could discuss medical history on equal terms. Osler was perceptive enough to understand the Australian psyche, labelling Cowlishaw the "bibliophile from the bush."[8] There are six letters from Osler to Cowlishaw in the archives of the Royal Australasian College of Surgeons (RACS) mentioning the purchasing of books; thanking him for sending him a book; and for correcting an article Osler had written. Osler was comfortable with Cowlishaw, offering him hospitality, and writing on 7 March 1916, to "come when you can . . . give a few days' notice as I am much away . . . stay at night. There are many things in my collection to interest you." In another letter, dated 8 August 1917, Osler writes: "I am devastated to miss you . . . do come to us direct your next leave." In yet another note, Osler writes: ". . . come here for a rest and bibliographic browse when you come back . . . I am struggling with my catalogue." Osler's influence on Cowlishaw added fuel to the fire of the latter who acquired the biggest collection of rare medical books in Australia, sold by his estate to RACS in 1943 upon his death. Cowlishaw followed Osler's example of not only collecting but also writing medical history. He presented a scholarly account of early printing presses and early medical books, many of which were in his possession.[9] Thornton correctly credits Cowlishaw with stating that the first medical book in English, *A litil boke the which traytied and reherced many gode things necessaries for the . . . pestilence . . . made by the . . . Bisshop of Arusiens*, was published in London by William of Machlinia in 1485.[10] Cowlishaw went on the write about the first 50 years of medicine in Australia and about many early medical practitioners of Australia.[11]

Another connection between Cowlishaw and Osler is in Osler's use of Australian publishing houses. A letter recently found from Osler to D. Appleton & Co., publisher of *The Principles and Practice of Medicine*, and dated 18 February1898, reads:

> I would like an arrangement made with publishing houses in India and Australia to issue special editions of my text-book in those countries . . .

Some more recent Australians with Osler connections[19]

Name	Relation to Osler	Notes
James Linklater Thomson Isbister (1870–1936)	A note, written by Scot Skirving inside a copy of Cushing's *Life of Sir William Osler*, in the Library of the Royal Australasian College of Physicians, states that he met Osler twice and that Isbister was said to be "impressed by his character and his influence on the young."	He worked as a surgeon and gynaecologist at the Royal North Shore Hospital. He was a reserved man and treated Sister Mary MacKillop, the first Australian Saint. He was the grandfather of James P. Isbister.
Oleg (Alec) Preda (b. 1941)	Dr. Preda privately printed 500 copies of his *The master-word of Dr William Osler*. He edited many of Osler's speeches, giving them modern, relevant titles removing gender-specific language and adding notes. The book added humanity and philosophy to the technical aspects of medicine. The small printing at his own expense was given to friends instead of making them available to a wider audience.	Born in Russia and educated at the University of Sydney, he worked at various hospitals and was in general practice. He was introduced to Osler when he told a doctor, who was doing his physical examination for his national service that he wanted to study medicine and was urged to read Osler's *The Student Life*. Dr. Preda made a pilgrimage to all the places Osler worked and lived. He was distressed when he saw Osler's brain at the Wistar Institute with gaps made by people cutting portions of his brain.
Michael O'Rourke (b. 1937)	Professor O'Rourke wrote an editorial in the *Medical Journal of Australia* in 1999[18] "we need to sit back, reflect and weigh knowledge, common sense and ethics in our daily practice, as Osler taught and practised."	Graduated from University of Sydney, worked in physiology at Johns Hopkins University before returning to Sydney as Professor of Medicine at the University of NSW. His main interest was in arterial haemodynamics.
James Paton Isbister (b. 1943)	In an editorial that posed the question "what would Osler say today?" in 1983,[19] Dr. Isbister wrote " In the Oslerian sense, it will be a collection of problem-oriented reviews aimed at bridging the gap between clinical and laboratory medicine." The author stressed the need not to interpret results in isolation but to weigh the possibilities and relating them to the clinical picture.	Dr. Isbister is a graduate of the University of New South Wales and specialised in clinical haematology. He set up the first blood cell separator (apheresis) unit and allogenic bone marrow transplant service in Australia.

I could even add if necessary a short supplement to the special edition dealing more fully with certain affections peculiar to those countries. I have so many friends in both places, many of them men in official and teaching positions that the book would be adopted in the schools—as it has been at Sydney . . . "[12]

This led to the eventual release in 1913, of a special eighth edition of his textbook for Australia which was used in Australian universities.[12] At that time there were three medical schools in Australia (Sydney, Melbourne and Adelaide), with a total enrolment of 957 medical students, while the number of doctors in Australia was less than 3000. These numbers were sufficient for Butterworth & Co. to publish a special Australian edition made up of American sheets.[12] Unfortunately Osler did not identify who his Australian friends were.

Robert Scot Skirving (1859–1956), of Scottish origin, travelled to Australia as a sailor and suffered beriberi on the return journey. His illness influenced him to study medicine at the University of Edinburgh, graduating in 1881. He returned to Australia as a ship's surgeon, later becoming a senior physician at Sydney's Prince Alfred Hospital and was chosen to review Cushing's biography

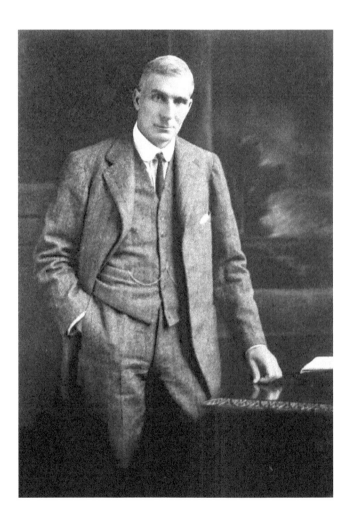

Figure 1. Robert Scot Skirving (1859–1956).
Credit: Ann McIntosh.

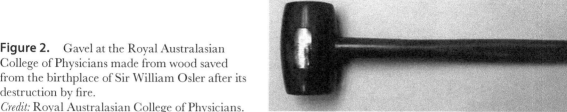

Figure 2.   Gavel at the Royal Australasian College of Physicians made from wood saved from the birthplace of Sir William Osler after its destruction by fire.
Credit: Royal Australasian College of Physicians.

of Osler. He wrote a delightfully thorough review.[13] He was full of praise for Osler's textbook, writing that it was "… absolutely sane, without faddism and with a perfect blending of scientific facts with their practical applications…." In another publication this physician wrote "I remember with personal pride that I myself was largely the means of making it [the textbook], the daily companion of the Sydney medical student."[14] It may well be that Osler was referring to him when he wrote that he had friends in Australia. Scot Skirving later wrote a short publication on the life of Osler for the Australian market.[15] His work was not widely distributed nor without error, as he wrote that Osler died at age 71 years instead of age 70.

A physical connection between Osler and Australia exists in the form of a gavel that was donated to the Royal Australasian College of Physicians in March 1950 by Dr. William C. Gibson a Canadian neuroscientist who worked with neurophysiologist John C. Eccles in Australia. This gavel was made from wood saved from Osler's childhood home in the parsonage at Bond Head, Ontario, Canada, and made up by Mr. Tom Jamison. It appears that Osler's nephew, Dr. Norman Gwyn, used wood from the Osler's home to make paper knives for the family and gavels which he gave to various associations.[16]

Osler's influence on Australia was similar to his influence on other countries. The Australian edition of his textbook taught the principle of medicine to a generation of doctors. Those fortunate enough to meet him took pride in the experience and were inspired to practice medicine with high ideals and humanity, as he had particular skill in being able to fuse the past and the present into a practical humanistic coherent whole. His writings and timeless sayings are often quoted because they have well-articulated wisdom, even in this age of molecular medicine. Australian doctors, medical teachers and writers continue to look to Osler's guidance in applying his principles to modern medical practice.[17] His cautious approach to medication ("man has an inborn craving for medicine") is a constant warning to those practising polypharmacy. He also highlighted the need for continuing medical education by stating "it is astonishing with how little reading a doctor can practice medicine, but it is not astonishing how badly he may do it." The employment of modern tests, be they chemical, imaging or pathological, do not lessen the need to be wise, well read, experienced, and compassionate towards the patient, in spite of the help given by computers and other technology.

Acknowledgments

I thank my daughter Emma Roxanas and Dr. Daniel Yardley for editorial assistance.

References

1. Osler W. *Aequanimitas, With other Addresses to Medical Students, Nurses and Prac-titioners of Medicine.* Third impression, London: H.K. Lewis; 1904.
2. Roxanas MG. Osler and his Australian associations—Part 1: During his life. *Medical Journal of Australia* 2010; 193(11–12): 686–689.
3. Osler W. The reserves of life. *St. Mary's Hospital Gazette* 1907; 13: 95–98.
4. Dunnill M. *The Plato of Praed Street: The Life and Times of Almroth Wright.* London: Royal Society of Medicine Press; 2000.
5. Osler W. Note on the relation of the capillary blood-vessels in purpura. *Lancet* 1909; 173(4472): 1385–1386.
6. Power D, Spencer WG, Gask GE. *Plarr's Lives of the Fellows of the Royal College of Surgeons of England.* Bristol: John Wright and Sons Ltd.; 1930.
7. Osler W. *The Evolution of Modern Medicine.* New Haven: Yale University Press; 1921.
8. Russell KF. *Catalogue of the Historical Books in the Library of the Royal Australasian College of Surgeons.* Melbourne: Queensbury Hill Press; 1979.
9. Cowlishaw L. Some early printed books: Their authors and printers. *Medical Journal of Australia* 1926; 2: 77–81.
10. Thornton JL. *Thornton's Medical Books, Libraries and Collectors.* Aldershot: Gower Publishing Company Limited; 1990: 33.
11. Cowlishaw L. The George Addington Syme Oration: The first fifty years of Medicine in Australia. *Australia and New Zealand Journal of Surgery* 1936; 6: 3–17.
12. Golden RL, Roxanas M. William Osler's textbook: The Australian edition. *Osler Library* 2007; 108: 4–6.
13. Scot Skirving R. Reviews—William Osler. *Medical Journal of Australia* 1925; 2: 457–458.
14. Scott Skirving R. *The Life of Sir William Osler* (review). *Australasian Nursing Journal* 1926; 24: 324–330.
15. Scott Skirving R. *The Life of Sir William Osler.* Sydney: Australasian Medical Publishing Company; 1926.
16. O'Rourke MF. William Osler: A model for the 21st century? *Medical Journal of Australia* 1999; 171: 577–579.
17. Isbister JP. Clinching the diagnosis: What would Osler say today? *Medical Journal of Australia* 1983; 15: 361–363.
18. MacDermott HE. On gavels. *Canadian Medical Association Journal* 1972; 106; 1109.
19. Roxanas MG. Osler and his Australian associations—Part 2: Continuing influence. *Medical Journal of Australia* 2010; 193(11–12): 690–693.

The Oslerian Legacy in the American South

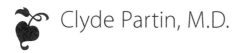 Clyde Partin, M.D.

In his courtesy and kindness to all with whom he came in contact, he surely had the characteristics of a Southern gentleman. His influence on the advancement of medicine in the South cannot be over-estimated and, in honor of his seventieth birthday, it seems only fitting that the SOUTHERN MEDICAL JOURNAL should publish an "Osler Number.

—Unsigned editorial from the July 1919 *Southern Medical Journal*, announcing "felicitations" to Osler.

In the pages of *The Southern Medical Journal*, William Osler's colleague Lewellys Barker published, in 1919, a curious piece entitled "Osler and the South."[1] With startling inaccuracy, Barker described in glowing terms Osler's relationship with the South and Southerners. This brief communication was essentially a happy birthday letter. If Osler held opinions on the Civil War, Reconstruction, or the Southern agrarian mindset, he never penned them, and a paucity of published information is available to support Barker's comments. Even though William Osler lived in Baltimore when he worked at Johns Hopkins, he was never particularly fond of that city. He rarely travelled further south but did find his way to Georgia, Florida, and South Carolina to do patient consults. When Osler did venture south, he sometimes left a literary or academic footprint. He gave his famous address, "The Fevers of the South," at the American Medical Association meeting in Atlanta in 1896. Osler's fascination with Thomas Moore's poem, "The Lake of the Dismal Swamp" inspired an excursion to Virginia's Dismal Swamp, which led to an enduring philological mystery. Renowned Emory University cardiologist J. Willis Hurst (1920–2011) was an inveterate writer, Osler fan, and devoted historian of medicine. In the late 1990s, Dr. Hurst and I were discuss-

Presented at the forty-seventh annual meeting of the American Osler Society, Atlanta, Georgia, on 10 April 2017. Portions of this paper were previously published in *Baylor University Medical Center Proceedings* 2019; 32(4): 538–543.

ing Sir William Osler when he suggested writing about Osler's trip to Georgia. Hurst's vague recollection was that Osler had come to Georgia for a meeting, then traveled to Americus, Georgia, by a special coach.

The AMA annual meeting comes to Atlanta

In 1896, the American Medical Association held in Atlanta, Georgia, its forty-seventh annual meeting. Cushing duly recorded Osler's attendance, as did *The Atlanta Constitution*. Travelling with the psychiatrist Henry Hurd, superintendent of the Johns Hopkins Hospital, he arrived in Atlanta on 3 or 4 May. Cushing reports Osler delivered opening remarks, said to be "given extemporaneously, in a charming and effective manner."[2] These remarks, were apparently "completely lost" in the subsequently published abstract of the *Proceedings*. As for the AMA convention, it was reported that "Atlanta with flowing speeches of welcome and a Georgia barbecue greeted and entertained for three days a thousand or more physicians."[2] On 6 May, Osler unleashed, to wide acclaim, his address, "The Study of the Fevers of the South." The first line of this oratory is the iconic and oft-quoted line: "Humanity has but three great enemies: fever, famine, and war; of these by far the greatest, by far the most terrible, is fever."[3]

The newspaper, on 7 May, recognized the AMA gathering with a full page of coverage (Figure 1). Osler's opinion on several administrative items elicited press scrutiny including his thoughts on replacing the AMA secretary. Another issue was Senate Bill 1552, which addressed rising antivivisectionist sentiment. Osler voiced a strong stand against this bill, fearing that progress in medical research would encounter constraints.[4] In five paragraphs under the subheading, "Dr. Osler's Splendid Paper," an innominate journalist wrote: "Dr. Osler dealt with fevers of all kinds in a technical way, but in an unusually lucid manner. . . .

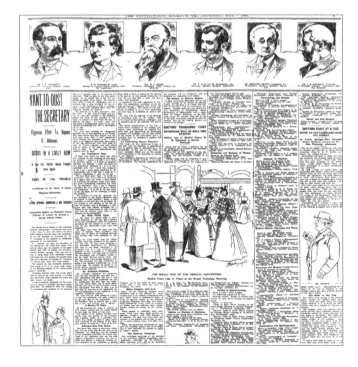

Figure 1.   The *Atlanta Constitution* newspaper coverage of the American Medical Association convention held in Atlanta, May 1896, with a full page devoted to the meeting.

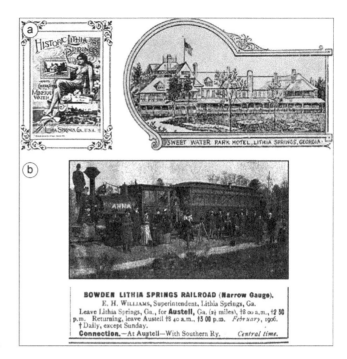

Figure 2. *Above:* Advertisements for the Lithia Springs spas and the Sweetwater Hotel, site of the AMA barbecue. *Below:* The narrow-gauge railroad Osler would have taken to the barbecue.

The paper was applauded frequently and when Dr. Osler was finished he was the recipient of the heartiest congratulations."[5] A century later, Charles Bryan from the University of South Carolina commemorated this oration in his 1996 Kass Lecture at the Infectious Diseases Society of America convention in New Orleans, noting: "Osler's address on "The Study of the Fevers of the South" at the 47th annual meeting of the American Medical Association in Atlanta, Georgia, in which he showed his appreciation of the history, epidemiology, management, and prevention of infectious diseases."[6]

The newspaper also devoted a column to the barbecue that followed:

> DOCTORS FEAST AT A 'CUE
> GIVEN AN OLD FASHIONED GEORGIA SPREAD
> At Lithia Springs—Two Thousand People Gathered
> Around the Tables Yesterday Afternoon

A reporter wrote: "The largest barbecue ever given on Georgia soil was that at Lithia Springs yesterday.... Everything that goes to make the Georgia barbecue the greatest feast of epicurean taste was there. Lithia water flowed freely, and other beverages of a more exhilarating type abounded."[7]

Did Osler go to Americus, Georgia?

In 1896 Americus, Georgia, 140 miles southwest of Atlanta, would have been easily accessible by three railroads, including a privately owned lavish rail line that catered to well-heeled vacationers. Visitors to Americus would have stayed in The Windsor Hotel, a Victorian edifice built in 1892 and marketed to Northerners as a winter destination. Osler could have departed Atlanta around May

10 and arrived in Americus in four hours. A letter to Henry V. Ogden that Osler penned at 1 West Franklin St. suggests that he returned to Baltimore at least by 20 May.[8] Osler's letter did not mention his recent Georgia trip. By July, he had travelled to the New England coast near Boston and sent a letter to William S. Thayer, again without epistolary recognition of his Georgia sojourn.[9]

In that era, the *Americus Times-Recorder* newspaper was published every day but Monday. Although Osler's arrival would likely have received mention in the paper, perusal of editions printed in the middle weeks of May 1896 revealed no reference to Osler. The Americus newspaper did offer one paragraph regarding the AMA meeting in Atlanta.[10] There were numerous newspaper stories describing various infectious illnesses from which the citizens of Americus were recovering. Had Osler gone to Americus, he would have encountered no shortage of fevers to challenge his diagnostic acumen, but no proof is available that he journeyed to Americus. Scrutiny of the chapter *Various Visitors* in a book about Americus was bereft of Osler's name but included many lesser lights.[11] The Windsor Hotel had no extant guest logs from that era.

Dr. Hurst's question and recollections about Osler's travels involving a train and a resort may have an explanation. The barbecue at Lithia Springs, about fifteen miles west of Atlanta, necessitated a train ride. Lithia Springs did feature spas at its resorts, and the therapeutic water was naturally infused with a touch of lithium. The train that conveyed over two thousand people to the barbecue was:

> Made up of two sections of about eight coaches each, and every coach was packed. From the depot in Lithia Springs, it was a half-mile walk to the springs, near the Sweetwater Park Hotel. Lofty descriptions of the affair hinted that Georgia invented the 'cue,' the tables were spread in the beautiful grove around the spring, which, since the days when the Indian tribes resorted to it to drink its healing waters.[7]

Perhaps Dr. Hurst conflated these two destinations in his mind and recalled the barbecue as being in Americus.

Osler and the American South

Osler promulgated a universal brotherhood of physicians that transcended political and geographical constraints. Nonetheless, for Osler the South, as a piece of the global pie, seems to have captured a lesser slice of the orb. Some might take exception that Osler never considered himself a Southerner, while others would note that Osler identified as British, and was never an American citizen. Slivers of southern recognition did exist, however. The iconic lecture alluded to above, "The Study of the Fevers of the South," was inspired by a practitioner in Alabama. Cushing wrote that this paper was "a by-product of which had been the discovery of the Alabama Student."[2] In that essay, Osler remarked:

> When looking over the literature of malarial fevers in the South, chance threw in my way Fenner's *Southern Medical Reports*, vols. i and ii, which were issued in 1849–50 and 1850–51. Among many articles of interest, I was particularly impressed with two by Dr. John Y. Bassett, of Huntsville, Alabama, in whom I seemed to recognize a 'likeness to the wise below,' a 'kindred with the great of old.'[12]

Osler simply did not travel that much to the Deep South. As a resident of Maryland, he lived in the South, though Maryland, a border state, had mixed proclivities during the Civil War.

A whimsical excursion with robust literary overtones took Osler to Old Point Comfort, Virginia. Travelling with his younger colleagues Thomas B. Futcher and Henry Barton Jacobs, in April 1920, they took a trip to the Dismal Swamp, featured in Tom Moore's poem, "The Lake of the Dismal Swamp." In a letter, Futcher observed Osler "had always been fascinated" by this poem.[2] Getting to the mystical lake was quite an ordeal that took most of the morning. Futcher noted further that: "On our way back, and while we were eating our frugal lunch, the Chief wrote a most imaginative account of our experiences for Revere on the blank pages in the back of Burton's 'Anatomy of Melancholy' which he had brought along with him." Despite Futcher's and Jacobs's encouragement, Osler never published "this amusing tale." That volume of Burton's work found its way into the collection at Christ Church, Oxford, and was later re-patriated to the Osler Library. The "added contents" had been quite a philological mystery until Futcher's letter was discovered and illuminated the activities of that outing.

Osler reported in his Autobiographical Notes that in 1901, "I twice went to the south—Fla. and Thomasville [Georgia]." His fee for the Thomasville patient was $3000. In May 1902, unable to respond to a consult request to go to Athens, Georgia, he sent Thayer.[13] Osler, in April 1905, was "in the south for consultation—in Columbus, Georgia, in Savannah, in Richmond."[2] George T. Harrell, in his paper on "Osler's Practice," mentions this trip, based on information obtained from Osler's 'Day Book,' a daily patient log.[14] Epistles from Osler to Lewellys F. Barker on 5 and 10 April 1905,[15,16] and to Francis J. Shepherd on 10 April 1905,[17] make no mention of this journey. Osler, abroad in Europe, did miss a prime opportunity to travel to Columbia, South Carolina, for the June 1890 wedding of Caroline Hampton and William S. Halsted.

Further scrutiny of Barker's 1919 letter feting Osler's birthday, reveals that: "In this impulse to honor Dr. Osler, Southern physicians delight to share." Acknowledging Osler's long tenure in Maryland, Barker ambitiously extrapolates that: "the South regards him peculiarly as its own."[1] More believably, Barker notes that Osler influenced many medical students and residents who migrated to Hopkins like disciples and then spread the Oslerian gospel in the South when they returned to their hometowns. With unwarranted reach, Barker concludes: "Osler had a peculiar understanding of the minds of the people of the South, and that Southerners generally have felt that they could share with him a kind of intimacy that they could not experience with other leaders." The remarkable hospitality of the Oslers gets well-deserved mention: "What greater praise in this regard could be given the Oslers than to admit that their genius for hospitality is worthy of the best traditions of the South?"[1] Little in Osler's published canon provides evidence to merit Barker's sappy Southern sentiments, although the Oslers' penchant for cordiality certainly ranks with the finest of this Southern custom. Barker's oleaginous comments were perhaps hastily written but with sincere intent. This remembrance of Barker's is immediately followed by a more reasoned tribute from Howard A. Kelly, who ends his remarks with, "In Osler, the South has renewed the best traditions of the past."[18]

Osler more likely shared feelings voiced by the fiery Sage of Baltimore, H.L. Mencken, with whom he was acquainted, but decorum and sensibility likely hindered Osler from openly embracing Mencken's inflammatory rhetoric. As his essay "The Sahara of the Bozart" attests, Mencken was no fan of the South. Osler, a humanist, took care of patients regardless of color or religion and assiduously avoided socio-political entanglements. The notable exceptions were his high-profile skirmishes with the political leadership of Baltimore, in which he chided them for their lack of attention to public health infrastructure. As Bliss observed: "Nor did he have much to say generally about the great racial divide in America and Baltimore."[19] Catching Osler in an anti-Semitic statement was also a lost cause. As news leaked that Osler was leaving Baltimore for England, Mencken later published, in the Interesting People section of *American Magazine*, six eloquent paragraphs lamenting Osler's departure:

> Say of one of them that he used to sit under Osler at the Johns Hopkins, and you are giving him high praise. Say of him, going further, that he promises, some day, to be worthy of his master, and you are at the limit of lawful eulogy. . . . Dr. Osler was solving problems that the textbooks put down as insoluble; he was ridding the art of medicine of cobwebs and barnacles; he was sending our parties of enthusiastic young men to explore the medical Farthest North and Darkest Africa. He observed things that no one else noticed, and he drew conclusions that violated the league rules.[20]

Perusal of the *Bibliotheca Osleriana*,[21] for southern literary connections, was minimally fruitful. Entries 1434 and 1446–1456 were devoted to Dr. Crawford W. Long, of Jefferson, Georgia, and the primacy question surrounding the discovery of anesthesia. John Y. Bassett, of "An Alabama Student" fame, garnered several entries (entries 3576, No. 166, page 319": Correspondence & 6748, Osler's book, *An Alabama Student*, page 578.)

American Osler Society meets in Atlanta, 1984 and 2017

The 1984 the American Osler Society (AOS) meeting took place in Atlanta and the venue was the Georgia World Congress Center. The one-day gathering featured Japanese Oslerian, Shigeaki Hinohara (1911–2017), who did some of his training at nearby Emory University. Hinohara gave the luncheon talk, "How Osler Came to Japan," at the Omni International Hotel. Jeremiah Barondess

United States Location by Region for Meetings of the American Osler Society—1971 through 2024*

Region	Number	Percentage
South (USA)	16	30.2
Midwest (USA)	11	20.8
West (USA)	9	17.0
Northeast (USA)	6	11.3
Canada	7	13.2
United Kingdom	4	7.5
Totals	53	100

*Numbers for 2020–2024 represent scheduled meetings and projected locations. The 2020 meeting scheduled for Pasadena, California, was canceled. Galveston, 2021, has been converted to zoom with 2022 returning to Galveston, hopefully in-person. For these two years, Galveston was tallied only once for this table.

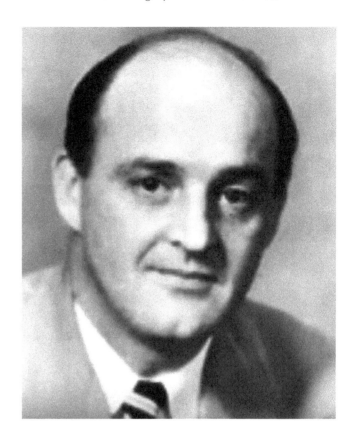

Figure 3.   Osler Almon Abbott (1912–1976),
a founding member of the Emory Clinic, who
performed the first intra-cardiac surgery in the
South in 1951, a mitral stenosis repair.

delivered the presidential address at the Piedmont Driving Club, on the topic of
the friendship between William Osler and Harvey Cushing. No presentation dealt
with any issue regarding the South, and a talk by William Bean turned north and
focused on Osler's Milwaukee connections. In 2017, 33 years later, the AOS again
met in Atlanta, this time on the Emory University campus. Fifty talks occurred,
and Joe Vander Veer gave a highly personal and moving presidential address
regarding a real-life encounter with *Aequanimitas*. Of the 53 AOS meetings from

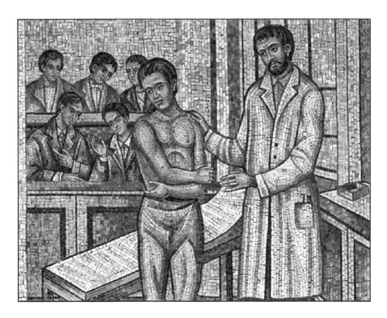

Figure 4.   Panel 23 of
the Emory University
History of Medicine
mural depicting
William Osler. In this
66-foot-long, 33-panel
mural, 2.5 million tiles
were used in the mosaic.
Italian-born Sirio
Tonelli (1922–2019) was
the artist.

1971 thru projected venues to 2024, the South has hosted the most meetings by region (16 meetings, or 30.2 percent of all meetings) (Table).

An Oslerian legacy at Emory University is that of Osler's grandnephew, Osler Almon Abbott, who was the grandchild of Charlotte (Aunt Chattie), William Osler's older sister.[22]

Abbott (1912–1976) (Figure 3), a founding member of the Emory Clinic, and a distinguished thoracic surgeon, performed the South's first intra-cardiac surgery, a mitral valve stenosis repair, in 1951. (I was privileged to care for his widow, Sarah, for a number of years. We both were devoted readers of the *New Yorker* magazine, and she annually graced me with a subscription as a holiday gift). Emory University has honored William Osler's achievements. The medical school at Emory is divided into four student houses, the Osler House being one. In the lobby of the medical school administration building a history of medicine mosaic, with over two million tiles and 3000 colors, depicts Osler on panel 23 (Figure 4). Stewart E. Roberts (1878–1941) (Figure 5), Georgia's first cardiologist, enjoyed an illustrious career at Emory and was known as "The Osler of the South."[23]

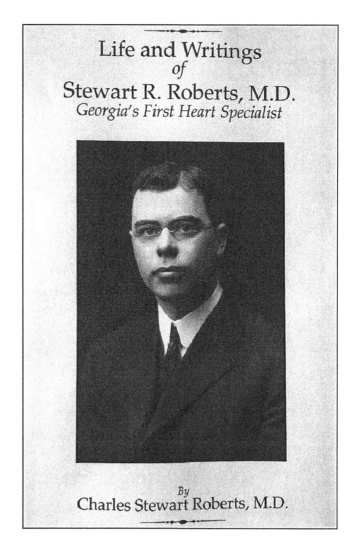

Figure 5. Biography of Stewart R. Roberts, also known as "the Osler of the South," written by his grandson and American Osler Society member Charles Stewart Roberts, whose father, William C. Roberts, is also an AOS member.

Conclusion

Why Osler traveled to the South so infrequently is a matter of speculation. One inescapable conclusion is that he did not have much need or desire to do so. His geographical sphere was Canada, the Northeastern US, England, and Western Europe. Medical centers in the South at the time were of marginal distinction and likely not attractive to him as destinations. Osler favored Europe for medical meetings. Holidays with his family included travelling to Northeastern cities, based on his wife Grace's heritage, and Canada, in view of his own roots. Overall, a limited but anecdotally rich body of evidence connects Osler to the South.

Acknowledgments

I thank Penny Merle Black, Michael Lubin, and Sally Wolff-King, all of Emory University, Charles S. Bryan of the University of South Carolina, and Daniel Pollock of CDC. Susan Kelen is the granddaughter of W.W. Francis, the first Osler Librarian and a second cousin (or first cousin once removed) of Sir William Osler. She is a practicing psychologist in Ottawa, Canada.

References

1. Barker LF. Osler and the South. *Southern Medical Journal* 1919; 12(7): 345–346.
2. Cushing H. *The Life of Sir William Osler*. Oxford: Clarendon Press; 1926, passim.
3. Osler W. The study of the fevers of the South. *Journal of the American Medical Association* 1896; 26: 999–1004.
4. Wants to oust the secretary. *Atlanta Constitution*, 7 May 1896, page 5.
5. Doctor's programme today. *Atlanta Constitution*, 7 May 1896, page 5.
6. Bryan CS. Fever, famine, and war: William Osler as an infectious diseases specialist. *Clinical Infectious Diseases* 1986; 23(5): 1139–1149.
7. Doctors feast at a 'cue [barbecue]. *Atlanta Constitution* 7 May 1896, page 5.
8. William Osler to Henry V. Ogden, 20 May 1896. Osler Letter Index, CUS417/92.13, Osler Library of the History of Medicine, McGill University.
9. William Osler to William S. Thayer, July 1986 ("Wednesday"), Osler Letter Index, CUS417/92.17, Osler Library of the History of Medicine, McGill University.
10. American Medical Association meets. *Americus* (Georgia) *Times-Recorder* 6 May 1896, page 1.
11. Anderson A. Various Visitors. In Anderson A. *Remembering Americus Georgia: Essays on Southern Life*. Charleston, South Carolina; History Press; 2006: 27–35.
12. Osler W. An Alabama Student. In Osler W. *An Alabama Student and Other Biographical Essays*. Toronto: Oxford University Press Canadian Branch; 1908: 1–18.
13. Bensley EH, Bates DG. Sir William Osler's Autobiographical Notes. *Bulletin of the History of Medicine* 1976; 50(4): 596–618.

14. Harrell GT. Osler's Practice. In Barondess JA, McGovern JP, Roland CG, Eds. *The Persisting Osler. Selected Transactions of the First Ten Years of the American Osler Society.* Baltimore, Maryland: University Park Press; 1985: 105–123.

15. William Osler to Lewellys F. Barker, 5 April 1905. Osler Letter Index, CUS417/102.42, Osler Library of the History of Medicine, McGill University.

16. William Osler to Lewellys F. Barker, 10 April 1905. Osler Letter Index, CUS417/102.46, Osler Library of the History of Medicine, McGill University.

17. William Osler to Francis J. Shepherd, 5 April 1905. Osler Letter Index, CUS 417/102.43. Osler Library of the History of Medicine, McGill University.

18. Kelly HA. A Tribute to Sir William Osler. *Southern Medical Journal* 1919; 12(7): 346–347.

19. Bliss M. *William Osler: A Life in Medicine.* New York: Oxford University Press; 1999.

20. Mencken HL. Interesting People: Dr. William Osler. *American Magazine* 1909; 68: 555.

21. Osler W. *Bibliotheca Osleriana: A Catalogue of Books Illustrating the History of Medicine and Science Collected, Arranged, and Annotated by Sir William Osler, BT. and Bequeathed to McGill University.* Oxford: Clarendon Press; 1929.

22. McFarland P. *The Descendants of Edward Osler (1734–1786) of Falmouth: In Britain, North America, South Africa and Australia—A Genealogy.* London, England; compiled 18 April 1993. Provided to the author by Paul McFarland, 22 November 2020.

23. Roberts CS. *Life and Writings of Stewart R. Roberts, M.D., Georgia's First Heart Specialist.* Spartanburg, South Carolina: The Reprint Company; 1993.

"The Doctor from North Carolina": William deBerniere MacNider and "The Way of a Teacher"

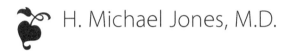 H. Michael Jones, M.D.

By the time of the American Civil War, North Carolinians were widely known as Tarheels, the origin of which is still in some doubt. One of its meanings is that of diligence and persistence in duty, due to the sticky tar (a North Carolina industrial product of the time) on one's heels. This is the story of a steadfast Tarheel, William deBernier MacNider (1881–1951), a key figure in the evolution of the University of North Carolina School (UNC) School of Medicine at Chapel Hill.[1]

Toward the end of his life, he wrote an essay on "The Way of a Teacher," which reflects the lasting impact a teacher made on him. The teacher was William Osler. Their interaction, although brief, illustrates the enduring power of mentoring.

The University of North Carolina School of Medicine— The early years

The story begins in 1879 with a short-lived UNC medical school headed by Dr. Thomas Harris; this lasted until 1885, when Thomas resigned to enter full-time private practice. During that venture, William Mallett was physician to the university and town of one thousand souls when his grandson William MacNider

Presented at the forty-second annual meeting of the American Osler Society, Chapel Hill, North Carolina, on 24 April 2012.

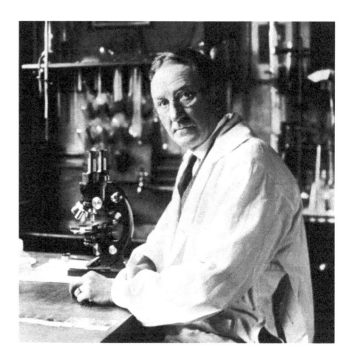

Figure 1.   William deBernier MacNider
(1881–1951).
Credit: Bayard Morgan Wootten Photographic
Collection #P0011, North Carolina Collection,
University of North Carolina at Chapel Hill
Library.

was born across the street. William McLendon, emeritus professor of pathology
and a 1953 graduate of the new four-year UNC medical school, knew MacNider
and illuminates MacNider's early years: "When William MacNider grew up in
Chapel Hill, NC, he was part of a family which had deep roots in Chapel Hill
and in the University. Although he was not part of a large family, it was a close-
knit family . . . enlarged by the many friends and distant relatives who would visit
with them. MacNider, as a boy, like William Osler, enjoyed the natural beauty
of the world, enjoyed hiking and hunting and observing nature.[2]

In 1890, when MacNider was nine, University president Kemp P. Battle
noted that over 200 young men were pursuing medical studies out of state.[3] That
year talented anatomist Richard Whitehead (Figure 2) agreed to become dean of
a new one-year program to prepare students for diploma-granting schools. Over
six years it grew into new quarters and expanded the curriculum to two years
(which lasted for over fifty years). Whitehead assumed Mallet's role of physician
to the village and often took young Will on professional visits. In 1899, while a
UNC senior, MacNider was given a faculty position as assistant in biology.[4]

Charles Jennette, chairman of the Department of Pathology and Laboratory Medicine at UNC, relates:

> If you look back on MacNider's career, it's clear that he became enthusi-
> astic about academic medicine early on, maybe in part because he actu-
> ally knew Dean Whitehead (who was the dean when he was a medical
> student) as a boy. So, he was well acquainted with Dean Whitehead . . .
> who was a true physician-scientist with multiple disciplines that he was
> interested in and knowledgeable about. For example, he taught anatomy,
> physiology, and pathology for a number of years . . . along with phar-
> macology. In fact, Will MacNider was his assistant as he was attending
> medical school. Undoubtedly Dean Whitehead was a tremendous influ-
> ence on Will MacNider.[5]

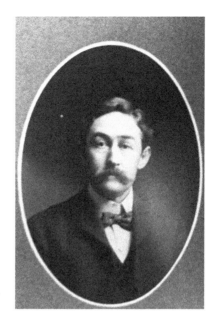

Figure 2. Richard Whitehead (1865–1916). *Credit:* North Carolina Collection Photographic Archives, University of North Carolina at Chapel Hill Library.

During MacNider's preclinical years, UNC President Preston Venable had been working with surgeon Hugh Royster (Figure 3) to establish a clinical department in larger Raleigh that would enable the institution to award MD degrees. The new program was in place by the time MacNider finished his preclinical years in Chapel Hill and he was the first student admitted to the new clinical program in Raleigh.[6, p. 240]

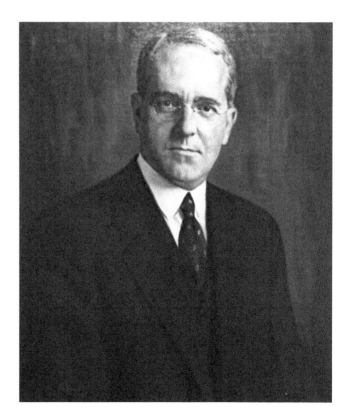

Figure 3. Hubert A. Royster (1871–1959). Author photograph of portrait haning in Bondurant Hall, University of North Carolina School of Medicine, Chapel Hill.

William Osler's influence on MacNider

Following graduation in 1903, MacNider began serving as instructor in diagnosis. Almost 50 years later, he would say that Royster was the "greatest student of medicine that I have ever known,"[4, p. 123] which was quite a compliment considering that MacNider had worked with William Osler. The Raleigh branch closed in 1910 primarily because of funding issues, just before release of the Flexner Report which led to closure of schools throughout the US.[7, p. 130] McLendon recalls:

> After graduating from the Raleigh school, Dr. MacNider realized that his clinical training had been very limited. . . . and so he wrote Dr. Osler and asked if he might spend the summer with him. Osler replied and MacNider made his first trip out of North Carolina by train to Baltimore and spent the summer in the clinics with Dr. Osler. . . . He described going up to the Johns Hopkins Hospital (since the taxi had let him off not at the front entrance) and he describes his amazement at seeing the 'statue of Jesus' in the lobby. He was overwhelmed by the immensity of the hospital and reputation of it. Soon someone came up and said, "Are you the doctor from North Carolina?"' and he said, "yes." He was taken immediately to see Dr. Osler and from that moment on, he felt very much a part of the institution.[2]

Wilburt C. Davison, before becoming dean of Duke University School of Medicine and befriending William MacNider, was an intimate friend of William and Grace Osler, having spent most of his time between 1913 and 1919 training in Oxford as a Rhodes Scholar. Davison publicly regaled a gathering with a humorous story about Osler's contact time with MacNider in the summer of 1904. Davison described MacNider as "one of the greatest characters in medicine I have ever known," and relates how Osler spent three hours teaching MacNider how to perform an autopsy on a patient who had died of typhoid fever. MacNider, covertly tongue in cheek, offered that Osler had been so "vulgar" that he "was ashamed to have even known him." When the shocked Davison asked what had happened, MacNider offered that the patient was being treated by Thomas B. Futcher (one of Osler's young assistants in medicine) with "intestinal antiseptics," whereupon Osler evaluated that treatment by saying, "treating typhoid fever with intestinal antiseptics is like trying to fertilize a ten-acre field with flatus."[8] And all enjoyed a good laugh!

MacNider's subsequent career at the University of North Carolina

MacNider, still incredibly young (24 years old), returned to the University of North Carolina School of Medicine to accept a post as professor of pharmacology. Over the next three years he spent summers with neurophysiologist A.F. Mathews in Chicago and pharmacologist Torald Sollman at Western Reserve, thereafter beginning a lifelong study of renal response to injury. Jennette, a renal pathologist, notes that MacNider "used renal pathology as one of the many modalities in his research."[5] MacNider was a faculty member until 1950, "teaching forty-four classes of medical students and carrying on an active and productive research career."[2] His life nurtured admiring students and close friendships as well as providing medical care to the community.

Contributions to scientific knowledge began with case reports before graduation and eventuated in three to six annual experimental reports for almost fifty years. McLendon notes, "at the time MacNider did research, it was pretty much a one-person project. He had a part-time janitor who helped with the research and... the animals, but he never had money enough to get an associate, other than a few times when he had enough money for a student research assistant, and one time for an assistant professor.... in general, his research was pretty much lonely—he did it by himself. His research was very meticulous and beautifully done."[2] Jennette expands:

> MacNider was an experimentalist. Much of his research centered around experimental models of disease in animals, especially dogs. He had some clinical scholarship, but much of his research focused on these experimental models. He used multiple approaches—biochemistry, physiology, pathology—to examine the effects of various toxins and drugs on tissues and organs and was very much focused on correlating functional abnormalities with changes in structure. Of course, the latter involved a tremendous amount of histopathologic examination of these models. He was clearly expert in this, based on the erudite descriptions in his publications. One might notice that many of the photographs of MacNider have a microscope in the field of view nearby. He clearly had an affinity for pathologic examination of tissues.[5, clip #1 min-00:00]

Chapel Hill was bucolic, yet with the most modern diversions, like the new-fangled movies and baseball games. Sadly, European conflicts soon claimed some faculty. MacNider attempted to enlist but was deferred so as not to "interfere with the manning of the medical schools."[9] Mary Kenan Flagler Bingham, whose fabulous wealth derived from Standard Oil, endowed the university to pay professors. "Dr. Billy" was teaching not only pharmacology, but also bacteriology, clinical diagnosis, and minor surgery. He was one of the first five Kenan professors in 1918, some fifteen years after his time with Osler. He then gave up student infirmary duties.

He continued practicing medicine in the community, however, and later that year he married Sallie Foard and built a house. McLendon recalls:

> After a few years they had one daughter, Sally Foard MacNider, who worked in the university and eventually married and moved elsewhere. So, he never had a large family, but he considered all the students and colleagues as part of his extended family... One of the classic stories is told about 24 hours in his life, when he spent one night with a woman in a rural community, who had eclampsia and a breech delivery. He delivered one of the two twins by forceps and the other was delivered without any further trouble. By this time, it was about 7 AM, so he returned to town, gave his 8 AM lecture in pharmacology and then returned back to check up on the patient.[2]

The 1920s roared with significant publications and recognition. He was elected to the presidency of the state medical society and the Mitchell Scientific Society, then the section chair on Pharmacy and Therapeutics of the AMA. Dr. Jennette reminds us, "Will MacNider was a true physician scientist at a time when many physicians were not scientists.... He also employed multidisciplinary research.... MacNider also had many interests and came up with seminal contributions to multiple fields of medicine—to nephrology, to hepatology, to pharmacology, even to geriatrics and in fact, he was one of the early physicians to recognize that great attention should be placed not only on developing younger individuals and middle life, but in fact, in older individuals. Some of his basic research addressed the underlying biological mechanisms that lead to aging in tissue."[5, clip #5 min-1:18, min 1:32, min 2:02]

McLendon recounts the numerous opportunities extended to improve Mac-Nider's academic career:

> He had a total of some eleven offers to go elsewhere, one of which was particularly important in that he was asked to become Professor and Chairman of Pharmacology at Jefferson Medical College in Philadelphia. He debated this a long time, and in fact, the story is told that he and Frank Porter Graham, the President, walked around the campus most of the night trying to decide whether he should take this, which would have given him the modern laboratory facility and assistance he could not afford at Chapel Hill. Finally, as he returned to his home as the dawn was arising, he told Graham, 'the MacNiders have been getting milk from the Sparrows for 30 years now and I'm not about to change this, and I will stay here in Chapel Hill.'[2, clip #2 min 2:23]

There had long been debate in North Carolina about the type and location of medical schools for the state. McLendon, who is extremely knowledgeable about the history of this subject, sheds further light on these events during MacNider's tenure, "In the 1920's, the Governor appointed a commission to study whether there should be a four-year medical school at Chapel Hill. President William Preston Few, of what was to become Duke University, proposed a joint school, with the two-year school in Chapel Hill and the clinical facilities in Durham at Duke University. This was thoroughly explored but was finally rejected... In retrospect, this was the best for all involved because it resulted in outstanding medical schools at Duke and Wake Forest and eventually at UNC."[2, clip #3 min 6:47, min 9:54]

Between 1937 and 1940 Will MacNider was dean of the medical school when the first building of today's modern medical campus was constructed. Dr. McLendon paints a more complete picture of MacNider, when he remembers that amid increasing demands, Dr. Billy did not forget the importance of friends, "Each year when the peak of the spring flowers was present in Chapel Hill, he would call up several friends and he and 'Miss Sally' (his wife) would get in the car, pick the friends up, and then they would drive through the countryside."[2, clip #1 min 22:29]

As Dr. MacNider entered the 1940s and more frequent invitations to speak arrived, his themes turned from the technical to the philosophical as audiences wanted the benefit of his experience. He was not flawless, however, and one bright student of that time, later to become a colleague, opined that Dr. MacNider's lectures were outdated, poorly organized, and frustrating. Chief remaining memories were descriptions of friendships with famous men. That observer also called MacNider "our school's shining star" and remarked on his kindnesses to many people, noting that his opinion of MacNider rose as time passed.[10, p. 144–145]

McLendon tells us of important contributions during the difficult war years, "One of the aspects of Dr. MacNider's research during the years included using uranium salts as a toxic agent.... It was not until the atomic bomb was dropped that he learned that uranium was being used during the Manhattan Project for the development of the atomic bomb and that he was one of the few scientists who was able in that day and time to talk to the Manhattan Project scientists about the toxic effects of uranium."[2]

It was the present author's privilege to interview Dr. McLendon, another of the "shining stars" at the University of North Carolina School of Medicine, and it was clear that he was touched by his personal friendship with Dr. MacNider as a young student, recalling for me, "he had a genius for fellowship and friendship, which again is a characteristic we associate with William Osler ... He invited me into his study, which was book-lined and photograph-lined, and we had an hour or two conversation about some of the medical and scientific greats, including Osler and Welch. He sent me at that Christmas an inscribed copy of a biography of Pasteur, which is one of my treasured books in my library to this day."[2]

MacNider's legacy

A tribute at MacNider's retirement epitomized his career, dubbing him "The Ambassador Extraordinary and Minister Plenipotentiary of the University of North Carolina." Dr. William Coppridge paid honor to MacNider after his death, summarizing his accomplishments, "This distinction is attested to by his member-ship in no less than twenty-nine medical and scientific societies. Notable among these are the National Academy of Sciences, the American Philosophical Society, and the American Academy of Arts and Sciences. He has been honored with the presidency of seven organizations and has served as editor or as a member of the editorial boards of four scientific journals."[4, p. xiv] McLendon recalls the events surrounding the death of William deBerniere MacNider, "When MacNider died in 1951, there was an outpouring of comments and responses from throughout the state, particularly in Chapel Hill ... Many people from around the state felt they had lost a close friend and an important person in the life of the state."[2] The hospital and four-year medical program, for which MacNider had prepared so diligently, opened the year after his death.

Some two years earlier, in his article "The Way of a Teacher," MacNider had reminisced about words on the sundial standing at the entrance to the Johns Hopkins Hospital, "One hour alone is in thy hands, the hour on which the shadow stands."[1, p.204] What a concise summary of Osler's principle of living life in "day-tight compartments." He was astonished that Osler treated him as an equal and recalls the epiphany, "The real teacher was at his best, not through a requirement nor by suggested research, but through a companionship that excited affection, respect, and an abiding yearning to go and do likewise[1, p. 204]. ... This student did not realize he was being instructed; these words were not labeled 'instruction' as the information came so freely and unconsciously from the master teacher. We were students together, learning and loving to learn with never a thought of an objective, an examination, a grade; ... And now, with the autopsy completed in perfect form ... the invitation came that we have Sunday dinner together, and we did."[1, p. 206] Dr. Billy's voice, thinking of his old teacher, fades from the page with a stanza from Matthew Arnold's "The Buried Life," where the poet had struggled with the unknowability of self and others. The good doctor had no such problem. He knew from whence he came, where he was, and where he was going. He caresses the meter, comparing a teacher like Osler to a great love that unlocks "the unregarded river of our life" so that,

> The eye sinks inward and the heart lies plain,
> And what we mean, we say, and what we would know.
> A man becomes aware of his life's flow
> And hears its widening murmur ... [1]

Dr. Jennette echoes the splashing impact of that ever-flowing river of mentoring, "His legacy arising from his research and scholarship is only, in some respects, a minor part of his overall legacy, which is primarily through his extremely important contributions to the establishment of the UNC School of Medicine as a leading academic medical center."[5] Dr. McLendon was an exemplar of that effect, saying all those years later when interviewed in 2012:

> Dr. MacNider was very influential in my early career and in the future choices I made in medicine. As well, he gave me the lasting gift of an interest in medical history, which I perhaps would not have had without that early exposure to him. He also gave me an interest in medical books and medical persons not only here of course, but throughout the world. As I look back at it, he probably had more impact on my career and my development that I had thought over the years . . . I am very grateful to him and in turn to Osler because I think that the several months that he spent with Dr. Osler obviously had a major impact on his life and in turn on the life of the students who were impacted by Dr. MacNider.[2]

He was visible for his research but venerated for his relationships. His last class honored him with a scroll saying, . . . "he has given to us a glimpse of the knowledge which is never found on the printed page of a text-book . . . He has taught us pride without snobbishness, and devotion to a concept without bigotry. With his own life, he has presented us with an ideal . . . of loyal friend and truly good physician."[4, p. xxiii]

And, one might add, one who followed "The Way of a Teacher."

Acknowledgments

This material was originally presented as a documentary film, now available in the archives of the University of North Carolina School of Medicine. I thank Conrad Fulkerson, who assisted with videography in the original documentary film and contributed the audio recording of Wilburt C. Davison.

References

1. MacNider W. The way of a teacher : Sir William Osler. *North Carolina Medical Journal.* 1949; 10(4): 203–206.
2. McLendon WW. Interview for video documentary about William deBerniere MacNider. In: Jones HM, ed. *American Osler Society Annual Meeting.* Chapel Hill, NC: H. Michael Jones; 2012.
3. Berryhill W, Blythe W, Manning I. *Medical Education at Chapel Hill: the First Hundred Years.* Chapel Hill: School of Medicine, University of North Carolina at Chapel Hill; 1979.
4. McLendon WW, ed. *The Good Doctor and other Selections from the Essays and Addresses of William de Berniere MacNider.* Chapel Hill: University of North Carolina Press; 1953.

5. Jennette CJ. Interview for video documentary about William deBernierre MacNider. In: Jones HM, ed. *American Osler Society Annual Meeting.* Chapel Hill, NC: H. Michael Jones; 2012.
6. Richards AN. William de Berniere MacNider: a Biographical Memoir. *Biographical Memoirs of the National Academy of Sciences* 1958: 239–272.
7. Wilson LR. *The University of North Carolina, 1900–1930: The Making of a Modern University.* Chapel Hill: University of North Carolina Press; 1957.
8. Lecture on William Osler by Wilburt Davison. Duke University Medical Center Archives, Duke University, Durham, North Carolina.
9. Martin F. Letter of deferral. In: MacNider W, ed. A Letter from the Council of National Defense deferring MacNider's application for military service ed. Chapel Hill, NC: #837, William deBerniere MacNider Papers 1905–1962, Southern Historical Collection, Wilson Library, University of North Carolina at Chapel Hill; 1918: 1.
10. Graham JB. *Memories & Reflections: Academic Medicine, 1936–2000.* Chapel Hill, North Carolina; 2002.

Earle Strain and William Osler: Coin Flips, Wood Ticks, and Rocky Mountain Spotted Fever

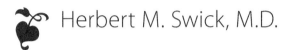 Herbert M. Swick, M.D.

Sir William Osler has long been revered and celebrated for his skills as a teacher and mentor.[1] Over his long and distinguished career at McGill University, the University of Pennsylvania, the Johns Hopkins University, and Oxford University, Osler taught thousands of medical students, acknowledging that "no bubble is so iridescent or floats longer than that blown by the successful teacher."[2] When one thinks of Osler's students, one thinks of the few who rose to prominence as deans, or department chairs, or research scientists. But most of his medical students became practicing physicians, often the "silent workers in the ranks, in villages and country districts."[3] For many of these physicians, even a brief time with William Osler etched a deep and lasting influence that shaped their careers, not only in what they had learned about the art and science of medicine but also in how they conducted their lives. One such student at the University of Pennsylvania was Earle Strain (1866–1953).

Presented at the forty-first annual meeting of the American Osler Society, Philadelphia, Pennsylvania, on 2 May 2011.

A long-floating bubble: Dr. Earle Strain

Born on 24 May 1866, Earle Strain (Figure 1) was the third of eleven children born to William and Eliza Strain. William was a farmer and implement store owner from Flesherton, Ontario, a small town which was quite near the Osler family home in Bond Head. Earle began medical school at the University of Toronto, but after two years, he transferred to the University of Pennsylvania, expressly so that he could study with William Osler. Strain's formative medical school experiences stayed with him. Five decades later, in 1944, Strain wrote to Henry Christian, then dean of the Harvard Medical School, "I had the great privilege of attending Dr. Osler's lectures in the Medical University of Pennsylvania in 1888 and 1889 and was one of a small group of students who sat at the bed sides of Old Blockley Hospital and listened to Dr. Osler classify and explain the different varieties of malaria showing examples of each. As I look back, I deem it a great privilege to have seen the beautiful dissections which he made at Blockley for the students."[4]

Following graduation from medical school in 1890, Strain set up practice in Minot, North Dakota, so that he could earn enough money to pay back his medical school debts. On 11 December 1894, Earle married Sara Elizabeth Wright, (Figure 1) who was also from Flesherton, Ontario. They had been childhood friends and sweethearts. Three weeks later, on January 2, 1895, the young newlyweds embarked on the steamship City of New York for a two-year visit to Europe, where Earle Strain spent time studying in Berlin, Vienna and London.

Earle and Sara kept a joint diary, and their contrasting entries are rather illuminating. Sara recorded excursions, tours, dinners, concerts and visits to museums such as the Louvre, where she noted that "the pictures are simply grand . . . Saw some famous paintings by Murillo [and] De,Vinci (*sic*) and the finest collection of Rubens paintings." While Sara filled her half of the diary with her impressions of European cultural treasures, Earle was recording in his half of the diary the appearance of various blood cells, amoebae and other microorgan-

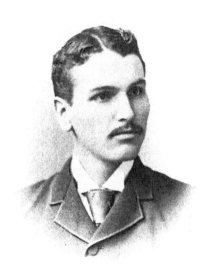
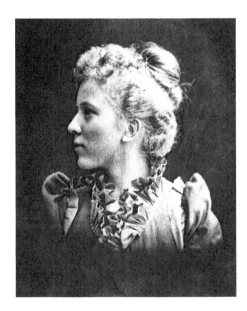

Figure 1.   Earle Strain as a medical student, circa 1890; Sara Wright Strain, undated. *Credits:* Montana Historical Society Research Center Photograph Archives, Helena, Montana, MHS PAc 94-18 1 and MHS PAc 94-18 4.

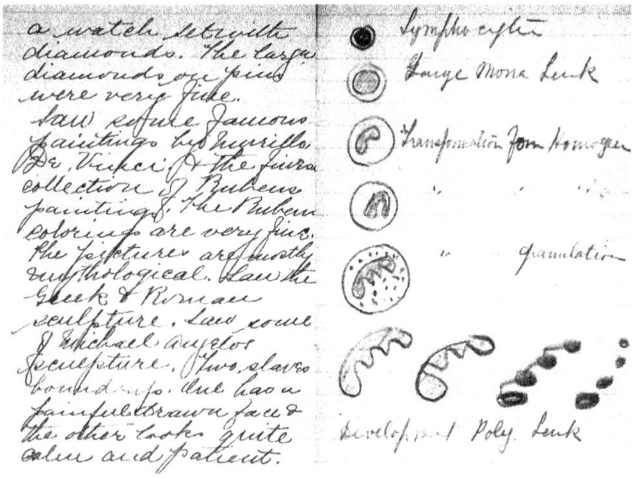

Figure 2. Diary entries by Sara and Earle Strain: Sara's notes on a museum visit and Earle's drawings on leukocyte development.
Credits: Montana Historical Society Research Center Photograph Archives, Helena, Montana, MHS MAC 249 B1 F13 and MHS MAC 249 B1 F13.

isms, as well as clinical descriptions of various diseases—not Michelangelo but microbes (Figure 2). On June 16, 1896, while the young couple was in London, Sara recorded: "South Kensington Museum. Lost Earle in the building had two policemen on his track but finally ran up against him and he seemed quite unconcerned being as he had all the money, or at least enough to pay bus fare home which I had not."[4]

On 14 February 1896, after the Strains had been in Europe for about a year, Sara wrote a delightful letter to a Canadian friend named Emma, in which she said, in part, "I think your rheumatism comes from poverty of the blood and of course that means take iron.... Well, I have to laugh when I think of the way Earle and Dr. Sippy laugh about my medical advice.... For the past year I have heard so much medicine and so many discussions.... Earle says that I will be able to assist in the practice of medicine when I get home."[4]

Later that year, the Strains returned to the United States and settled in the new frontier town of Great Falls, Montana. Founded only in 1883 near the Great Falls of the Missouri River to take advantage of hydroelectric power, the city soon became a railroad hub and industrial center. In 1894, Great Falls was described by naturalist Vernon Bailey as a "very good town" with about 15,000 inhabitants that appeared "prosperous and booming."[5] Two of Strain's brothers had already established a successful mercantile business there.

For a short time after moving to Great Falls, Earle Strain was employed as the camp physician for a large smelter owned by the Anaconda Copper Company. But he soon entered private practice, where for over 50 years, he earned "the love and gratitude of manifold hearts."[6] One indication of that gratitude is a photograph in the Strain Family archives, a photograph that one of his patients went to the effort to acquire and that Strain had obviously kept for the remainder of his life. It is an undated publicity photograph of the heavyweight boxer Jack Dempsey and the wrestler known as "Wildcat" Pete, inscribed "Happy New Year to Dr. Earle Strain from Geo. 'Wildcat' Pete and Jack Dempsey" (Figure 3). There is no information about who presented this photograph to Strain, or when, although it seems to have been taken some time during the 1930s.

At the time of his death in 1953 at the age of 87, Earle Strain was "the oldest doctor in point of service in Great Falls."[7]

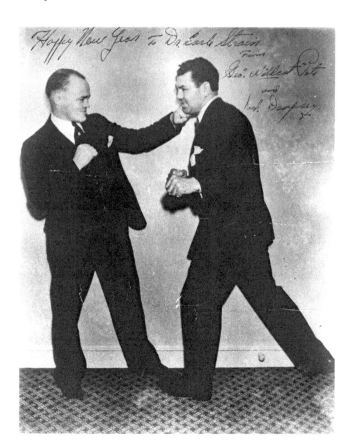

Figure 3.   George "Wildcat" Pete and Jack
Dempsey pretending to box. Inscribed: "Happy
New Year to Dr. Earle Strain from Geo.
'Wildcat' Pete and Jack Dempsey."
Credit: Montana Historical Society Research
Center Photograph Archives, Helena, Montana.
MHS PAc 94-18 36.

"... add your mite to the store of medical knowledge"[8]
—Earle Strain and wood ticks

At the turn of the last century, a disease known as "spotted fever" was a serious
problem in regions of the Rocky Mountain west, especially Idaho and Montana.
It was most common and most serious in the Bitterroot Valley just south of Missoula, where every spring brought outbreaks of what was commonly known as the
"black measles." The disease typically occurred in young men and the mortality
rate approached 80 percent, but the cause remained a mystery. There had been
earlier unsubstantiated reports of isolated patients with rashes and fevers, but
the first published reports of spotted fever as a mild disease with a low mortality
rate were from Idaho in 1896. These reports suggested that spotted fever was
a water-borne disease, or it was attributed to miasmas arising from the earth.
Ticks were never mentioned.[9] People in the Bitterroot Valley wondered if the
much more serious disease seen in that region came from drinking melted snow
water from the nearby canyons or breathing sawdust during timber operations
in the dense forests.

Soon after the Montana State Board of Health was created in April 1901,
with a lavish annual budget of $2000, an urgent appeal from the people of the
Bitterroot Valley led the governor to charge the board's first director, Dr. Albert F.
Longeway (1865–1953), with solving the "black measles" problem.[10] In April 1902,
Longeway invited his close friend, Earle Strain, to travel with him by train over
200 miles, from Great Falls, where both men practiced, to Stevensville, located
in the heart of the Bitterroot Valley. They made the trip to collect snow water

samples.[11] While in Stevensville, the two men visited a physician who happened to be removing several wood ticks embedded in the back of a young man with the "black measles." Perhaps Strain remembered William Osler's admonition to "never forget to look at the back of a patient."[12]

In 1889, as a student at the University of Pennsylvania, Strain had attended a guest lecture about mosquitoes being the possible carriers of yellow fever. The speaker was Dr. Juan Guitéras (1852–1925), himself a graduate of the University of Pennsylvania. Guiteras had been appointed to the first American Yellow Fever Commission in 1879, and in this position, he worked in Havana with Dr. Carlos Finlay (1833–1915), the Cuban physician who suggested that yellow fever could be carried by mosquitoes. In 1904, more than a decade later, while standing at the bedside of a patient in Sevensville, Montana, Strain immediately recalled this lecture. This knowledge, along with the clinical observation and reasoning skills that he had learned while studying under William Osler, gave Strain the insight and impetus to identify ticks as the vector for Rocky Mountain Spotted Fever.

Strain suggested his idea about ticks not only to Longeway, but also to two pathologists from the University of Minnesota—Louis B. Wilson (1866–1943) and William M. Chowning (b. 1873)—who had been invited to Montana by Longeway to study "black measles." Wilson and Chowning agreed that a tick was a likely vector of an infectious agent, although they hypothesized that the causative organism was a protozoan parasite.[13]

The idea of a tick-borne disease met immediate, vocal, even vehement resistance. In November 1904, Charles Wardell Stiles (1867–1941), an eminent zoologist from the US Public Health Service gave the Middleton Goldsmith Lecture to the New York Pathological Society, during which he attacked the work by Wilson and Chowning and refuted their findings.[14] He also published a long paper in 1905, denying that ticks could be the carrier and arguing that Rocky Mountain spotted fever came from drinking melted snow water. He wrote: "The tick theory has caused serious financial loss to the Bitter Root Valley and has produced an effect which in a few cases bordered on hysteria. In justice to the property interests of the valley and peace of mind of the inhabitants," he urged that no time be lost in reassuring the public that he, Stiles, had "absolutely and totally failed to confirm [the tick] hypothesis."[15] Entrepreneurs, land speculators and powerful mining interests were all concerned that news of a disease carried by insects would scare away homesteaders, settlers and investors from Chicago and other urban areas.

It was Howard T. Ricketts (1871–1910) some five years later who finally isolated the organism that causes Rocky Mountain spotted fever (later named *Rickettsia rickettsii* in his honor) and confirmed that the disease was transmitted by ticks.[16] The Strain archives contain no information concerning whether Strain and Ricketts were ever in contact, but it seems unlikely because by the time Ricketts arrived in Montana, Strain had returned to his busy practice in Great Falls.

The flip of a coin: William Osler and Albert Longeway

In 1873, William Osler traveled to Europe to spend several months studying in Berlin and Vienna. In Berlin, he was met "very graciously" by the eminent physician and scientist Rudolf Virchow, even though Osler was "just another foreign medical student" sitting in the large, tiered lecture hall.[1, pp. 76–77] Even though Osler's interactions with Rudolf Virchow were brief and limited, he made a strong and lasting impact on the young physician. Osler returned to Berlin in 1884, in part to revisit the sites—including the lecture hall—where once again he was able "to listen to the great master."[1, p. 123] It was during this visit in 1884 that Osler received an invitation to move to Philadelphia to become the Chair of Clinical Medicine. He flipped a coin to decide whether to accept the offer.[1, p. 130]

Albert F. Longeway, the first director of the Montana Board of Health, was, like Earle Strain, a Canadian. Longeway was born in Dunham, Quebec on April 6, 1865. After graduating from Bishops Medical School in Montreal in 1886, Longeway was looking for a place to practice, and he finally narrowed his choices to El Paso, Texas or Butte, Montana. He quite literally flipped a nickel to decide, and Butte it was. But when he arrived in Butte on 4 July 1887, he learned about the new city of Great Falls and decided to move there. In Great Falls, he contracted to take care of the poor for a low fixed fee, and he led a drive to establish a house to care for indigent women and orphans. Longeway was also instrumental in establishing the State Board of Health. After a long career as a surgeon and obstetrician, Longeway died in Great Falls on September 4, 1933.[17]

"... life outside the narrow circle"[18]—Earle Strain in his community

William Osler counseled students that because they would be members of both a polite and a liberal profession, "the more you see of life outside the narrow circle of your work the better ... "[18] As a practicing physician, Earle Strain exemplified this principle.

He was a long-standing member of The Round Table, comprising business, civic and professional leaders of Great Falls. The Round Table was founded in 1916 as "an informal dinner club which should meet once a month for dinner followed by a [free and understanding] discussion of some topic." Earle Strain gave ten presentations at the Round Table between September 1917 and February 1934. His topics reveal the breadth of his interests, ranging from a talk on the Irish political party Sinn Fein in 1919, to one on insulin in 1923, not long after insulin had first been described by Banting and Best. And from one titled "Religion—Medicine and Magic" in 1927, to one titled "Modern Trends in Scientific Thought" in 1934. Two of his lectures must have been truly forgettable, because the club records show the dates of the talks but not their topics![4]

Also reflecting his involvement in and commitment to the community, Earle Strain was an active member of the Royal Arch Masonic Lodge in Great Falls, one of whose missions was to spread knowledge. He was elected a life member in 1943.[7]

"To hold him who taught me this art equally dear to me as my parents"[19]—Earle Strain's other mentors

Since the days of Hippocratic medicine, physicians have acknowledged the importance of their teachers. Earle Strain followed this ancient precept.

In 1944, on the fiftieth anniversary of the Johns Hopkins University School of Medicine, Strain wrote to the dean Alan M. Chesney: "It was a great pleasure to have had as teachers for one-year Drs. William Osler and Howard Kelly," both of whom were to become founding professors at Hopkins.[4]

More than 50 years after Earle Strain had studied with Kelly in Pennsylvania, he wrote to him expressing his sympathy on the recent death of the medical illustrator Max Brödel. Kelly replied on 11 December 1941: "Thank you for such a nice kindly letter and its memories. Did not Broedel do fine work and how he did transform all our American medical art. His death was very sad. I had him for many years. . . . My one distress was that he rejected Xian faith and left us utterly rejecting it. I wonder how you are in that calling! I am most thankful to be now nearing my own end with faith in Christ. What is life without it; just nothing to hope for and with it so much to hope for. Faithfully, Howard A. Kelly"[4]

It is likely that Strain heard William Osler speak of his own experiences in Berlin and Vienna in 1873 and 1884, so it is not surprising that when he went to Europe to study fifteen years later, in 1895, he also spent time in those two cities. In Berlin, Strain studied with Rudolf Virchow's son, Hans, professor of anatomy at the University of Berlin. A few years after Strain settled in Great Falls, he sent some photographs of the city and its people to Virchow. Virchow replied on 23 March 1902: "I have only today been able to look with true enjoyment at the pictures you sent to me. There seems to be much sorrow and melancholy in those western figures. It was a great joy to me that you—so far away—thought enough of me to send me such a lovely remembrance and I thank you and Mrs. Strain." Virchow's letter was addressed simply to Dr. Earle Strain, Great Falls, Montana.[4]

Another of the famous physicians with whom Strain studied was Professor Friedrich Kovacs in Vienna, who was later to become Gustav Mahler's cardiologist as Mahler lay dying of subacute bacterial endocarditis. After the ravages of World War, I, Vienna's population faced economic hardship and starvation. Learning that his old teacher Friedrich Kovacs was in desperate straits, Earle Strain sent him some money, and received this reply, dated 3 December 1922: "Heartfelt thanks for your gift! The acceptance of which is only made possible by the awareness that you wanted to express with it your friendly feelings and memories of your former teacher. The current sad situation of Austria . . . leaves us reliant on foreign aid. Unfortunately, we cannot hope for improvement in the present unnatural isolation and. . . . Only changing the views of the current world powers can create or effect true improvement! Thank you once again. Yours, Prof Kovacs."[4]

Summary

Earle Strain's journey took him from Flesherton, Ontario, to the University of Pennsylvania to study with William Osler, to major clinics and laboratories in Europe, and finally to the small frontier town of Great Falls, Montana. His clinical skills, honed at the bedside with William Osler, were employed to serve individual patients in Great Falls, Montana for fifty years. His keen observational skills advanced the science of medicine by helping to solve the challenging riddle of Rocky Mountain spotted fever.

Acknowledgments

I thank Dr. Michael Cater, whose interest in Earle Strain and Rocky Mountain spotted fever was sparked by a brief hallway conversation at the AOS meeting in Rochester in 2010. Dr. Cater's own research was key to the preparation of this manuscript. I also thank the staff of the Montana Historical Society Research Center, Helena, Montana, for their assistance with access to the Strain Family Papers and for their permission to publish the images.

References

1. Bliss M. *William Osler: A Life in Medicine.* Oxford: Oxford University Press; 1999: 498.
2. Osler W. The pathological institute of a general hospital. *Glasgow Medical Journal* 1911; 76:321–333. Cited in Silverman ME, Murray TJ, Bryan CS, eds. *The Quotable Osler.* Philadelphia: American College of Physicians; 2003: 215.
3. Osler W. The master-word in medicine. In Osler W. *Aequanimitas, With other Addresses to Medical Students, Nurses and Practitioners of Medicine.* Third edition; Philadelphia: P. Blakiston's Son & Co., Inc.; 1932: 347–371.
4. Earle and Sara Wright Strain Family Papers, 1889–1953, Montana Historical Society Archives, Helena, Montana.
5. Bailey V. *Journal: Belt to Great Falls, August 31, 1894. In the Smithsonian Institution Archives,* https://siarchives.si.edu/collections/siris_arc_217424. *Record Unit 7267, Folder 9.*
6. Osler W. Introductory address at the opening of the forty-fifth session of the medical faculty, McGill College. *Canada Medical and Surgical Journal* 1877–1878; 6: 193–210. Cited in Silverman et al., eds., *Quotable Osler,* 79.
7. Earle Strain obituary. Montana Historical Society Photograph Archives, MC 249 B1 F2.
8. Osler W. Valedictory address to the graduates in medicine and surgery, McGill University. *Canada Medical and Surgical Journal* 1874–1875; 76: 321–333. Cited in Silverman et al., eds., *Quotable Osler,* 57.
9. Hardin V. *Rocky Mountain spotted fever: history of a twentieth-century disease.* Baltimore: The Johns Hopkins University Press; 1990: 18–19.
10. Hardin V. Rocky mountain spotted fever research and the development of the insect vector theory, 1900–1930. *Bulletin of the History of Medicine* 1985; 59: 449–466.
11. Steele V. *Bleed, Blister, and Purge: A History of Medicine on the American Frontier.* Missoula, Montana: Mountain Press Publishing Company; 2005: 270.
12. Bean WB, ed. *Sir William Osler: Aphorisms.* Cited in Silverman et al., eds., *Quotable Osler,* 99.
13. Wilson LB and Chowning WM. Studies in pyroplasmosis hominis ("spotted fever" or "tick fever" of the Rocky Mountains). *Journal of Infectious Diseases* 1904; 1: 31–57.
14. Stiles CW. Zoological pitfalls for the pathologist. *Proceedings of the New York Pathological Society* 1905. Cited in Harden: *Rocky Mountain Spotted Fever,* 49.
15. Stiles CW. *Annual Report, Public Health and Marine Hospital Service*; 1904; 363.

16. Aikawa JK. *Rocky Mountain Spotted Fever*. Springfield, Illinois: Charles C. Thomas; 1966: 14–15.

17. Phillips PC. *Medicine in the Making of Montana*. Missoula: Montana State University Press; 1962: 356, 359.

18. Osler W. After twenty-five years. In Osler, *Aequanimitas* (third edition), 289–206.

19. The Hippocratic Oath. https://www.nlm.nih.gov/hmd/greek/greek_oath.html, accessed 7 March 2021.

Osler, *The Fixed Period,* and Science Fiction

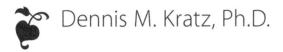 Dennis M. Kratz, Ph.D.

Sir William Osler's approving mention, in his 1905 farewell address to colleagues at the Johns Hopkins University, of Anthony Trollope's "charming novel" *The Fixed Period* (1882) has received considerable attention—much of it focused on the controversy that his remarks provoked.[1-5] Although Osler clearly intended his praise of "college and chloroform" in jest, serious concerns often underlie humorous remarks. Trollope's novel clearly resonated both with Osler's fear of a useless old age and with his conviction that human beings have a physiologically fixed life span. As Michael Bliss has observed, "Osler did not foresee the great payoff of modern medicine . . . an extension of our life span also enriched by better health at every stage, including old age;"[6] and yet that extension arguably reinforces the continuing relevance of Osler's concern. Physical health and mental acuity eventually decline in all of us. Technological advances beyond the capacity of Osler (or perhaps any of his contemporaries) to imagine, such as cloning and genetic manipulation, already exist. What if scientific and medical advances were to produce sentient beings, perhaps indistinguishable from humans, by artificial means? Would it be morally acceptable to impose a fixed period of life on them? Meant humorously or not, Osler's remarks raise intriguing questions; moreover, although he rarely referred to contemporary fiction, he drew his inspiration from a novel. This essay, then, has three modest goals: first, to examine once more the intent and implications of Osler's reference to *The Fixed Period*; second, to survey some of the most important works of Science Fiction that deal directly or obliquely with the notion of a governmentally imposed Fixed Period on the life of its citizens; third, to reconsider Osler's concern in light of those fictions.

Presented at the forty-fourth annual meeting of the American Osler Society, Oxford, United Kingdom, on 12 May 2014.

Why stories? Because we are, after all, story-telling beings. We share information, ideas and emotions most often and most effectively by shaping them as narratives.[7] The essential role of science, as the physicist Brian Greene eloquently states, is "to pull back the veil obscuring an objective reality," fixing on results that transcend the experience of any given individual."[8] Stories have a different concern: "They illuminate the richness of our ineluctably circumscribed and thoroughly subjective existence."[8, p. 181] While Science helps us understand the processes at work in the natural world, it is primarily through stories that we endow our lives with meaning and significance.

Why Science Fiction? Because it integrates science, art, and the humanities by weaving compelling tales from extrapolated or plausible developments in science, technology, and medicine. It is fitting that this essay originated in a presentation delivered at Oxford. Some would trace the origin of the genre to the publication of Mary Shelley's *Frankenstein: or The Modern Prometheus* (1816). In my mind, the true founder of modern philosophic Science Fiction is H.G. Wells, born less than 100 kilometers from Oxford. Both these foundational writers dealt with medical themes: Shelley with the artificial creation of life, and Wells, in *The Island of Dr. Moreau* (1896), with the transformation of animals into humans through vivisection and conditioning. At its best, Science Fiction confronts the reader with new and imagined developments that challenge our ethical assumptions, including our concept of what constitutes human.

Osler citing Trollope

Published in 1882 and set in 1980, *The Fixed Period* is a satirical novel about euthanasia as a solution to the problem of aging. It is presented as the memoir of John Neverbend, first President of Britannula, a fictional island near New Zealand founded by idealistic young rebels who have declared independence from Britain. Neverbend had led the enactment of a law obligating men upon reaching their sixty-seventh birthday to retire to a college for a year of contemplation before committing voluntary suicide. The justification for this policy, Neverbend explains, was solely to prevent the suffering and calamities of old age. The mandate, however, has generated increasing opposition as its citizens age toward their legislated demise. Before the first citizen to reach sixty-seven could fulfill his obligation, a British warship arrives to depose Neverbend, overthrow the government and re-annex Britannula.

Among the most striking characteristics of Osler's reference to *The Fixed Period* is its inaccuracy. The "admirable scheme" at the center of the novel that he describes as retirement to a college at age sixty for "a year of contemplation followed by a peaceful departure by chloroform"[1] is doubly inaccurate: The age was sixty-seven and the ritual suicide did not involve chloroform. Osler also neglects to mention that the policy was never enacted. Just as jests often reflect a serious concern, however, so "mistakes" often reflect purposeful changes by an author. Osler was, after all, an accomplished lecturer who had paid considerable attention to the design and content of this address. He may well have considered "college and chloroform" a more memorable phrase than "college and ritual suicide." He modifies his approbation of the concept, moreover, by admitting that he had become a "little dubious" regarding its wisdom of as his own time was getting so short. He was at the time fifty-five—much closer to sixty than the actual age of "departure" in Britannula. Finally, as an occasional satirist and self-professed jokester, Osler may have chosen this novel because of his impish sense of humor. While it is impossible to estimate how many in the audience would have been familiar with *The Fixed Period*, given its publication date and relative obscurity, the number surely was small. Those who took the trouble to read it would discover that, whether by accident or subtle irony, Osler—about to leave North America for England—had called attention to a fictional former British colony that had acted with sufficient foolishness to justify invasion and re-annexation.

Fixed Periods in Science Fiction

Fixed-Period Science Fiction—defined here as the depiction of imagined societies that have adopted compulsory suicide or execution at the conclusion of an arbitrarily allotted lifetime—has had a sporadic afterlife in the Science Fiction literature. The narratives range from short stories to novels, an episode of a popular television series to full-length films. Most are set in a dystopian future where an oppressive government enforces a Fixed Period of life for its citizens. Some are satirical, others use the subject as the frame for generic adventure tales, and several offer thoughtful commentaries on the concept. American authors tend to imagine the impulse for such a policy less on minimizing the horrors of aging than on maintaining economic abundance or controlling the population. Several stories pointedly serve as warnings against the loss of freedom under authoritarian governments. Freedom and Consumption, often conjoined, are the philosophic bedrock of American popular culture.

Most American narratives also make use of the conventional plot device of heroic efforts by an idealistic or revolutionary hero to strike a blow for liberty and the pursuit of personal happiness. Among the earliest narratives of this sort is *Pebble in the Sky*,[9] the first novel published by the scientist-author Isaac Asimov. It imagines Earth tens of thousands of years into the future as ecologically devastated and despised by the other planets that form a Galactic Empire. The Empire requires all humans be executed at age sixty-one of many humiliations reflecting Earth's lowly placement in the galactic caste system. The novel itself focuses on Earth's rebellion against the Empire.

Variations of the Fixed Period theme flourished most intensely during 1965–1976—an era of American history where the appearance of stories about rebellion and rage against conformity hardly comes as a surprise. In 1965, Harlan Ellison published in *Galaxy Magazine* the immensely popular short story "Repent, Harlequin, Said the Tick-Tock Man!"[10] A Fixed Period, with an additional dimension, is central to this tale. Ellison depicts the failed rebellion of one Everett C. Marm (in the guise of the heroic Harlequin) to disrupt his totally regimented society, where citizens not only are allotted a fixed lifespan, but also where crimes (along a spectrum from robbery to arriving late for work) are punished by deductions of time from that allotted span. Ellison's tale extends the Fixed Period theme to encompass the dangers of mindlessly accepting order over adventure, regimented safety over joy. It invites interpretation also as a parable about the exploitation of workers for the benefit of the wealthy and powerful—some lives shortened by the dangers of work so that others can be extended.

In this same period of imaginative florescence, Philip K. Dick published *Do Androids Dream of Electric Sheep?*[11] that introduced "replicants," or genetically modified androids, into literature. Dick's replicants are designed specifically for environments and work (for example, mining on asteroids) impossible for humans. Since the replicants were powerful and could be distinguished from natural humans only with difficulty, the creators had purposely and severely limited their lifespan to limit their individual and collective power. Although the limited lifespan is a relatively minor element, Dick embedded within the plot (efforts by a human detective to capture rebellious replicants) a deeply philosophic exploration of "humanness."

In 1967, William Nolan and George Clayton published the novel *Logan's Run*.[12] In the world of 2116, citizens are allotted a fixed life span of 21 years. The justification has obviously moved away from preventing the agonies of old age: 21 as the onset of senility is a radical notion even for a youth-centric era known for admonishing against trusting anyone over 30. In *Logan's Run* the early deaths assure the availability of resources needed for a "good life" for everyone. The novel offers an early and intriguing contribution to critiques of American obsession with both consumption and control, though the culturally critical element of the story is diminished by a conventional plot about the attempt of the eponymous hero Logan to escape his allotted fate by joining a rebellion against the state.

Generally regarded as the best of American mid-century dystopian novels is Ira Levin's *This Perfect Day*,[13] although it too falls back on the conventional depiction of an oppressively regimented society and a small band of freedom-seeking rebels. In the future imagined by Levin, a world government has been established. A computer (known as Uni) has programmed everything for efficiency. Uni not only monitors the behavior of every individual but also provides all of humanity's needs: food, shelter, employment, medical care, and monthly sedatives. Even the vagaries of nature are controlled and predictable—it only rains in the evening, and everyone dies at the arbitrarily set age of sixty-two. Levin revives the justification of preventing the ravages of age, but automatic euthanasia is just one among many aspects of the society's complete regimentation. The novel ends with a symbolic indication that the rebels have won: a rain shower in the middle of the afternoon.

Finally, two narratives that place a Fixed Period at their center rise above the rest to demonstrate the power of science fiction as a vehicle for philosophic speculation. The first is an episode of the highly regarded television series *Star Trek: Next Generation*. The episode "Half a Life"[14] depicts an encounter of the Starship *Enterprise* with a planet, Kaelon, where ancient custom and common assent have established that every person must commit ritual suicide at age sixty. This imagined society has adopted forced euthanasia for both economic and medical reasons: to prevent the suffering of old age and the burdens that caring for the aged would place on the limited resources of the planet and the lives of the young. The policy has become embedded as an unquestioned thread of the social fabric.

The *Enterprise* has arrived to help the planet deal with an imminent threat to its existence: its sun is dying. On board is the planet's greatest scientist, Timicin, who has devoted his life save his planet from destruction. He is on the verge of finding a successful solution; unfortunately, he is also on the verge of turning sixty. He has sought refuge on the *Enterprise* to accelerate his work in the limited time remaining him. The episode consists primarily of conversations and debates about the Fixed Period. Although Timicin initially defends the custom, the realization that he is so close to achieving his goal leads him to seek an "extension." His request is denied; in fact, he is informed that any discoveries or solutions that he reaches after his sixtieth birthday will not be implemented. In the pivotal scene, his daughter beams aboard the *Enterprise* to tell her father that she is ashamed of him—and that "every day past sixty that you are alive will be an insult to all that we believe in."

The episode concludes with Timicin having decided return to his death—and leaving questions for the viewer to decide. The often-simplified distinction between individual liberty and government oppression here receives a more nuanced expression—fulfilling the artistic goal of raising questions rather than providing solutions. The practice has not been imposed by an autocratic government, but rather is part of the social fabric. Is the governing outlook of the inhabitants a barbaric custom that inhibits not only scientific progress but also—more disastrously—their very survival? Or is it a ritual that gives structure, cohesiveness and meaning to the lives of the inhabitants? The episode breathes new life into a too often predictable theme by replacing the easier emphasis on heroic disobedience with a more nuanced exploration of the power of "the web of values of our own creation in which we are suspended" to guide behavior.[15]

Finally, a major work of Science Fiction by Kazuo Ishiguro, the 2017 Nobel Laureate in Literature, uses a Fixed Period (related to function rather than time) to explore issues of medicine and human value. In the brilliant and disturbing novel *Never Let Me Go* (2005),[16] Ishiguro (who was born in Japan and educated in England) describes an alternate twentieth-century world where the demand for organ transplants, coupled with dramatic advances in cloning technology, has led to the creation of a sub-class of cloned beings who exist for the purpose of donating organs at regular intervals until they die. The clones are "students" of an institution designed to prepare them for their lives of "service." He avoids the generic emphasis on rebellion against oppression to focus on the lives, friendships, loves and sorrows of three clones, whom we meet as adolescents and slowly discover, with them, the truth of their origin and fate.

Never Let Me Go invites direct comparison to both *Frankenstein* and *The Island of Dr. Moreau*. Central to all three is the creation of artificial life and a focus on the "education" of those creations. Ishiguro's novel establishes an especially meaningful connection, however, with the central theme of Wells' novel: the danger of the quest for truth detached from considerations of moral principles or human kindness. Wells uses a chilling soliloquy by Moreau to justify his experiments with animals:

> You see, I went on with this research just the way it led me. That is the only way I ever heard of research going. I asked a question, devised some method of getting an answer, and got—a fresh question.... To this day I have never troubled about the ethics of the matter. The study of Nature makes a man at last as remorseless as
> Nature. I have gone on, not heeding anything but the question I was pursuing.[17]

Ishiguro includes a similar justification of subordinating the ethical implications of medical research to the benefits of success—perhaps more disturbing because it is couched in language of kindness and benevolence. Confronted by her former students, a retired administrator of the school thus explains the context:

> After the war, in the early fifties, when the great breakthroughs in science followed one after the other so rapidly, there was not time to take stock, to ask the sensible questions. Suddenly there were all these new possibilities laid before us, all these ways to cure so many previously incurable conditions. And for a long time, people preferred to believe these organs appeared from nowhere, or at least that they grew in a kind of vacuum ... There was no way to reverse the process. How can you ask a world that has come to regard cancer as curable, how can you ask such

a world to put away that cure, to go back to the dark days? There was no going back.[16, p. 262]

Ishiguro's extraordinary novel weaves together multiple threads to create the most intellectually provocative of all the fictions mentioned in this essay: scientific curiosity, the human desire to control nature, the lure of improving life spans and the quality of life for the many through the exploitation of the vulnerable, and the temptation of permitting ignoble actions if they produce noble—that is, popular and profitable—results.

As so often happens, examining one idea leads to another, more profound one: in this case, Osler's insistence on the complementarity of Science and the Humanities. In his lecture "The Old Humanities and the New Science" Osler employs the compelling metaphor that Science and Humanities are "twin berries one stem, grievous damage has been done to both" in regarding them in any other way.[18] Ishiguro this separation addresses by questioning the moral implications of shortening the length and quality of some lives so that others can be longer and more pleasant. In the same lecture, Osler expressed his concern whether a love of the "higher and brighter" aspects of life can thrive "in a civilization based on a philosophy of force." Nonetheless, he ends that lecture on a note of optimism. Leaving behind thoughts of "college and chloroform," he finds in Hippocrates' fusion of *philanthropia* and *philotechnia* (love of humanity joined to love of one's work) "perhaps the subtle suggestion that perhaps in this combination the longings of humanity may find their solution." Symbolically appropriate, he spoke those words at Oxford—in May 1919, as his seventieth birthday approached.

Summary

Although meant humorously, Osler's apparent approval of Trollope's *The Fixed Period* anticipates ethical dilemmas that could arise from the separation of scientific research and medical innovation from moral considerations. Authors of Science Fiction subsequently have explored the implications and dilemmas associated specifically with attempts to enhance the quality or extend the length of some lives at the expense of others. In his final lecture, "The Old Humanities and the New Science," Osler emphasized the complementary relationship of Science and the Humanities, concluding with a statement on the importance of combining technical knowledge with philanthropy.

References

1. Osler W. The Fixed Period. In Hinohara S. and Hisae N., eds. *Osler's A Way of Life and Other Addresses*. Durham and London: Duke University Press; 2001: 287–304.
2. Trollope A. *The Fixed Period*. Leipzig: Bernard Tauchnitz; 1882.
3. Bliss M. *William Osler: A Life in Medicine*. Oxford: Oxford University Press; 1999: 321–328.
4. Ambrose CT. William Osler and the "fixed period" of creativity. *Journal of Medical Biography* 2019; 27(4): 187–197.

5. Bryan CS. Osler goes viral: "The fixed period" revisited. *Baylor University Medical Center Proceedings* 2018; 31(4): 550–553.
6. Bliss M. *The Making of Modern Medicine. Turning Points in the Treatment of Disease.* Chicago: University of Chicago Press; 2011: 90.
7. Bruner J. *Actual Minds, Possible Worlds.* Cambridge MA: Harvard University Press; 1986: 15–16.
8. Greene B. *Until the End of Time.* New York: Alfred A. Knopf; 2020: 180.
9. Asimov A. *Pebble in the Sky.* New York: Doubleday; 1950.
10. Ellison H. "Repent Harlequin! Said the Tick-Tock Man." *Galaxy Science Fiction Magazine*; December 1965.
11. Dick P. *Do Androids Dream of Electric Sheep?* New York: Doubleday; 1968
12. Clayton G. and Nolan W. *Logan's Run.* New York: Doubleday; 1967.
13. Levin I. *This Perfect Day.* New York: Random House; 1970.
14. "Half a Life." *Star Trek: Next Generation.* Season 4. Episode 22; 1991.
15. Geertz C. *The Interpretation of Cultures.* New York: Basic Books; 1983: 38.
16. Ishiguro K. *Never Let Me Go.* New York: Random House; 2005.
17. Wells H. *The Island of Dr. Moreau.* In *Seven Famous Novels by H. G. Wells.* New York: Knopf; 1934: 116.
18. Osler W. *The Old Humanities and the New Science.* Boston: Houghton Mifflin Company; 1920.

SECTION V

 Osler's Afterlife—Moving Forward

Chester R. Burns and the Origins of the American Osler Society

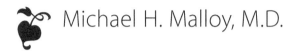 Michael H. Malloy, M.D.

The American Osler Society (AOS), one of the premier organizations devoted to the history of medicine, medical biography and more broadly, the humanities as related to medicine, traces its origin to a symposium held in Spring of 1970 at the Flagship Hotel in Galveston, Texas.[1,2] Attendees included some several notable physicians who had been proteges of Sir William Osler (1849–1919) at Oxford including the pediatrician Wilburt Cornell Davison (1892–1972), the vascular surgeon Emile Frederic Holman (1890–1977), and the neurosurgeon Wilder Graves Penfield (1891–1976). The symposium generated sufficient enthusiasm to prompt the formal organization of the AOS, which held its first official meeting in Denver, Colorado, on 1 April 1971. Papers from the symposium in Galveston were later published as a monograph to which the introduction begins:

> Why is William Osler revered as a medical humanist? . . . What are
> the relationships or lack thereof between studies in the humanities and
> the development of humane and humanistic attitudes? Is the future
> of humanism in medicine a matter of teaching humanities in medical
> schools or a matter of defining desired attitudes and determining ways to
> cultivate these attitudes or both?[1]

The introduction was signed by John P. McGovern (1921–2007) and Chester Ray Burns (1937–2007). Charles G. Roland (1933–2009) in his account of the origins of AOS recognizes McGovern as the driving force and mentions Burns only in

Accepted for presentation at the fiftieth annual meeting of the American Osler Society, Pasadena, California, 26–30 April 2020, which was canceled due to the Covid-19 pandemic. Portions of this manuscript are, at the time of this writing, in press at the *Journal of Medical Biography*.

passing.[3] However, McGovern introduced Burns at the 1970 symposium as the only attendee possessing doctoral degrees in both medicine and the humanities.[4]

Chester Ray Burns

Chester Burns (Figure 1) was born in Nashville, Tennessee, and received his undergraduate and medical degrees (1959 and 1963, respectively) from Vanderbilt University in that city. As an undergraduate he majored in philosophy, was president of the Debate Club, and belonged to the Glee Club, the Skull and Bones Pre-Med Club, and other organizations.[5] He received his undergraduate degree with honors but finished medical school in the lower third of his class. The dean of students at Vanderbilt, however, noted that his academic record "does not represent his scholastic ability," and that while he "experienced considerable difficulty . . . during his first two years" his work during the third and fourth years showed "progressive improvement." The dean of students further noted that he got on well with fellow students and served as president of his medical fraternity and president of the Vanderbilt Historical Society. These attributes served him well during his subsequent career as a physician-humanist.

Burns did an internship in pediatrics at the University of Oklahoma, during which he applied to become a doctoral candidate in the History and Philosophy

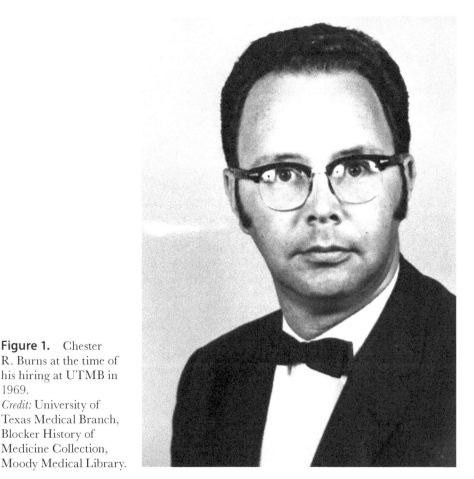

Figure 1.   Chester R. Burns at the time of his hiring at UTMB in 1969.
Credit: University of Texas Medical Branch, Blocker History of Medicine Collection, Moody Medical Library.

of Medicine at Johns Hopkins. No record of his application exists apart from its approval by Owsei Temkin (1902–2002), director of the Institute of History of Medicine at Hopkins.[6] In 1969 Burns became the first American-born physician to receive a doctorate in the history of medicine from Johns Hopkins. (Of the four previous persons to receive Ph.D. degrees in the history of medicine from Johns Hopkins, two were non-physicians and two were physicians born outside the U.S.) His doctoral dissertation was on "Medical Ethics in the United States before the Civil War."[7] The dissertation was not published but has been frequently cited in the literature and formed the basis for some of Burns's later work.

In August 1969 Burns was hired fresh out of his doctoral program by Truman Blocker (1909–1984) to become director of a new History of Medicine Division at the University of Texas Medical Branch (UTMB) in Galveston. Burns spent the rest of his career at that institution and eventually wrote its centennial history. He noted that some of the original professors at UTMB, which was founded in 1891, lectured in medical history, ethics, and jurisprudence although none had specific training in these areas.[8] In 1952 Chauncey D. Leake (1896–1978), who was then dean of UTMB, hired Patrick Romanell (1912–2002), who had a doctorate in philosophy from Columbia University, to teach ethics and philosophy. Romanell left the UTMB in 1962 and teaching in the humanities lay fallow until Blocker became chief executive officer and, in 1965, invited Leake to come back to lecture in the history and philosophy of medicine. Blocker later obtained funding from the Rockwell Foundation in Houston to endow a professorship in the history of medicine. Burns was thus the first person to fill that position (Figure 1).

Burns and the founding of the American Osler Society

Concern that science and technology were eroding the humanistic dimensions of medicine accelerated during the 1960s, prompting McGovern and Alfred R. Henderson (1920–2019) to consider a new organization to address this problem. They envisioned a symposium on "Humanism in Medicine" as a trial balloon.[9] McGovern hoped to hold the symposium in Houston, and to that end worked with H. Grant Taylor (1903–1995), dean of the Graduate School of Biomedical Sciences at the University of Texas Medical School at Houston (now the John P. and Kathrine G. McGovern Medical School at the University of Texas Health Sciences Center, Houston). Taylor encountered obstacles at his institution and therefore consulted Blocker at UTMB, who agreed to hold the meeting in Galveston. Blocker instructed Taylor to ask McGovern to contact Chester Burns to begin planning for the symposium on Humanism in Medicine.[10]

McGovern and Burns already knew of each other if only by correspondence. The link dates to 1968 as evinced by correspondence filed at the John P. McGovern Historical Collections and Research Center at the Texas Medical Center in Houston. McGovern was looking for a good copy of the second edition of *The Principles and Practice of Medicine* by Osler. How Burns learned of McGovern's need remains a mystery—perhaps McGovern asked someone at Johns Hopkins for a recommendation, and was referred to Burns—but at any rate McGovern offered Burns $6.00 for the book plus payment for the postage.[11]

Burns apparently agreed to do most of the legwork for the symposium on Humanism in Medicine, including a meeting of the Program Committee held in Galveston on 7 January 1970. Shortly thereafter, on 7 February, McGovern signed the Articles of Incorporation of the AOS in Houston.[12] The five original trustees were William Bennett Bean (1909–1989), George T. Harrell (1908–1999), Thomas M. Durant (1905–1977), McGovern, and Henderson. Bean, Harrell, and Durant consented to serve as president, first vice president, and second vice president, respectively. Edward C. Rosenow, Jr. (1909–2002) became the sixth officer as secretary-elect.

The symposium on Humanism in Medicine took place 21–22 April 1970 at the Flagship Hotel in Galveston, hosted by McGovern and Burns.[1] The stated aims were to address how humanism is manifested in the history of medicine, "whether humanism has a place in the construction of goals and priorities in medicine," and "why William Osler is revered as a medical humanist." Three of the 13 papers were given by the honored guests who had known Osler—Davison, Holman, and Penfield—who discussed their understanding and experience of

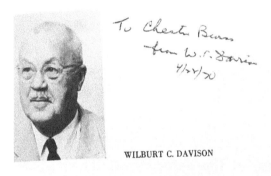

Figure 2. Photographs and autographs of Wilburt C. Davison (1892–1972), Emile F. Holman (1890–1977), and Wilder G. Penfield (1891–1976)—all of whom were among the last surviving protégés of Sir William Osler—from the 1970 symposium on Humanism in Medicine. *Credit:* University of Texas Medical Branch, Blocker History of Medicine Collection, Moody Medical Library.

WILBURT C. DAVISON

EMILE F. HOLMAN

WILDER G. PENFIELD

Osler's effect on medical humanism (Figure 2). Six other presentations further described Osler's influence on the humanities and the persons who had influenced Osler. The remaining four presentations dealt with various aspects of humanism in the medical past and the impact of humanism on the education of the physician.

McGovern received most of the credit for the symposium, as evinced by a letter from Bean congratulating him on the "magnificent program, magnificent in conception and in execution."[13] There is no written documentation that any attendees acknowledged Burns for having done most of the organizational work, although some, including Emile Holman and Wilburt Davison, thanked him for kindnesses and courtesies that helped make the meeting so enjoyable and memorable.[2]

Burns did not become a charter member of the AOS even though he did much and perhaps most of the organizational work for the symposium. The trustees had met in February 1970, two months before the symposium, and elected 30 charter members from a pool of 60 nominees. McGovern expressed his regrets to Burns: "I did put your name into the pot but unfortunately, we didn't make it this go-round, as the majority wished to select individuals who had demonstrated a long-time interest in Osleriana and related aspects. I have little doubt, however, that you will be elected at the next general membership meeting next year as I am on the nominating committee."[14] Burns was elected into the second class of inductees and introduced at the May 1972 meeting, which took place in Montreal.[15]

Burns's subsequent career

Burns co-edited with McGovern *Humanism in Medicine* (1983), a monograph containing all of the papers presented at the 1970 symposium. Again, it is unclear how much of the work was done by McGovern and how much by Burns. Burns went on to become a major force in developing the humanities program at UTMB. He was largely responsible for obtaining systems approval and financial support, including a grant from the National Endowment for the Arts of which he was principal investigator, to establish an Institute for the Medical Humanities.[16]

This institute has now provided educational programs at the undergraduate and graduate levels at the UTMB Schools of Medicine, Nursing, and Allied Health Professions for nearly half a century.[17]

William B. Bean, the first president of the AOS, was appointed the first Director of the Institute for the Medical Humanities at UTMB, with Burns being appointed co-director.[18] Bean resigned his Directorship in 1979, and Burns was appointed as Acting Director through January 1981.[19] Burns became interested in Osler as a result of the 1970 symposium and continued that interest, eventually serving as the thirty-fifth president of the AOS (2004–2005) (Figure 3).[20] He published actively in ethics and philosophy as well as in the history of medicine and supervised graduate students in these areas. He retired from UTMB shortly before his unexpected death in 2006.[21 26]

The questions posed in the introduction to the symposium on the Humanism in Medicine still resonate in medical education. What do we mean by "humanism"? Are the humanities necessary for "humanism"? How can we best balance detached objectivity with empathic caring in medical education? Burns worried about these issues and tried as best he could to integrate the humanities into the process of educating future physicians and keeping these issues in front

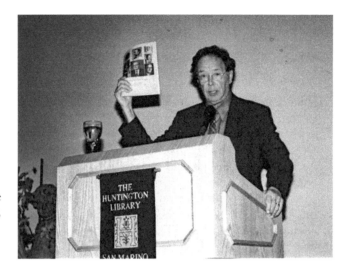

Figure 3.   Chester R. Burns as president of the American Osler Society, Pasadena, California, 2005. *Credit:* Charles S. Bryan.

of his colleagues. After all, his first student in developing the curriculum for this process was himself.[27] Chester Burns's dedication to the humanities and medicine is made manifest by the life he lived. The hope in presenting this brief narrative of his life is that others will remember him as a contributor to the early evolution of the American Osler Society and as a staunch advocate for the integration of the humanities into medical education and the practice of medicine.

Acknowledgments

I thank librarians and archivists at the John P. McGovern Historical Collections and Research Center at the Texas Medical Center in Houston, Texas, Vanderbilt University and Vanderbilt University School of Medicine, both in Nashville, Tennessee, and The Institute of the History of Medicine, The Johns Hopkins University, Baltimore, Maryland, for invaluable assistance.

References

1. McGovern JP, Burns CR. *Humanism in Medicine.* Springfield, IL: Charles C Thomas; 1973.
2. Burns, CR. Oslerians Gather in Galveston, April 1970. University of Texas Medical Branch, Blocker History of Medicine Collection, Moody Medical Library. Institute for the Medical Humanities Records (1969–1983); MS79; Box 2, File 15.
3. Roland CG. The formative years of the American Osler Society. *The Persisting Osler III Selected Transactions of the American Osler Society 1991–2000.* Malabar, Florida: Krieger Publishing Company; 2002: 189–201.
4. McGovern JP. Introductory notes to Humanism in Medicine Symposium, April 21, 1970. John P. McGovern Papers at John P. McGovern Historical

Collections and Research Center, Texas Medical Center Library, Houston. MS115; Box 1, File 3.

5. Personal communication, History of Medicine Collections and Archives Vanderbilt University Libraries, 2019.

6. Personal communication, Alan Mason Chesney Archives of the Johns Hopkins Medical Institutions, 2019.

7. Burns CR. *Medical Ethics in the United States Before the Civil War.* 1969. Institute of the History of Medicine Rare Books—Vault 1, third floor, William H. Welch Medical Library, the Johns Hopkins Medical Institutions; INST Diss.B967 1965 c.1.

8. Burns CR. *Saving Lives, Training Caregivers, Making Discoveries: A Centennial History of the University of Texas Medical Branch at Galveston.* Austin, TX. Texas State Historical Association; 2003: 223–236.

9. Boutwell, B. *John P. McGovern: A Lifetime of Stories.* College Station, TX. Texas A&M University Press; 2014: 174–181.

10. Truman R. Blocker to H. Grant Taylor, 20 October 1969. University of Texas Medical Branch, Blocker History of Medicine Collection, Moody Medical Library. Institute for the Medical Humanities Records (1969–1983); MS79; Box 2, File 16.

11. Chester R. Burns to John P. McGovern, 26 September 1968. University of Texas Medical Branch, Blocker History of Medicine Collection, Moody Medical Library. Institute for the Medical Humanities Records (1969–1983); MS 79; Box 2, File 16.

12. William Bean to John P. McGovern, 27 April 1970. John P. McGovern Papers at John P. McGovern Historical Collections and Research Center, Texas Medical Center Library, Houston. MS 115, Box 220.

13. John P. McGovern to Chester Burns, 25 February 1970. John P. McGovern Papers at John P. McGovern Historical Collections and Research Center, Texas Medical Center Library, Houston. MS 115, Box 220.

14. William Bean to John P. McGovern, 5 February 1972. John P. McGovern Papers at John P. McGovern Historical Collections and Research Center, Texas Medical Center Library, Houston. MS 115, Box 220.

15. Burns, Chester R. NEH: Original Grant Proposal, 1974–1979. University of Texas Medical Branch, Blocker History of Medicine Collection, Moody Medical Library. Institute for the Medical Humanities Records (1969–1983); MS79; Box 17, File 127.

16. Jones AH and Carson R. Medical humanities at the University of Texas Medical Branch at Galveston. *Academic Medicine* 2003; 78: 1006–1009.

17. Ed Brandt to William Bean, 15 July 1974. University of Texas Medical Branch, Blocker History of Medicine Collection, Moody Medical Library. Institute for the Medical Humanities Records (1969–1983); MS79; Levin, Box 16, File 3.

18. William Bean to Bill Levin, 25 July 1979. University of Texas Medical Branch, Blocker History of Medicine Collection, Moody Medical Library. Institute for the Medical Humanities Records (1969–1983); MS79; Levin, Box 16, File 3.

19. Burns CR. In search of wisdom: William Osler and the humanities. *Medical Education* 2003; 37: 165–167.

20. Burns CR. History in medical education: the development of current trends in the United States. *Bulletin of the New York Academy of Medicine* 1975; 51(7): 851–869.

21. Burns CR. Richard Clarke Cabot (1868–1939) and reformation in American medical ethics. *Bulletin of the History of Medicine* 1977; 51(3): 353–368.
22. Burns CR. Fictional doctors and the evolution of medical ethics in the United States, 1875–1900. *Literature & Medicine* 1988; 7: 39–55.
23. Burns CR. Writing the history of medical ethics: a new era for the new millennium. *Medical Humanities Review* 2000; 14(1): 35–41.
24. Burns CR. The development of hospitals in Galveston during the nineteenth century. *Southwestern Historical Quarterly* 1993; 97: 238–263.
25. Burns CR. The University of Texas Medical Branch at Galveston. Origins and beginnings. *Journal of the American Medical Association* 1991: 266(10): 1400–1403.
26. Burns CR. A journey in the borderlands of medicine and the humanities. *Medical Humanities Review* 2001; 15(2): 9–20.

An Osler-Centered Undergraduate Course in Medical Humanities

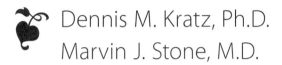

Dennis M. Kratz, Ph.D.
Marvin J. Stone, M.D.

Some medical schools and graduate courses on medical humanities—notably, at Penn State,[1,2] the University of Texas Medical Branch in Galveston,[3] and Dalhousie Medical School in Nova Scotia[4,5]—have integrated the life and writings of Sir William Osler into their curricula. However, Osler seems to be essentially absent from American undergraduate education. The present authors sought to address that absence by developing an undergraduate course at The University of Texas at Dallas (UT Dallas) that uses Osler's career and writings to explore current issues, challenges, and ethical concerns of health care.

The idea for the course emerged from a team-taught course that Dr. Marvin Stone had created for Texas A&M Senior medical students rotating at Baylor Hospital in Dallas. That course included sessions dedicated to Osler's life, thoughts, and contributions to medical practice and education. Dr. Stone approached Dr. Dennis Kratz, a member of the teaching team who was then serving as Dean of the UT Dallas School of Arts and Humanities, about adapting the Texas A&M course for undergraduate instruction.

After much discussion, Kratz and Stone decided to build a separate undergraduate course around Osler's life, writings, and contributions to medical practice. They based this decision on three factors: First, Osler is arguably the role model par excellence of the clinician-educator in the history of modern medicine.

Presented in part at the forty-seventh annual meeting of the American Osler Society, Atlanta, Georgia, on 11 April 2017.

Second, Osler was not only internationally recognized as a physician and educator but also "much more than a physician, Osler was a literate, inspiring, humanist in science."[6] Third, his career provides a valuable entrance point for examining issues of current ethical and cultural importance. The last half of the nineteenth century signaled the acceleration of progress in medicine. Other eras, both before and after Osler, could also be good starting points for medical history-humanities, depending on one's interest, but they did not seem to offer the same opportunities for discussion as the last 170 years.

UT Dallas provided a fertile academic environment to introduce such a course. The university has a historic commitment to education and research in the fields now identified as STEM (Science, Technology, Engineering and Mathematics); moreover, it attracts large numbers of students interested specifically in pursuing medical and other health-centered professions. As is the case nationally, these students gravitate toward science-focused degree programs such as Biology, Neuroscience and Bioengineering. While students had also expressed interest in the ethical and cultural aspects of medicine, the requirements of science-focused majors restrict the number of opportunities for students to enroll in Humanities courses.

Fortunately, the university also has a long-standing commitment to interdisciplinary education that encourages Science-Humanities collaborations—among them the establishment in 2007 of a Center for Values in Medicine, Science and Technology. To help students balance their educational experience, the University Honors Program (known as Collegium V) offers a group of special, focused seminars, each limited to fifteen students. The goal of these popular seminars is to encourage students to broaden their academic vision and enhance their studies by exploring new subjects and fields. Since they require only one fifty-minute class session per week and generate only one semester credit hour, students can add them to otherwise full schedules. The convergence of these factors led Kratz and Stone to submit the course proposal to the Honors program. It was accepted, first offered in the Fall 2012 semester—and has been offered at least once in every subsequent academic year.

The underlying and unifying theme of the course finds expression in Osler's description of Science and the Humanities as "twin berries on one stem, grievous damage has been done to both in regarding the Humanities and Science in any other light than complemental."[7]

Elaborating on Osler's important observation, the course presents Science and Humanities, not as separate "fields" or bodies of knowledge that need to be connected, but rather as two activities representing the innate human desire to make sense of the world and our experience of it. Science is the most advanced and nuanced form of seeking explanations for the natural forces at work in the world. The Humanities are the most advanced and nuanced study of the ways that human beings invest the world and our experience of it with meaning, significance, and values. This "active" notion of that relationship reflects Osler's emphasis on medicine as a "way of life" and his approving reference to the interaction of "*philanthropia* and *philotechnia*—the love of humanity associated with the love of his craft"—as the essence of medical practice.[7, p. 97]

The course uses Osler's life and writings as a lens through which to explore that interaction in the history, current ethical concerns, and future of medical practice. With some modifications and refinements each year of subjects and readings, the course has retained the same design. That basic design (with the associated reading from Osler listed where appropriate) is as follows:

SESSION 1. Introduction: Who are we and why are we here?
SESSION 2: Who was William Osler and why is he important?
    FILM: "Sir William Osler: Science and the Art of Medicine"
SESSION 3: Osler II: Film discussion
    READING: Osler, "A Way of Life"
SESSION 4: Osler III: The Reserves of Life
    READING: Osler, "The Reserves of Life"
SESSION 5: The Decision to Become a Physician
    READING: Osler, "The Student Life"
SESSION 6: Medicine and Philosophy
    READING: Osler: "Aequanimitas"
SESSION 7: Science and Humanities "Twin Berries on the Same Stem"
    READING: Osler: "The Old Humanities and the New Science"
SESSION 8: Medicine in Literature and Film
SESSION 9: Medicine and Death I: The "Fixed Period"
    READING: Osler: "The Fixed Period"
SESSION 10: Medicine and Death II: Extended or Immortal Life
SESSION 11: Women in Medicine
SESSION 12: Medical Education for the Future
    READING: Osler: "The Master Word in Medicine"
SESSIONS 13–15: STUDENT PRESENTATIONS AND FINAL DISCUSSION

The course unfolds, as the template syllabus suggests, in three parts. First, it introduces the students to Osler—person, physician, humanist—and his era. It then focuses on specific cultural and historic issues suggested by Osler's writings. The course at UT Dallas inevitably reflects the expertise and interests of the two instructors—an experienced physician and a classicist-medievalist who also studies the interaction of science with the humanities. For most sessions, supplementary readings are assigned. The introductory session, for example, assigns Stone's essay, "The Wisdom of Sir William Osler."[8] The supplementary reading for the session dedicated to Medicine and Philosophy includes excerpts from Greek and Roman philosophic texts that shed light on the origins of Osler's emphasis on *aequanimitas*. The session that focuses on extending human life draws heavily on contemporary works of Science Fiction, as of course does the session that deals with Osler's mention of Anthony Trollope's novel, *The Fixed Period*.

Often current events provide the focus of class discussions. The pandemic of 2019–2020, for example, invited comparisons with the outbreaks of smallpox and the great flu epidemic of 1918. The rise of genetic manipulation and other therapies has heightened interest in the moral implications of medical research. (A recent class included an excellent student report on "The Ethical Dilemma of CRISPR Through the Eyes of Sir William Osler.") Finally, the fact that every semester the majority of students are women led to the addition of a session devoted to the history and status of women in medical practice.

The course design reflects three primary, desired learning outcomes—two immediate and susceptible to objective evaluation, the third long range and subjective: At the conclusion of the course the students will be able to explain, using specific examples, Osler's contributions to the medical profession; second, they will be able to examine a medically related issue raised by their reading of Osler and/or through class discussion. The student presentations at the end of the course provide an opportunity for the students to display their realization of those goals. The third desired outcome is that the students will integrate Osler's persisting and eloquent emphasis, mentioned above, on combining science and humanities, attention to one's humanity as well as one's craft, in their future studies and careers.

Educators realize that every course is a work in progress that changes and evolves each time it is offered. The course has its challenges—chief among them Osler's mode of expression. Modern students find his writing style—complex sentences featuring a profusion of classical and Biblical references—difficult to understand. Often the cultural assumptions of a man with Edwardian sensibilities and assumptions strike them as odd, almost alien. Nonetheless, the UT Dallas medical humanities seminar has, in every important respect, proved successful. Indeed, the perceived "alien-ness" of Osler and his world has increased their fascination for many students.

As of the 2020 academic year, the course has been offered twelve times— always to maximum enrollment; moreover, the Student Evaluation forms have been uniformly positive. The two instructors have also received, over the years, numerous personal notes from students thanking us for the atmosphere and content of the course. The experience of the instructors has confirmed the original expectation, mingled with hope, that Osler's vision—its limits as well as its grandeur—can still illuminate and inspire students in the twenty-first century.

References

1. Harrell GT. Humanities in medical education: A career experience. *Perspectives in Biology and Medicine* 1985; 28(3): 382–401.
2. Hawkins AH, Ballard JO, Hufford DJ. Humanities education at Pennsylvania State University College of Medicine, Hershey, Pennsylvania. *Academic Medicine* 2003; 78(10): 1001–1005.
3. Hudson Jones A, Carson RA. Medical humanities at the University of Texas Medical Branch at Galveston. *Academic Medicine* 2003; 78(10): 1006–1009.
4. Murray TJ. Why the medical humanities? *Dalhousie Medical Journal* 1998; 26(1): 46–50.
5. Murray TJ. *Dalhousie Society for the History of Medicine, 1981–2020.* Halifax, Nova Scotia: Dalhousie University Faculty of Medicine; n.d.: 1–46.
6. Bliss M. *William Osler: A Life in Medicine.* Oxford: Oxford University Press; 1999: x.
7. Osler W. The Old Humanities and the New Science. In Hinohara S, Hisae N., eds. *Osler's 'A Way of Life' and Other Addresses.* Durham, North Carolina: Duke University Press; 2001: 82.
8. Stone MJ. The wisdom of Sir William Osler. *American Journal of Cardiology* 1995; 75(4): 269–276.

The Osler Student Societies of the University of Texas Medical Branch: A Medical Professionalism Translational Tool

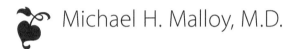 Michael H. Malloy, M.D.

As "translational medicine" seeks to move basic scientific research to practicable diagnostic procedures and therapies with meaningful improvements in physical, mental, or social health outcomes, so I use the term "translational" to indicate the attempt to transmit, interpret, and integrate the cognitive base of medical professionalism attributes into the educational process of medical students. The importance of doing so resides in the extensive attempts over the past 20 years to re-define medical professionalism as it relates to the medical ethics and moral values of the physician-healer and the obligations of the medical professional in contemporary society.[1-6] How to best transmit these attributes to medical students and to integrate them in the process of identity transformation associated with the socialization process of medical school remains a process in evolution.[4,7,8]

Experiential learning and reflection on the experience have been and continue to be important modes of learning in the medical education process.[4] Gaining that experience in small group problem-based learning environments through the use of clinical cases provide those opportunities. Reflecting on clinical science and professionalism issues that arise in paper-cases as well as exposure to actual patients at the bedside also offer those learning opportunities. These

Presented in part at the forty-third annual meeting of the American Osler Society, Tucson, Arizona, on 8 April 2013. Portions of this paper were previously published in *HEC Forum* (2012; 24[4]: 273–278) and are reprinted with permission.

methods engage the mind. If the intent of the medical professionalism education movement is "to produce humanistic and virtuous physicians," engagement of the heart to internalize the attributes of a virtuous physician is also necessary.[9] The ability to recite lists of characteristics offered in various definitions of medical professionalism[10] provides the cognitive material that medical students must be aware of in order to become virtuous physicians. Nevertheless, it does not offer medical students the opportunities to incorporate those characteristics into their identity formation as physicians. In contrast, Coulehan[9] proposes a narrative-based approach to professionalism in the medical education process. This narrative-based approach is dependent on role-modeling of professionalism by medical school faculty; providing the opportunity for students to develop a greater self-awareness of their own "beliefs, feelings, attitudes, and response patterns,"[9] promoting the development of narrative competence among students which includes "the ability to acknowledge, absorb, interpret, and act on the stories and plights of others"[11] and by providing the opportunity for students to engage in community service.

If engagement of the heart is considered an appropriate goal of the medical education process such that virtuous and humanistic physicians result, the study and incorporation of the ideals of historically significant physicians of the past has merit. Sir William Osler (1849–1919) was a Canadian-born physician who progressed through the ranks of academic medicine holding leadership positions at the University of Pennsylvania (1884–1889) and the Johns Hopkins Medical School (1889–1905) during periods of innovation in the education of medical students.[12] He was instrumental in bringing medical students to the bedside for clinical teaching and emphasized the importance of treating the patient and not just the disease. Osler completed his career as the Regius professor of medicine at Oxford University (1905–1919). He appreciated the importance of engaging both the mind and the heart in the process of educating physicians. "The practice of medicine is an art, not a trade; a calling, not a business: a calling in which your heart will be exercised equally with your head," so said Osler in an address at the University of Toronto in 1903.[13] The use of historical perspective, figures, and codes may reek of traditionalism and sentimentality to postmodern ethicists.[14,15] Nevertheless, the incorporation of the historical traditions and ideals of medicine in conjunction with transmission and discussion of contemporary normative issues in the professional roles of physicians has gained favor as an acceptable means of the teaching and learning of medical professionalism at the undergraduate level.[3]

The John P. McGovern Academy of Oslerian Medicine and the Osler Student Societies

To address the preservation and transmission of the historical ideals of medicine, The John P. McGovern Academy of Oslerian Medicine at the University of Texas Medical Branch was founded in 2001 by a generous grant from the John P. McGovern Foundation that recognizes physicians who provide highly compassionate care and to encourage the teaching and practice of such care to medical students in the tradition of William Osler. At its origin, the Academy funded eight Oslerian Faculty Scholars nominated by clinical faculty of the University of Texas Medical Branch (UTMB) to learn, review, and transmit Oslerian ideals through educational seminars and special projects.

The Osler Student Societies are an outgrowth of a pilot project undertaken by one of the Osler Scholars. In 2005, Dr. Mark Holden, an internist and Oslerian Faculty Scholar, developed a pilot project in which he invited 18 freshmen medical students to participate during their first year of medical school in developing a community service project and provided the resources to facilitate group activities in the presence of a senior faculty mentor. At the conclusion of the pilot year, focus group interviews of the participating students determined that the activities of the group and the relationship formed between the students and its primary mentor were valuable experiences. As a result, the John P. McGovern Foundation that funded the Academy of Oslerian Medicine at UTMB agreed to fund the development of Student Societies that would enroll the entire entering freshman class in 2006. Eight Student Societies thus evolved with approximately 30 new freshmen assigned to each Society, though participation in the Societies was and is entirely voluntary. Five faculty mentors were assigned to each Society, one of whom was an endowed Oslerian Scholar.

The vision of the Osler Student Societies is to provide developing physicians insight into "A Way of Life," as described by Sir William Osler,[16] not through formal lectures, but through the guidance of faculty mentors in contact with students within and outside their academic setting. The goals of the Student Societies are to enhance faculty-student interaction, to promote professionalism and humanism, to promote community service, and to promote the development of mentoring skills and comradery among students. Thus, the Osler Student Societies offer the components of Jack Coulehan's narrative-based approach[9] to medical professionalism. Professionalism role-modeling comes through the exposure of medical students to the faculty mentors of each Society who are chosen on the basis of their qualities as outstanding teachers and humanistic clinicians; opportunities for the promotion of self-awareness and self-reflection come through non-graded interactions between faculty and students that occur on an informal basis; narrative competence is promoted through the use of reflections on humanistic literature; and all Societies engage in community service projects that range from food drives, to volunteering for free clinics, and to fund raising.

The promotion of narrative competence is a particularly interesting component of the professionalism narrative-based approach that is being addressed in the Osler Student Societies through the use of reflection on literature-in-medicine sessions facilitated by Osler Student Society faculty mentors and faculty members of the UTMB Institute for the Medical Humanities. The goals of these sessions are to promote opportunities for self-awareness and reflection through the review of great literature related to the human condition and medicine. Whether or not these sessions have resulted in the narrative skills of "recognizing, absorbing, interpreting, and being moved by the stories of illness" which Charon[17] uses to define narrative medicine is uncertain as no valid assessment tool has been used. That this exercise results in greater empathy which may lead to mature sympathy and altruistic behavior upon the part of the medical students participating in this process may be only a hope at this point. As extensive reviews of the "literature induced empathy-altruism hypothesis" suggest, the ability to determine the extent of the occurrence of such a relationship remains a complex issue to examine.[18] Nevertheless, listed below are samplings of the literature that have been reviewed in these sessions. For the most part these excerpts of great literature come from readings assembled by Leon Kass in his book *Being Human: Core Readings in the Humanities*[19] assembled for use by the President's Council on Bioethics in 2003.

The topics covered in the literature-in-medicine sessions follow Kass's book chapters. Literature dealing with the search for perfection included excerpts from Gerard Manley Hopkins's poem "Pied Beauty"; Lewis Thomas's essay "The Wonderful Mistake"; and Andrew M. Niccol's screenplay, *GATTACA*. Human perfection or imperfections are issues that physicians will come in contact within their interactions with patients. Gaining a greater understanding of how humanity may strive for perfection to the detriment of individuals and populations is an important exercise for the medical student to experience.

Healing and comforting, essential topics for evolving physicians to gain a greater appreciation for, were addressed in excerpts from Albert Camus's *The Plague*. In *The Plague*, the physician Rieux is questioned by the journalist, Tarrou, about spirituality and healing. Contemporary physicians must also deal with these issues. Richard Selzer's *The Surgeon as Priest* examined how physicians care for the human body and their attitudes towards it. W.H. Auden's poem "The Art of Healing" discusses the limitations of healing and the "art of wooing nature." How we inhabit our bodies and view our material being was discussed in a group session that reviewed Chitra Banerjee Kivakaruni's essay "What the Body Knows." In this essay a young woman confronted with a surgical complication of a cesarean delivery learns her body carries on in different directions from her wishes, but she comes to appreciate how to recognize and incorporate her bodily cues into her conscious existence. In an excerpt from Leo Tolstoy's *War and Peace: Cannon Fodder and The Operating Tent*, Prince Andrew sees the bodies of his men as mere cannon fodder but is brought to compassion for humanity when he suffers bodily wounds himself. Walt Whitman, in his poem "I Sing the Body Electric," offers an appreciation of the human body and its relationship to the soul. Might not the young medical student gain a greater understanding of their patients through the appreciation of such a relationship? The stages of life were examined from a translation by Lane Cooper of *The Rhetoric of Aristotle*, in which Aristotle takes a cynical look at the aging process. Similarly, an excerpt from Francis Bacon's *Of Youth and Age* examines the defects of both the young and old, taking a dim view of the perfection of any stage of life. In an excerpt from Shakespeare's *As You Like It*, Jaques reviews the seven ages of man in a disparaging manner. In reflecting on these readings, the medical students took a much more compassionate view of the ages of man based on the quixotic turns of life and injustices to which some humans are subject. Generations and the transmission of life across generations and the impact of childbirth on a relationship were reflected upon through discussion of Tolstoy's *Anna Karenina*, in which a new father is confronted with disturbing feelings of repulsion, fear, and then tenderness towards his newly born son. How loyalty in relationships plays out when opportunities are missed was reviewed through an excerpt from George Eliot's *Silas Marner*; and coming to terms with a deceptive relationship was dealt with in Geoffrey Wolff's memoir of his father, *The Duke of Deception*.

In this age of accountability and attempts to measure an outcome as a result of an exposure to a learning experience it will be extremely difficult to measure and/or validate the utility of these reflections on literature on the formation of medical students' professional identity.[20–22] I, for one, would worry that such an attempt would ruin the experience by being intrusive and perhaps modifying the experience. If the goal is to provide the medical students an opportunity to be exposed to human conditions and great literature from which they might derive some insight into humanity, perhaps the exposure is meritorious enough. How will we recognize the impact of the exposure? It is doubtful that all the evaluative instruments designed to measure medical student progress will do any better than the subjective assessment of the patient who experiences an interaction with a humane physician.

Summary

The Osler Student Societies at the University of Texas Medical Branch offer an ideal vehicle to promote a narrative-based approach to medical professionalism. Mentor role-modeled professional behavior; opportunities for self-reflection and self-awareness; the development of narrative competence through reflection on literature; and community service—these are all vital components of the Student Societies. The good fortune of having an endowment to fund many of these efforts is a gift bestowed on few medical schools and will hopefully provide the incentive to continue the translational process of integrating the cognitive base of medical professionalism into the identity of the medical student.

References

1. Castellani B, Hafferty FW. The complexities of medical professionalism. In Wear D, Aultman JM, eds. *Professionalism in Medicine: Critical Perspectives* (pp. 3–23). New York: Springer; 2006: 3–23.
2. Cohen JJ, Cruess S, Davidson C. Alliance between society and medicine: the public's stake in medical professionalism. *Journal of the American Medical Association* 2007; 298(6): 670–673.
3. Cruess SR, Cruess RL. The cognitive base of professionalism. In Cruess RL, Cruess SR, Steinert Y, eds. *Teaching Medical Professionalism*. New York: Cambridge University Pres; 2009: 7–27.
4. Cruess RL, Cruess SR. Principles for designing a program for the teaching and learning of professionalism at the undergraduate level. In Cruess RL, Cruess SR, Steinert Y, eds. *Teaching Medical Professionalism*. New York: Cambridge University Pres; 2009: 73–91.
5. Lesser CS, Lucey CR, Egener B, Braddock CH, Linas SL, Levinson W. A behavioral and systems view of professionalism. *Journal of the American Medical Association* 2010; 304(24): 2732–2737.
6. Relman AS. Medical professionalism in a commercialized health care market. *Journal of the American Medical Association* 2007; 298(22): 2668–2670.
7. Hafferty FW. Professionalism and the socialization of medical students. In Cruess RL, Cruess SR, Steinert Y, eds. *Teaching Medical Professionalism*. New York: Cambridge University Pres; 2009: 53–70.
8. Inui TS, Cottingham AH, Frankel RM, Litzelman DK, Suchman AL, and Williamson PR. Supporting teaching and learning of professionalism—changing the educational environment and students' navigational skills. In Cruess RL, Cruess SR, Steinert Y, eds. *Teaching Medical Professionalism*. New York: Cambridge University Press; 2009: 108–123.
9. Coulehan J. Today's professionalism: engaging the mind but not the heart. *Academic Medicine* 2005; 80(10): 892–898.
10. American Board of Internal Medicine and European Federation of Internal Medicine Medical professionalism in the new millennium: a physician charter. *Annals of Internal Medicine* 2002; 136: 243–246.

11. Charon R. Narrative medicine. A model for empathy, reflection, profession, and trust. *Journal of the American Medical Association* 2001; 286: 1897–1902.

12. Bliss M. *William Osler: A Life in Medicine.* New York: Oxford University Press; 1999.

13. Osler W. The master-word in medicine. In *Aequanimitas, With other Addresses to Medical Students, Nurses and Practitioners of Medicine.* Third edition, Philadelphia: P. Blakiston's Son & Co., Inc.; 1932: 347–371.

14. Baker RB, McCullough LB. What is the history of medical ethics? In Baker RB, McCullough LB, eds. *The Cambridge World History of Medical Ethics* New York: Cambridge University Press.; 2009: 3–20.

15. Thomasma DC Theories of medical ethics: the philosophical structure. https://www.semanticscholar.org/paper/Chapter-2-THEORIES-OF-MEDICAL-ETHICS-%3A-THE-Thomasma/79d2c5d6f7bf010f4e1c5c14c4a4066ce891665a#paper-header. Accessed November 23, 2020.

16. Osler W. A way of life. In Hinohara S, Niki H, eds. *Osler's "A Way of Life" and Other Addresses, with Commentary and Annotations.* Durham, North Carolina: Duke University Press; 2001: 3–18.

17. Charon R. The sources of narrative medicine. In Charon R, ed. *Narrative Medicine: Honoring the Stories of Illness.* New York: Oxford University Press; 2008: 3–15.

18. Keen S. *Empathy and the Novel.* New York: Oxford University Press; 2007: vii–xxv.

19. Kass L. *Being Human: Core Readings in the Humanities.* New York: W.W. Norton; 2004.

20. Hafferty FW. Professionalism—the next wave. *New England Journal of Medicine* 2006; 355(20): 2151–2152.

21. Huddle TS. Teaching professionalism: is medical morality a competency? *Academic Medicine* 2005; 80: 885–891.

22. Stern DT, Papadakis M. The developing physician—becoming a professional. *New England Journal of Medicine* 2006; 355(17): 1794–1799.

Proving Osler Wrong: Mary Stults Sherman and Jacqueline Perry, Pioneering American Women Academic Orthopaedic Surgeons

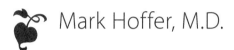 Mark Hoffer, M.D.

As is well known, William Osler like most male physicians of his era was ambivalent about women in medicine. In 1889, as a condition to fund the Johns Hopkins Medical School, he voted reluctantly to accept women students. He softened his views over time, and was of enormous help to individual women medical students and women physicians. He kept his opinion, however, that women were poorly suited for certain areas of medicine, notably the rough-and-tumble of surgical practice. Addressing students and faculty of the London School of Medicine for Women in 1907, Osler suggested three principal avenues for their work: in sciences such as bacteriology, histology, and pathology; in institutions such as schools and asylums; and in general practice, especially in dealing with diseases of women and children.[1]

Osler apparently never considered the possibility of women in orthopaedic surgery. To be sure, he had no examples before him in this regard. As late as 1940 no women were listed in the American Academy of Orthopaedic Surgeons directory of more than 2,000 persons practicing orthopaedic surgery in the United States.[2] The first woman to complete orthopaedic training was Ruth Jackson. She passed her boards in 1937 and became the first woman admitted to the

Presented at the forty-eighth annual meeting of the American Osler Society, Pittsburgh, Pennsylvania, on 14 March 2018.

American Academy of Orthopaedic Surgeons a few years later. Jackson enjoyed a long career in private practice in Dallas, was a founding member of the Texas Orthopaedic Association (1974), described her experience treating more than 15,000 neck injuries in a monograph, and is memorialized by the Ruth Jackson Orthopaedic Society, founded in 1983 as a networking and support group for women in orthopaedic surgery.[3]

Two of the next few women to do so began remarkable careers as academic clinician–surgeon–scientists: Mary Stults Sherman in 1946 and Jacqueline Perry in 1958. They were both unique because of their surgical experience and their academic scientific contributions. Here, I shall give brief biographical sketches and discuss their importance.

Mary Stults Sherman (1913–1964) (Figure 1)

Mary Stults was born and raised in Evanston, Illinois. She attended local public schools, received her undergraduate degree in 1934 from Northwestern University, and in 1935 received a Master of Arts degree and spent the next two years teaching at the French Institute in Paris. She then entered medical school at the University of Chicago, graduating in 1941. A marriage to Dr. Thomas Sherman, a US Army physician, unfortunately led to years of wartime separation and divorce. Mary Sherman started postgraduate training as an intern in pediatrics

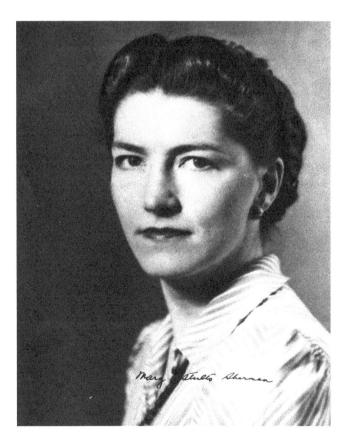

Figure 1. Mary Stults Sherman (1913–1964). *Credit: Journal of Bone and Joint Surgery.*

and then pursued a residency in orthopaedics with Drs. Dallas Phemister and Howard Hatcher at the University of Chicago. She completed that training in 1946 and became an assistant professor in Chicago by 1947.

She eventually focused her orthopaedic work in Chicago in three areas: poliomyelitis, fracture healing, and necrosis of bone. In 1944 she published a review of 75 cases of polio.[4] In 1947 she helped clarify the problem of non-union of femoral neck fractures by studies of the pathology of this condition.[5] There followed a number of papers and national presentations along these lines.

In 1952 Drs. Guy Caldwell and Harry Morris asked her to join them at the Ochsner Clinic and Tulane University in New Orleans. Dr. Sherman was eventually appointed associate professor as she continued her clinical-surgical-research career. She had a rural outreach clinic for children with deformities. Children were brought to Oschner Clinic for surgical correction of deformities. Fractures were followed in Oschner Clinic and at the Charity Hospital of New Orleans, where she rotated for emergency call.

Dr. Sherman developed in New Orleans a world-famous bone laboratory. Hers was the largest referral practice for musculoskeletal tumors in the southeastern United States. She continued her interest in bone necrosis. She worked with the Ochsner team at the Decompression Chamber for treatment caisson's disease among Gulf Coast oil-rig divers. She developed an interest in the inflammatory reactions of the musculoskeletal system with particular focus on synovia and giant cells. Her paper on synovial reaction is considered unique.[6] She involved residents (house staff) in most of her research. She conducted weekly teaching sessions in bone pathology. She wrote classic papers on the pathology of clubfoot and radiation necrosis.[7,8] She became the principal examiner for the pathology portion of the American Orthopaedic Boards. In 1954, she was the first woman accepted in the American Orthopaedic Association. That society founded in 1887, invites only the highly recognized academic members of the specialty. In 1963 she received the prestigious annual research award (Kappa Delta) by her colleagues. She also continued her interest in the arts and was a favored guest in the New Orleans art community.

In 1964 at age 51 Dr. Sherman was fatally stabbed in the heart while in her home. The building was destroyed by fire and the killer never discovered.[9] A memorial lecture series was established in her name.

Jacqueline Perry (1918–2013) (Figure 2)

Jacqueline Perry was born in Denver and raised in Los Angeles. She attended the local public schools and was noted to be an outstanding athlete scholar. She remained a vigorous athlete most of her adult life. She received her undergraduate degree in 1940 from the University of California, Los Angeles, with a dual major in English and physical education. She was recruited by the US Army for physical therapy school at Walter Reed Hospital and served rest of World War II as a physical therapy officer. Dr. Perry was proud of her five-years of service in the military and served as a consultant to the Armed Forces throughout her career. After the war, she attended medical school at the University of California, San Francisco (UCSF), and trained in orthopaedic surgery at the same institution. At UCSF she was involved in Dr. Vern Inman's gait studies as they applied to veterans with amputations and prostheses. When she was examined for her Orthopaedic Boards in 1958, she was surprised to meet another woman as her

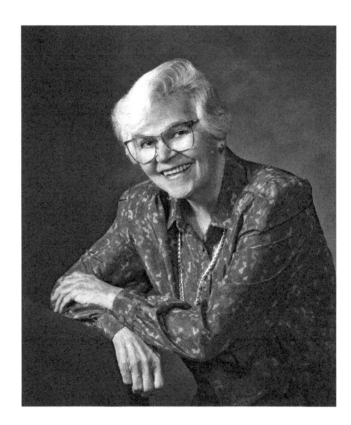

Figure 2. Jacqueline Perry (1918–2013). *Credit: Journal of Bone and Joint Surgery* and EA photographers, Anaheim, California.

examiner—Dr. Sherman. Dr. Sherman said of that meeting "I was equally surprised to meet another woman in the specialty."

In 1955 Dr. Perry was asked by Drs. Vern Nickel and John Apfeld to join the Rancho Los Amigos Hospital–University of Southern California staff. There she became chief of one of the largest polio services in the United States, and also of a large spinal deformity program. She was eventually named full professor in both the University of Southern California Medical School and Physical Therapy department. Her weekly routine included teaching anatomy to the residents, lecturing at the physical therapy school, two full days of operating (one for complex spinal fusions and another for paralytic limb surgery), conducting grand rounds, and working in clinics. In the midst of all these challenges she found time for clinical research, focusing mainly on novel procedures. She did important work on spinal fusion in paralytics,[10] and her paper on the development of the Halo device for cervical spine deformity is considered a classic.[11] In 1970 she was invited into the American Orthopaedic Association as a highly recognized academic orthopaedic surgeon.

As she became more senior, she made time for her basic science interest in the normal and pathological gait. Dr. Perry helped develop gait study tools to define normal and pathological variations. These were then applied to spastic deformities caused by stroke and cerebral palsy.[12] She summarized her observations and approach to gait disorders in a classic textbook.[13] In 1977 Dr. Perry received the prestigious annual research award (Kappa Delta) from her orthopaedic colleagues.

Dr. Perry died at age 94. In spite of decades long problems with Parkinson's disease she continued to attend clinics for her old polio paralytic patients. Some of her students organized the Perry Initiative to direct young women into careers in orthopaedic surgery. In 2020 she was named "One of the Eight Pillars of the Orthopaedic Profession" by the American Orthopaedic Association.

Discussion and conclusions

In 2012 Mark Gebhardt commented on data from the previous five years provided by the American Board of Orthopaedic Surgery. He found that of the 21,954 qualified Orthopaedic Surgeons fewer less than ten percent were women. This was close to the percentage of applicants for Orthopaedic training. This was one of the lowest percentages in all the board specialties. In those years 48 percent of the graduating medical students and 35 percent of residents were women.[14]

In 2017 there were 33,812 orthopaedic Surgeons in the national American Academy of Orthopaedic Surgeons of which 2,307 are women. This represents an increase of women but in 2018 they were only 5.8 percent of the Academy membership. There are few full-time women academic professors of orthopaedic surgery and only two department chairs. The Orthopaedic Academy Diversity Board and Ruth Jackson Women's Orthopaedic Society have recently designed programs to encourage women to apply for orthopaedic training. Mentors are believed to be one of the important factors.

Mary Sherman and Jacqueline Perry were the pioneers to open doors for women in academic research-oriented orthopaedic surgery. They were the early mentors and their disciples have already reached out to students with the Mary Sherman Lectureships and the Jacquelin Perry Initiative. Sir William Osler in 1897 declared medicine free of distinctions of "race, nationality, colour, and creed."[15] Today he might declare medicine and *surgery* free of distinctions of race, nationality, colour, creed and *gender*.

References

1. McIntyre N. Women in medicine, William Osler on. In Bryan CS, ed. *Sir William Osler: An Encyclopedia*. Novato, CA: Norman Publishing/Historyof-Science.Com; 2020: 847–849.
2. American Academy of Orthopaedic Surgeons. A snapshot of US Orthopaedic Surgeons—AAOS published yearly and re-accessed 22 July 2020.
3. Manring MM, Calhoun JH. Biographical sketch: Ruth Jackson, MD, FACS 1902–1994. *Clinical Orthopaedics and Related Research* 210: 468: 1736–1738.
4. Sherman MS. The natural course of poliomyelitis: A report of 70 cases. *Journal of the American Medical Association* 1944; 125(2): 99–102.
5. Sherman MS. Phemister DB. The pathology of ununited fractures of the neck of the femur. *Journal of Bone and Joint Surgery* 1947; 29(1): 19–40.
6. Sherman M.S. The non-specificity of synovial reactions: *Bulletin of the Hospital for Joint Diseases* 1950; 12: 110–125.
7. Irani RN, Sherman MS. The pathological anatomy of club foot. *Journal of Bone and Joint Surgery* 1963; 45–A: 45–52.
8. Goodman AH, Sherman M. Post radiation fracture of femoral neck. *Journal of Bone and Joint Surgery* 1963; 45–A: 723–727.
9. Mary Stults Sherman, 1913–1964 (obituary). *Journal of Bone and Joint Surgery* 1964; 46–A: 1824–1826.

10. Perry J, Nickel VL. Total cervical spine fusion for neck paralysis. Journal of Bone and Joint Surgery 1959; 41–A: 37–60.

11. Nickel VL, Perry J, Garrett A, Heppenstall M. The halo. A skeletal traction fixation device. *Journal of Bone and Joint Surgery* 1968; 50–A: 1400–1409.

12. Perry J, Hoffer M. Preoperative and postoperative dynamic electromyography as an aid in planning tendon transfers in children with cerebral palsy. *Journal of Bone and Joint Surgery* 1977; 59–A: 531–537.

13. Perry J. *Gait Analysis: Normal and Pathological*. Thorofare, New Jersey: Slack Incorporated; 1992.

14. Gebhardt M. Board of Medical Specialties Combined meeting BOC/BOS 2012.

15. Medical Professionalism, William Osler on. In Bryan CS, ed. *Sir William Osler: An Encyclopedia*. Novato, California: Norman Publishing/History of Science.Com; 2020: 662.

The Making of
Encyclopedia Osleriana

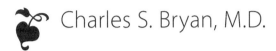 Charles S. Bryan, M.D.

Sir William Osler (Figure 1), the most iconic physician in the history of North American medicine, died at his home in Oxford on December 29, 1919, from hemorrhage into an empyema cavity that had been drained several days earlier. At the time of his death, he was by far the most famous physician in the English-speaking world on account of his textbook of medicine, his inspirational addresses and essays, his participation in organizations, and his influence on a generation of physicians and medical students. After he died contemporaries could not find enough good things to say about him. Over the ensuing century he has been the subject of at least 17 biographies and quasi-biographies and more than 2,000 articles in the medical literature. To consolidate this mass of information, to facilitate future "Osler studies" including critical re-assessments, and to encourage scholarship in the history of medicine and the medical humanities, 138 scholars throughout the world contributed 1,145 articles to a forthcoming encyclopedia.[1,2] Here we address three questions:

- How did Osler become so nearly emblematic of the "Heroic Age" of medicine, the period that gave birth to scientific, evidence-based medicine as we know it today?
- What was Osler really like, what made him unique to his contemporaries, and was there a deep, underlying melancholy beneath the saintly countenance?
- What would he say to us were he here today?

Accepted for presentation at the fiftieth annual meeting of the American Osler Society, Pasadena, California, 27–29 April 2020. (The meeting was cancelled because of the Covid-19 pandemic.) Presented at the one hundred thirty-second meeting of the American Clinical and Climatological Association, Clear Point, Alabama, 19 October 2019. The manuscript was previously published in the *Transactions of the American Clinical and Climatological Association* (2020; 131: 335–355) and is reprinted with permission.

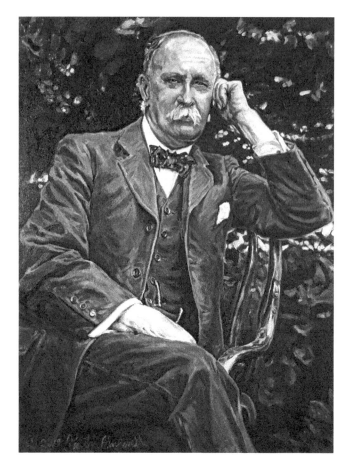

Figure 1.   *Sir William Osler*, by Tarleton Blackwell. 1999. Oil on canvas, 48 × 36 inches. Collection of Charles S. Bryan. This painting was commissioned for the frontispiece of the forthcoming *Sir William Osler: An Encyclopedia*. *Credit:* Collection of Charles S. Bryan.

How did Osler become emblematic of the "Heroic Age" of Medicine?

In 2016 North American physicians were asked to name "the most influential physician in history." Osler beat out Hippocrates for first place.[3] Osler has become emblematic, at least in North America, of what has been called the "Heroic Age" of medicine, the period between roughly 1880 and 1920 to which we trace the emergence of science-based medicine as we know it today. As Harvard physiologist Lawrence J. Henderson (1878–1942) famously put it, "Sometime between 1910 and 1912 in this country, a random patient, with a random disease, consulting a doctor chosen at random had, for the first time in the history of mankind, a better than fifty-fifty chance of profiting from the encounter."[4] Osler's recent biographer Michael Bliss observed that it is difficult to study this period "without bumping into Osler."[5] One reviewer suggested Osler has become the subject of "a body of serious hagiography larger than that of any other physician except, possibly, St. Luke."[6] Why does Osler's name stand out so saliently? How did he escape what Sir Thomas Browne (1605–1682), whom he called his "lifelong mentor," described as "the iniquity of oblivion"?

This question has been asked many times and answered in various ways. Here we consider it through the lens of Malcolm Gladwell's 2008 bestseller, *Outliers*.[7] Gladwell argues that people who stand out conspicuously in any field possess certain commonalities. These include focused hard work, a favorable family of origin, and luck.

Osler if he were here with us this morning would seize the first of these commonalities: *work*, which he called "the master-word of medicine."[8] Gladwell's outliers not only worked harder than other people; they worked *much* harder. The magic formula seemed to be at least 10,000 hours of goal-directed work spread over about 10 years. This formula accords perfectly with Osler's second Montreal period (1874–1884) during which he led a semi-monastic life while teaching, writing, and performing nearly 800 autopsies. These activities gained him sufficient recognition to become professor of clinical medicine at the University of Pennsylvania (1884–1889). In Philadelphia he possibly worked even harder and drew enough recognition to become inaugural professor of medicine at Johns Hopkins. In Baltimore, his capacity for work astounded colleagues when he wrote in about 18 months a definitive textbook, *The Principles and Practice of Medicine* (1892).

Gladwell supports his second commonality—favorable family of origin—by citing the Terman Study of individuals with IQs above 140 when tested as schoolchildren.[9] Lewis M. Terman (1877–1956) and his colleagues at Stanford stratified their cohort into three groups by socioeconomic status of family of origin. Those who enjoyed great success as adults came overwhelmingly from middle- or upper-class homes that brimmed with books. Horatio Alger "rags to riches" stories occur in real life but are rare. Even the most gifted struggle without favorable families of origin.

The Reverend Featherstone Lake Osler (1805–1895) and his wife, Ellen Free Pickton Osler (1806–1907), were the most successful parents in Upper Canada (present-day Ontario) judged by their offspring's accomplishments. This would have been the case even without their youngest son, William, whose older brothers included one of Canada's leading jurists, a leading businessman and philanthropist, and Canada's most famous trial lawyer.[10,11] After six years in the Royal Navy, during which he survived several shipwrecks, Featherstone Osler received a divinity degree from Cambridge only to be told he was just the right man to minister to some 2,000 unruly Scotch-Irish immigrants scattered over 240 square miles. The life of an Anglican traveling missionary in the 1830s was at least as hard as that of a Methodist circuit rider, whose life expectancy was less than 40 years.[12] Featherstone's sponsors later wrote that "few Missionaries have had severer hardships to endure than Mr. Osler." He would travel up to nine miles through woods and swamps, sometimes at night, often leading his horse over corduroy roads, occasionally encountering a wolf, to provide hope of salvation to a single dying parishioner. Few missionaries have been more successful than Featherstone Osler, who eventually established 28 congregations in 20 townships and lived to be ninety.[13–16] Ellen Pickton Osler was equally successful in her ministry to the youth and women of the Canadian backwoods. She started Sunday schools, taught domestic skills, modeled piety, cheerfulness, and equanimity, and lived to be one hundred. Featherstone and Ellen Osler had "the right stuff" to pass on to their children.

Gladwell's third commonality is luck. It is well and good to "hitch your wagon to a star," as Ralph Waldo Emerson (1803–1882) wrote in "Civilization" (1870), but it helps to have a constellation of stars align in your favor. In 1874 William Osler returned from 18 months abroad to learn McGill had no job to offer. He was sorting out what to do when Joseph Morley Drake (1828–1886), professor of the Institutes of Medicine (basically, physiology and pathology), took leave of absence due to heart trouble. Osler was appointed lecturer and then professor when Drake retired for good. However, he could not teach and practice at the Montreal General Hospital because clinical positions were scarce and coveted. In 1878 a clinical position opened but ahead of Osler was a friend who was slightly older and clinically accomplished. The friend, John Bell (1845–1878), applied but died within two weeks from pneumonia. The clinical position made Osler a credible candidate to succeed William Pepper (1843–1898) at the University of Pennsylvania when Pepper became provost of the university.

In 1884 Osler arrived in Philadelphia ambitious to impact medical education by combining the best features of the German and English systems—the German hierarchical organization of a hospital within a university and the British model of clinical teaching on the wards. Penn's rich tradition and bureaucracy posed formidable obstacles to a 35-year-old outsider. He watched what was happening farther south in Baltimore where plans called for a teaching hospital under the administrative umbrella of a research-oriented university and where the service-line chiefs at the hospital would double as department heads at the university. There he might be able to popularize bedside teaching. There he might be able to incorporate senior medical students into the hospital machinery as clinical clerks. But he still had to get the job and John Shaw Billings (1838–1913) had another man in mind: Thomas Lauder Brunton (1844–1916) of London, introducer of amyl nitrite for angina pectoris. Lauder Brunton said no. Osler got the job and arrived in Baltimore in May 1889 in time for the opening ceremonies of the Johns Hopkins Hospital.

His lucky streak was not over. Had the Johns Hopkins Medical School opened soon after the hospital, we would probably remember Osler as we remember, for example, Frederick Shattuck (1847–1929) of Boston, Francis Delafield (1841–1914) of New York City, or James Tyson (1841–1919) of Philadelphia—a leading physician of his time and place but hardly emblematic of an era. Osler's next break had two components. The authors of the leading textbooks of medicine on both sides of the Atlantic, Sir Thomas Watson (1792–1882) of London and Austin Flint (1812–1886) of New York City, had died within the decade. The railroad stock in which the estate of Johns Hopkins (1795–1873) was heavily invested plummeted in value, delaying by four years the opening of the medical school. Osler had ample time to write the book, which spread his fame throughout the English-speaking medical world and twelve years later helped him become one of the two top candidates to succeed John Burdon-Sanderson (1828–1905) as Regius professor of medicine at Oxford. Lady Luck smiled again: the other top candidate, Sir Patrick Manson (1844–1922), "father of tropical medicine," was perfectly happy in London. In 1905 Osler, burned out in Baltimore by demands on his time, escaped to Oxford, and lived happily ever after.

Well, not quite. His luck ran out on August 29, 1917, when his only surviving child, Edward Revere Osler (1895–1917), was mortally wounded by a German artillery shell. He wrote in his diary: "The Fates do not allow the good fortune that has followed me to go with me to the grave—call no man happy till he dies."[17]

What was Osler really like?

Focused work, favorable family of origin, and lucky breaks made Osler an outlier, but it was his personality that made him so special to contemporaries. They admired his accomplishments but raved about his personality. Sir Arthur Keith (1866–1955), co-discoverer of the sinoatrial node, wrote: "A future generation will never understand the love which Osler's own generation lavished on him, and the respect in which it held him," making him "the central pivot" whereby "the international medical wheels turned with an easy movement."[18] How was Osler's personality unique? What was he really like?

Birth order explains a lot. Osler's personality resembles that of Benjamin Franklin (1706–1790) in some respects, which is not surprising since both benefitted from being the youngest son among many siblings (nine in Osler's case, 17 in Franklin's) whose parents prized education and industry. Watching older siblings gave Osler, as it did Franklin, daily lessons in interpersonal dynamics, how to "read the vibes," how to size up situations, and, more broadly, emotional intelligence. Osler emerged from adolescence with a delightful personality, a remarkable equanimity, a penchant for mischief, and the ability to defuse tension with humor. Birth order also explains in part how Osler became his mother's darling, her "Benjamin," which, as Sigmund Freud (1856–1939) pointed out, confers a triumphant self-confidence that often leads to actual success.[19]

To understand what made Osler special, I analyzed reminiscences and tributes by 205 of his contemporaries using the classification of character strengths developed by members of the American Psychological Association during the Values in Action Project (VIA).[20] The VIA investigators concluded that virtues and character strengths fall into six broad categories (clusters) corresponding to the seven classic virtues of antiquity—the four cardinal virtues (wisdom, justice, temperance, and courage) articulated by Plato in *The Republic* and elsewhere, and the three "theological" virtues (faith, hope, and love) named by St. Paul in 1 Corinthians 13:13. (The researchers combined faith and hope as strengths of transcendence.) Within the six categories (clusters) they identified 24 specific character strengths (Table 1). The VIA Character Strengths Survey instrument is available online for self-administration.[21]

From the reminiscences and tributes of 205 of Osler's contemporaries, I tabulated 1,441 mentions of individual character strengths. Strengths of humanity (551 of the 1,441 mentions) and strengths of courage (423 mentions) headed up the categories (clusters) of strengths (Table 1). Vitality (313 mentions) and kindness (305 mentions) headed up the individual strengths (Table 2). These tabulations

Table 1.   William Osler's character strengths, by category, based on the reminiscences of, or tributes to, Osler by 205 contemporaries (number of mentions, by category)*

Category	Individual character strengths	Mentions
Humanity	Love, kindness, social intelligence	551
Courage	Bravery, persistence, integrity, vitality	423
Wisdom and knowledge	Creativity, curiosity, open-mindedness, love of learning, perspective (wisdom)	134
Transcendence	Appreciation of beauty and excellence, gratitude, hope/optimism, humor/playfulness, spirituality	123
Temperance	Forgiveness and mercy, humility and modesty, prudence, self-regulation (self-control)	113
Justice	Citizenship (social responsibility, loyalty, teamwork), fairness, leadership	97
Total number of mentions		1,441

*After Peterson and Seligman.[20]

Table 2.   William Osler's top 12 character strengths, based on the reminiscences of, or tributes to, Osler by 205 contemporaries (number of mentions, by category)*

Strength	Mentions	Strength	Mentions
Vitality**	313	Humor/playfulness	63
Kindness†	305	Love of learning	48
Social intelligence‡	140	Persistence	40
Love of fellow humans§	106	Curiosity	31
Self-regulation	81	Hope/optimism	21
Integrity	64	Humility and modesty	18

* After Peterson and Seligman.[20]

** Osler's vitality as observed by others included charm/charming (38 mentions), enthusiasm (37), personality as his predominant strength (31), lovability (22), magnetic/electromagnetic (19), and energy/energetic (13 mentions).

† Osler's kindness as observed by others included encouragement (44 mentions), sympathy (44), kindness/kindliness/kindhearted (37), generosity (32), inspiring/inspirational (28), hospitality (20< and stimulating/stimulation of others (18 mentions).

‡ Osler's social intelligence as observed by others included human/humanist, humaneness/humanitarian (32 mentions), interest in others (27), and insight into others (14 mentions).

§ Osler's love of fellow humans as observed by others included friend/friendliness/friendship (53 mentions; "genius for friendship" was a common observation); love of fellow humans (36), and "Abou ben Adhem"-like (nine mentions).

probably carry substantial margins of error, since assigning observations to specific character strengths was arbitrary in some instances, but the extent to which vitality and kindness dwarf the other strengths (Table 2) indicate that it was these that most impressed contemporaries.

Let us imagine what would happen should Osler show up at the present meeting His arrival at would resemble that of a patriarch at a family reunion. None could fail to notice his dapper appearance and energetic gait; descriptors included "quick," "active," "springing," "elastic," and "swinging." None could fail to notice the sparkling eyes; descriptors included "merry," "twinkling," "sharp," "piercing," "bright and smiling," "laughing," "humorous," and "never inquisitive but always searching and comprehending." Those who previously knew him would swarm around him as he entered the room. He would say just the right thing to each in turn, his measured words delivered in a voice described as quiet, deep, and resonant. Banalities would be conspicuously absent. He would often resume a conversation precisely where it had left off even if years had intervened.

If you did not already know him, you would certainly know him before the meeting adjourns. He would seek you out. You would bask in his penetrating gaze for several minutes feeling like his only concern. As he slipped away to introduce himself to someone else, you would feel you had just made a friend for life. In fact, you had. When your next paper appeared in print, you would receive a postcard saying something like, "Great paper—please send me a reprint—Osler." If you failed to send him a reprint of a subsequent paper, he would give you a humorous scolding. During the holiday season you might receive a book, possibly a rare one, tailored to your interests. From this meeting forward, you would strive to do your best if only to please William Osler.

The results shown in Tables 1 and 2 would differ had Osler self-administered the VIA Character Strengths Survey instrument. His top strengths, the ones to which he credited his success, might have included love of learning, curiosity, persistence, self-regulation, and hope/optimism. In my opinion, Osler's outstanding character trait—the trait that best explains his phenomenal success and popularity—was a preternatural ability to manage time.[22] He had an uncanny ability to balance sociability and solitude—sociability for enhancing the self-esteem of others, solitude for academic productivity. He excelled at "mindfulness" (to use current jargon), the ability to be fully focused and engaged in the present moment. He also had the rare ability to rivet his focus on another person without diverting his own agenda. Sir Arthur Keith reflected, "There was much of the Will-o'-the-Wisp about him; you put out your mental hand to catch him, as it were, and before you could touch him he was gone."[18] Henry V. Ogden, who knew him well, observed that Osler's ability to affirm people without sidetracking his own agenda was "instinctive with him and so noticeable, that more than once it provoked the remark that he was 'among us but not one of us.'"[23]

The latter remark evokes descriptions of Jesus of Nazareth (John 17:14 and elsewhere) and indeed some saw Osler as a Christ-like figure. One of the few criticisms of Osler by contemporaries was that he sometimes seemed "too sweet"[24]—an image he tried to defuse with unpredictable humor and practical jokes that did not always sit well. However, and again like Benjamin Franklin,[25] Osler's cheerfulness and optimism sometimes masked reservations about humanity, as when he referred in his last public address to "the depth and ferocity of primal passions which reveal the unchangeableness of human nature."[26]

A few have suggested that beneath Osler's charm and upbeat personality lurked a deep sorrow. Physician-historian Charles J. Singer (1875–1960) wrote that "despite his gaiety, Osler always appeared to me as profoundly and essentially melancholy," appearing as "one who has passed through some tragedy to a life of human service, one who is always whispering to himself, '"Down, thou climbing sorrow.'"[27] Psychiatrist James A. Knight (1918–1998) concurred, suggesting Osler had a psychological wound from which his healing flowed.[28]

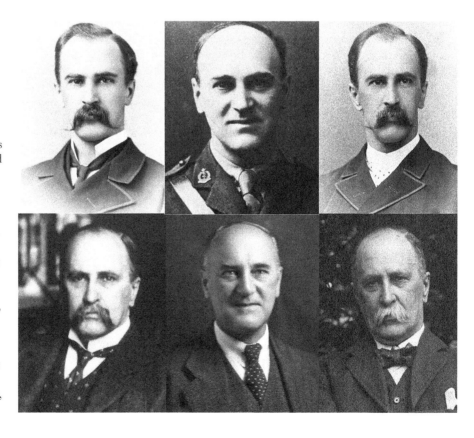

Figure 2. Photographs of Sir William Osler and W.W. Francis at various ages. Top row (left to right): Osler at age 32, Francis at age circa 34, and Osler at 35. Bottom row (left to right): Osler at age 56, Francis at age 60, and Osler at age 64. *Credits:* Osler Library of the History of Medicine, McGill University (all except bottom row, right); Alan Mason Chesney Archives of the Johns Hopkins Medical Institutions (bottom row, right).

There were rumors that Osler harbored a psychological wound, a deep sorrow, from an affair with an older first cousin, Marian Osler (Bath) Francis (1841–1915), that produced William Willoughby Francis (1879–1959), Marian's fifth son and the sixth of her nine children. Most but not all relatives of Osler and W.W. Francis have discounted the rumors, as did Michael Bliss: "I have read thousands and personal letters by, to, and about Osler, the Francises, and the rest of their family circle, and I cannot find the slightest hint than an affair took place between Marian and Willie. . . . Moreover, neither Bill Francis nor any of his sisters [there were also rumors that Osler fathered one or more of Marian Francis's daughters] resembled William Osler physically, intellectually, in work habits, or in strength of character."[5, pp. 394–396]

Bliss's judgment of W.W. Francis is unnecessarily harsh. Francis was highly intelligent, industrious, upright, and widely admired. Moreover, Francis bore at least some physical resemblances to Osler (Figure 2). A. Salusbury MacNalty (1880–1969), who knew them both, wrote that Francis "bore a close family resemblance to Sir William Osler in features, in dark eyes flashing with humour, in olive complexion, in stature and gesture."[29]

Evidence supporting the rumors Osler may have been W.W. Francis's father, not just his first cousin-once-removed and godfather, is reviewed in detail elsewhere[30] and includes the following:

- Romances between cousins were not uncommon during the Victorian era. William Osler's first romantic attachment was to a first cousin.
- There were ample opportunities for mating. In 1866 the recently widowed Marian Osler Bath spent several months in the Osler household, when William was 17, and it was rumored she introduced several Osler boys to sex. Osler during his second Montreal period (1874–1884) visited her household nearly every day and sometimes lived there. Marian's second husband, George Grant Francis, Jr., was out of town more often than not.
- In 1889 Osler began his courtship of the recently widowed Grace Revere Gross (1854–1928) with a trip to New Brunswick, where Grace was vacationing, and took with him 11-year-old Billy Francis. He apparently told Grace that Francis would always be a part of his household.[31]
- In 1895 Osler brought W.W. Francis to Baltimore where he lived most of the next eight years in the Osler household at 1West Francis Street while Osler financed his undergraduate and medical education at Johns Hopkins.
- On December 29, 1919, Francis was among the eight persons in Osler's bedroom when he died. On January 2, 1920, Francis was among the seven persons who attended the committal service for Osler at Golders Green Crematorium in London.
- Beginning in 1922, Francis devoted his life to preserving Osler's memory. He spent nearly six years organizing and cataloging Osler's books, during which time he caused Lady Osler great discomfit and frustration. He then became "the Keeper of the Shrine" at the Osler Library of the History of Medicine at McGill, where his ashes now reside in the same vault with those of Sir William and Lady Osler.

The most compelling evidence for Osler's paternity of W.W. Francis consists of provisions in Lady Osler's last will and testament, made out shortly before her death. Despite her troubles with Francis, she left him 5,000 pounds (equivalent to $416,927 in 2021 US dollars), her largest bequest to any individual. And she divided furniture that did not stay in Oxford between her own relatives and

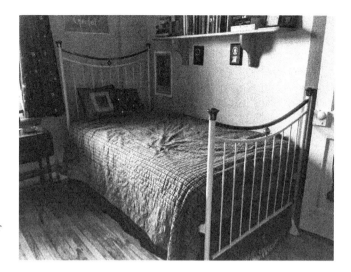

Figure 3. The bed in which Sir William Osler probably died. *Credit:* Wendy Kelen.

Francis (Wendy Kelen, personal communication, 2 June 2019) (Figure 3). Thus, although Lady Osler was closer to other young people, notably T. Archibald Malloch (1887–1953), who became a surrogate son, she apparently felt compelled to do as her late husband would have wanted her to do.

The truth will never be known barring a definitive DNA-based study. Should rumors that Osler fathered W.W. Francis be true, however, we might ask whether Osler represents a medical counterpart of the fictional Spanish priest described by Miguel de Unamuno (1864–1936) in *San Manuel Bueno, Mártir* (1931), who sublimates inability to believe in the divinity of Jesus through relentless service to his parishioners. Osler, like Unamuno's protagonist, was presumed to have taken as a motto, "Do the kind thing and do it first."[32] Edith Gittings Reid (1863–1954) described her friend William Osler in a way evocative of Unamuno's protagonist: "The deep, sad eyes of his soul watched a little cynically the light humor of his mind."[33]

In summary, we will never know for sure what Osler was really like—it is arguable whether we really know ourselves, after all—but we can safely conclude that few if any physicians have been so special to so many contemporaries, and that this largely reflected his vitality and his genuine interest in, and concern for, fellow humans.

What would Osler say to us were he alive today?

In 1949 Sir Robert Hutchison (1871–1960) predicted that "as members of our calling tend to become more and more merely expert technicians it is improbable that we shall look upon his [Osler's] like again in another century."[24] Proliferating technologies breed new specialties, cause balkanization, and make it almost inconceivable that anyone, even one with Osler's attributes, could "bestride the medical world like a Colossus" as he did. In 1999 the French medical historian Danielle Gourevitch predicted wide replacement of physicians by technicians and called Osler "the last *maître à penser* of a noble-minded general medicine."[34] Hence, the question, "What would Osler say to us were he alive today?"

Some would like to see a twenty-first-century Osler restore humanism to medical practice. Concerns during the 1960s that technology was eroding the humanistic dimension of medicine prompted a 1970 symposium on "Humanism in Medicine" that resulted in the American Osler Society.[35] Osler is often seen as an avatar for humanism and advocate for "the medical humanities." He is sometimes seen as the quintessential caring doctor, the author of such aphoristic advice as, "Care more particularly for the individual patient than for the special features of the disease."[36] However, if we define humanism as the promotion of human flourishing, it follows that appropriate and beneficent use of technology is as "humanistic" as "caring," which does not require a medical degree. Moreover, we should also note that Osler's posthumous reputation for caring was not based on a large and hectic clinical practice.

Others would like to see a twenty-first-century Osler restore power and prestige to the medical profession. Concerns during the 1980s that the twin forces of business and government were eroding the status of physicians as "professionals" spawned a burgeoning literature on "medical professionalism." Osler is sometimes seen as an avatar of "professionalism,"[37] a term he never used. However, "professionalism" presumes "a profession," and Osler's greatest gift to physicians was a sense of belonging to a noble, cohesive profession, which he sometimes conceptualized as an apostolic succession of cultured physicians dating back to Hippocrates. This image strikes us today as decidedly naïve.[38] Moreover, because science and technology progressively change the nature of medical practice, each generation of physicians must re-define what it means by "profession" and "medical professionalism."

Osler were he alive today would probably weigh in on how to balance empathic caring with technology, and he might say a word or two about "professionalism," but he would say a lot more about issues that far transcend medicine.

Osler's interests changed considerably after he left North America. During his Oxford period (1905–1919) he seldom gave inspirational addresses to medical students and physicians, the major exception being a 1907 address to students at St. Mary's Hospital in London.[39] Historians Elizabeth Fee and Theodore Brown make a compelling case that "in leaving behind his Hopkins commitment to the history of medicine as a tool for shaping the medical profession, Osler at Oxford turned toward a grander intellectual mission."[40] His book collecting prompted him to integrate the history of medicine into the broader history of science as evinced by the titles in his posthumously published *Bibliotheca Osleriana*.[41] The Great War prompted him to enter a debate over whether the sciences deserved more emphasis in British public schools and universities even at the expense of the humanities. These concerns coalesced in Osler's last public address, delivered on May 16, 1919, as president of the Classical Association on "The Old Humanities and the New Science."[26,42]

"The Old Humanities and the New Science" is usually read as a call for more interaction between liberal-arts faculty and science faculty, anticipating by forty years the 1959 Rede Lecture at Cambridge by C.P. Snow (1905–1980) on "The Two Cultures and the Scientific Revolution."[43] It is also cited as a paean to the Hippocratic maxim, "Where there is love of humanity (*philanthropia*), there also is love of the art (*philotechnia*)," eloquently restated in Osler's closing paragraph. However, Osler's major concern that day was the question of human survivability. Aspects of Osler's thoughts on human survivability include the question whether science will ultimately prove a source for good or evil; the relationship of the sciences to the humanities; and the need for a different model of civilization, which in today's terminology would be called globalization.

On the question whether science would ultimately prove a source for good or evil, Osler's thinking can be traced through sequential lectures, notably "The

Leaven of Science" (1894), "Man's Redemption of Man" (1910), and "Science and War" (1916). In "The Leaven of Science" he suggests that science benefits "the whole social fabric" and promotes reliance on reason rather than emotion (passion) in decision-making.[44] In "Man's Redemption of Man" he endorses medical science as a form of secular religion and concludes by quoting from "Queen Mab" by Percy Bysshe Shelley: "Happiness and Science dawn though late upon the earth; / Peace cheers the mind, health renovates the frame . . . "[45] In "Science and War," delivered as the Battle of Loos raged across the English Channel, he conveys a grim view of human nature:

> And some of us had indulged the fond hope that in the power man had gained over nature had arisen possibilities for intellectual and social development such as to control his morals and emotions, so that the nations would not learn war any more. We were foolish enough to think that where Christianity had failed Science might succeed, forgetting that the hopelessness of the failure of the Gospel lay not in the message, but in its interpretation . . . .[46]

Now, in "The Old Humanities and the New Science," Osler confesses: "Two years changed me into an ordinary barbarian. . . . it has yet to be determined whether Science, as the embodiment of a mechanical force, can rule without invoking ruin."

On the question of the relationship of the sciences and the humanities, Osler's thoughts reflect a debate among British educators. Science teachers justified demands for more time in the curriculum by the Great War's demonstration that Britain lagged behind Germany in science and technology. Classicists sought to defend their dominance—in 1919 only 51 of the 257 Heads and Fellows of the 23 colleges at Oxford were scientists, even including the mathematicians. Various stakeholders formed interest groups, held conferences, and drew up petitions. At the center of these activities was Osler's friend Sir Frederic Kenyon (Figure 4), who averred that the scientific method should pervade all branches of knowledge.

Osler was caught in the middle. Having been made president of the Classical Association on nomination by his friend Gilbert Murray (Figure 4), he fretted over what to say to the classicists without making enemies. In 1916, as president of the Association of Public School Science Masters, Osler had supported the science teachers' quest for more time in the curriculum. A peacemaker by nature, he inadvertently signed petitions both for and against compulsory Greek as a requirement for admission to Oxford. He substituted "The Old Humanities" for "The Old Humanism" in the title of his last address after reading a paper on "The Humanities" by his Oxford colleague P.S. Allen (Figure 4). Allen had reviewed the organization of knowledge through the centuries, pointed out that "humanism" and "the humanities" have many meanings, and called for revival of "the humanities" as an appropriate term for the classics.

In "The Old Humanities and the New Science," Osler asserts that "the humanities are the hormones" but that "all educated men" should stay abreast of developments in science. He calls for "recognition of a new philosophy—the *scientia scientiarum*," which we would now call the philosophy of science. He alludes to "the New Humanism" being developed by George Sarton (Figure 4), with whom he had corresponded. Sarton's ideas about the organization of knowledge, fully articulated after Osler's lifetime,[47] might be compared to that of a three-piece golf ball: The scientific method comprises the core around which all human activities are wound, but humanism makes up the scuff-resistant outer cover. Sarton pushed for "humanized science." He expressed confidence that "the New Humanism . . . will confirm the oneness of mankind."

On the question for a new model of civilization, Osler, perhaps embracing Sarton's ideas, asserts in this his last address: "Two things are clear: there must be a very different civilization or there will be no civilization at all; and the other is that neither the old religion combined with the old learning, nor both with the new science, suffice to save a nation bent on self-destruction." The latter statement reflects "the suicide of Germany" during the Great War, but the former statement reflects Osler's distrust of nationalism, which he had called in 1902 "the great curse of humanity."[48] He saw beneficent science, notably medical science, as offering "fuller hope for humanity than in any other direction."[49] Osler's remark that "there must be a very different civilization or there will be no civilization at all" is eerily redolent of a 1946 report entitled *One World or None* by scientists and opinion leaders in the wake of the atomic bomb.[50]

"The Old Humanities and the New Science" was well received. Lady Osler wrote her sister three months later, "there is reconstruction in every branch of Education & all people come for his [Osler's] opinion & advice."[51]

It seems reasonable to suggest that Osler if alive today would endorse the original definition of "bioethics" proposed in 1970 by Van Rensselaer Potter (1911–2001): a science of human survival integrating biology, ecology, medicine, and human values.[52] It seems reasonable to suggest he would frown on those who look askance at science when, for example, they deny human contributions to global warming.[53] It seems reasonable to suggest he would find a glimmer of hope in the recent writings of certain thought leaders. In 2018, for example, the Canadian American cognitive scientist Steven Pinker argued in *Enlightenment Now* that reason, science, and humanism acting in concert will result in human flourishing[54]—which was Osler's basic argument in "The Old Humanities and

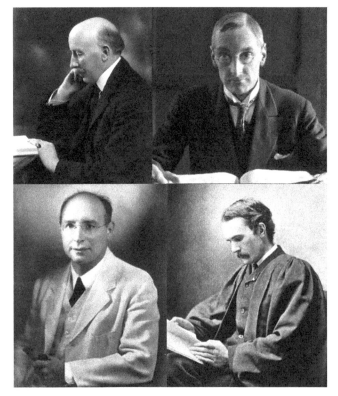

Figure 4. Younger contemporaries who influenced Sir William Osler during his last years through their interactions included (clockwise from upper left) Sir Frederic Kenyon (1863–1852), director of the British Museum; Percy Stafford Allen (1869–1933), a classicist at Oxford; Gilbert Murray (1866–1957), Regius Professor of Greek at Oxford; and George Sarton (1884–1956), a Belgian-born chemist and historian who is often considered "the father of the history of science."
Credits: National Portrait Gallery, London (upper row); Alamy Stock Photo (bottom row).

the New Science" and elsewhere. In 2019, the Spanish-born intellectual Felice Fernández-Armesto after reviewing the history of thought concluded that "sooner or later . . . we shall have only one worldwide culture."[55] Also in 2019, the Canadian social theorist Todd Dufresne after reviewing "the fiction of human exceptionalism" predicted that a global catastrophe will ere long create "a democracy of suffering" which will bring about the realization that we must act collectively if the species is to survive.[56]

Osler in the end was a "despairing optimist."[57] He liked to quote a statement by the Greek philosopher Prodicus that he had learned from the classicist Gilbert Murray: "That which benefits human life is God."[58,59]

References

1. Bryan CS, ed. *Sir William Osler: An Encyclopedia*. Novato, California: Norman Publishing/HistoryofScience.Com; 2020.
2. Bryan CS, Toodayan N. Osler studies enter second century. *Journal of Medical Biography* 2019; 27(4): 186–187.
3. Rourke S, Ellis G. The most influential physicians in history. [art 4: The top 10. https://www.medscape.com/features/slideshow/influential-physicians-part-4
4. Strauss MB, ed. *Familiar Medical Quotations*. Boston: Little, Brown and Company; 1968: 302.
5. Bliss M. *William Osler: A Life in Medicine*. New York: Oxford University Press; 1999: 496.
6. Madison DL Review of *Osler: Inspirations from a Great Physician*, by Charles S. Bryan. *New England Journal of Medicine* 1997; 337(18): 1324–1325.
7. Gladwell M. *Outliers: The Story of Success*. New York: Little, Brown and Company; 2008.
8. Osler W. The master-word in medicine. In: Osler W. *Aequanimitas, With other Addresses to Medical Students, Nurses and Practitioners of Medicine*. Third edition, Philadelphia: P. Blakiston's Son & Co., Inc.; 1932: 347–371.
9. Terman LM, Oden MH. *The Gifted Group at Mid-Life*. Stanford, California: Stanford University Press; 1959.
10. Gidney RD, Millar WPJ. *Professional Gentlemen: The Professions in Nineteenth-Century Ontario*. Toronto: University of Toronto Press; 1994: 377–378.
11. Wilkinson A. *Lions in the Way: A Discursive History of the Oslers*. Toronto: The Macmillan Company of Canada Limited; 1956.
12. Beeson JF. *John Wesley and the American Frontier*. Maitland, Florida: Xulon Press; 2007: 173.
13. Unsigned. *Records of the Lives of Ellen Free Pickton and Featherstone Lake Osler*. Oxford: Oxford University Press; 1915.
14. Unsigned. *The First Report of the Upper Canada Clergy Society for Sending out Clergymen, & C. to that Province with a Statement of the Design and Constitution of the Society*. London: G. Norman; 1838.
15. Unsigned. *The Second Report of the Upper Canada Clergy Society for Sending out Clergymen, & C. to that Province. . . .* London: G. Norman; 1839.
16. Fahey C. *The Anglican Experience in Upper Canada, 1791–1854*. Ottawa, Canada: Carleton University Press; 1991: 45–47.
17. Cushing H. *The Life of Sir William Osler*: Oxford: Clarendon Press; 1926; ii: 577–578.

18. Keith A. Osler and the medical museum. In [Abbott ME, ed.] *Bulletin No. IX of the International Association of Medical Museums and Journal of Technical Methods. Sir William Osler Memorial Number. Appreciations*; 1926; 5–6.

19. Lella JW. An archeology of two Oslerian dreams and a perspective on Sir William Osler's historical significance. In Barondess JA, Roland CG, eds. *Persisting Osler—III. Selected Transactions of the American Osler Society, 1991–2000.* Malabar, Florida: Krieger Publishing Company; 2002: 27–42.

20. Peterson C, Seligman ME. *Character Strengths and Virtues: A Handbook and Classification*: New York: Oxford University Press; 2004.

21. https://www.authentichappiness.sas.upenn.edu/user/login?destination= node/434. accessed March 14, 2020.

22. Bryan CS. Manage time well. Chapter 1 in Bryan CS. *Osler: Inspirations from a Great Physician.* New York: Oxford University Press; 1997: 3–30.

23. Weistrop L. *The Life & Letters of Dr. Henry Vining Ogden, 1857–1931.* Milwaukee: Milwaukee Academy of Medicine Press; 1986: 14.

24. Hutchison R. William Osler. *Quarterly Journal of Medicine* 1949; 18: 275–277.

25. Bosco RA. "He that best understands the world, least likes it": The dark side of Benjamin Franklin. *Pennsylvania Magazine of History and Biography* 1987; 111: 525–554.

26. Osler. The old humanities and the new science. *British Medical Journal* 1919; 2: 1–7.

27. Singer C. Osler: some personal reminiscences. *British Medical Journal* 1949; 2: 47–48.

28. Knight JA. William Osler's call to ministry and medicine. *Journal of Medical Humanities* 1986; 7: 4–17.

29. MacNalty AS. Obituary. W.W. Francis, A.B., M.D. (1878–1959). *Medical History* 1960; 4: 163–166.

30. Bryan CS, Wright JR. Sir William Osler (1849–1919) and the paternity of William Willoughby Francis (1878–1959): review of the evidence. *Journal of Medical Biography* 2019; 27(4): 229–241.

31. Harrell GT. Foreword. In Wagner FB. *The Twilight Years of Lady Osler: Letters of a Doctor's Wife.* Canton, MA: Science History Publications; 1985: xi–xiii.

32. Emerson CP. Reminiscences of Sir William Osler. In [Abbott ME, ed.] *Bulletin No. IX of the International Association of Medical Museums and Journal of Technical Methods. Sir William Osler Memorial Number.* Appreciations; 1926; 294–303.

33. Reid EG. *The Great Physician: A Short Life of Sir William Osler.* New York: Oxford University Press; 1931.

34. Gourevitch D. The history of medical teaching. *Lancet* 1999; 354 Supplement: SIV 33.

35. McGovern JP, Burns CR, eds. *Humanism in Medicine.* Springfield, Illinois: Charles C. Thomas; 1973.

36. Osler W. Address [to the students of the Albany Medical College, February 1, 1899]. *Albany Medical Annals* 1899; 20: 307–309.

37. Bryan CS. Medical professionalism in the new millennium: a neo-Oslerian perspective. In Byyny R, Paauw DS, Papadakis M, Pfiel S, ed. *Medical Professionalism: Best Practices.* Aurora, Colorado: Alpha Omega Alpha Honor Medical Society; 2017: 41–57.

38. Bryan CS, Podolsky SH. Sir William Osler (1849–1949)—The uses of history and the singular beneficence of medicine. *New England Journal of Medicine* 2019; 381(23): 2194–2196.

39. Osler W. The reserves of life. *St. Mary's Hospital Gazette* 1907; 13(November 6): 95–98.

40. Fee E, Brown TM. Using medical history to shape a profession: The ideals of William Osler and Henry E. Sigerist. In Huisman F, Warner JH, eds. *Locating Medical History: The Stories and Their Meanings.* Baltimore: The Johns Hopkins University Press; 2004: 139–164.

41. Osler W. *Bibliotheca Osleriana: A Catalogue of Books Illustrating the History of Medicine and Science Collected, Arranged, and Annotated by Sir William Osler, Bt., and bequeathed to McGill University.* Oxford: Clarendon Press; 1929.

42. Bryan CS. The centenary of 'The Old Humanities and the New Science,' the last public address of Sir William Osler (1849–1919). *Journal of Medical Biography* 2018; 27: 197–204.

43. Snow CP. *The Two Cultures and the Scientific Revolution.* New York: Cambridge University Press; 1959.

44. Osler W. The leaven of science. In Osler W. *Aequanimitas, With other Addresses to Medical Students, Nurses and Practitioners of Medicine.* Philadelphia: P. Blakiston's Son & Co., Inc.; 1932: 73–95.

45. Osler W. *Man's Redemption of Man. A Lay Sermon, McEwan Hall, Edinburgh, Sunday, July 2nd, 1910.* New York: Paul B. Hoeber; 1913.

46. Osler W. On science and war. *Lancet* 1915; 186: 795–801.

47. Sarton G. *The History of Science and the New Humanism.* Cambridge, Massachusetts: Harvard University Press; 1937 [1931].

48. Osler W. Chauvinism in medicine. In Osler W. *Aequanimitas, With other Addresses to Medical Students, Nurses and Practitioners of Medicine.* Philadelphia: P. Blakiston's Son & Co., Inc.; 1932: 263–289.

49. Osler W. Unity, peace and concord. In Osler W. *Aequanimitas, With other Addresses to Medical Students, Nurses and Practitioners of Medicine.* Philadelphia: P. Blakiston's Son & Co., Inc.; 1932: 425–443.

50. Masters D, Way K. *One World or None: A Report to the Public on the Full Meaning of the Atomic Bomb.* New York: McGraw-Hill Book Company, Inc.; 1946.

51. Grace Revere Osler to Susan Revere Chapin, circa 22 August 1919, Harvey Cushing fonds, 417/41.15, Osler Library of the History of Medicine, McGill University.

52. Potter V. Bioethics, the science of survival. *Perspectives in Biology and Medicine* 1970; 14(2): 127–152.

53. Alighieri D. Into a climate ever vexed with storms. *Inferno* 1320; 4: 147.

54. Pinker S. *Enlightenment Now: The Case for Reason, Science, Humanism, and Progress.* New York: Penguin Books Limited/Viking.

55. Fernández-Armesto F. *Out of Our Minds: What We Think and How We Came to Think It.* London: OneWorld Publications; 2019: 402.

56. Dufresne T. *The Democracy of Suffering: Life on the Edge of Catastrophe, Philosophy in the Anthropocene.* Montreal, Quebec, & Kingston, Ontario: McGill-Queen's University Press; 2019.

57. Dubos R. The despairing optimist. *The American Scholar* 1977; 46(1): 10–18.

58. Murray G. *The Rise of the Greek Epic. Being a Course of Lectures Delivered at Harvard University.* Second edition, Oxford: Clarendon Press; 1911: 2.

59. Osler W. *The Evolution of Modern Medicine. A Series of Lectures Delivered at Yale University on the Silliman Foundation in April, 1913.* New Haven: Yale University Press; 1921: 62.

✿ Index

Dent, Marmaduke H., 109
De Perac, Etienne, 220
Dercum, Francis Xavier, 201, 202
Diabetes mellitus, 227–228
Dick, Philip K., 227–228
Dock, George, 120
Doudna, Jennifer A., 183
Douglas, Sylvester (Lord Glenbervie), 125
Dozinghem Commonwealth War Cemetery, 158, 162–163
Drake, Joseph Morley, 307
Drummond, Lady Julia, 21
Duchess of Connaught Canadian Red Cross Hospital, Cliveden, 13–26
Duckworth, Sir Dyce, 186
Dufresne, Todd, 317
Dumas, Alexandre, 4
Dundas Grammar School, 51
Durant, Thomas M., xiii, 284

E
Early, Jubal A., 134
Eberth, Karl Joseph, 8
Eccles, John C., 239
Edward VII of England, 219
Ehrlich, Paul, 11, 230
Einstein, Albert, 74
Eisenbrey, Arthur Bradley, 158–161
Eliot, George, 296
Ellison, Harlan, 273
Emerson, Ralph Waldo, 307
Episcopal Theological School, 65
Erasmus, Desiderius, 71
Ewelme Almshouse, 91–97
Ewelme Church, 93–96
Exposition Universelle (World's Exposition), 3–6

F
Fallot, Étienne Louis Arthur, 168–178
Fallot, Tetralogy of, 167–175
Fairchild, Helen, 160
Farrar, Frederic William, 185
Fee, Elizabeth, 314
Fenwick, Samuel, 231
Féréol, Louis Henri Félix, 7
Fernández-Armesto, Felice, 317
Few, William Preston, 256
Finlay, Carlos, 265
Finney, John M.T., 160, 177–182
Fisher, Herbert, 126
Fleming, Alexander, 236
Fletcher, Charles Robert Leslie, 19

Flexner Report (1910), 254
Flint, Austin, 7, 40, 231, 308
Flower, Sir William, 125
Forbes, William S., 198
Fordyce, George, 124
Fowler, Orsen, 201
Fox, Charles James, 123
Fracastorius, Hieronymous, 119–120
Francis, George Grant, 151
Francis, Hilda Colley, 151, 153
Francis, Marian Grace. See Kelen, Marian Francis.
Francis, Marian Osler (Bath), 151, 312
Francis, William Willoughby, 48, 50–51, 55–56, 57, 88, 95, 141–153, 162, 311–313
Franklin, Benjamin, 195, 309, 311
Freud, Sigmund, 309
Friedenwald, Aaron, 178–179
Friedenwald, Harry, 184
Fuller, William Henry, 184
Fulton, John, 144
Fulton, Lucia, 144
Futcher, Thomas B., 186, 187, 245, 254

G
Gaisford, Thomas, 70
Gall, Franz Joseph, 201
Gardner, William, 230
Garrett, Mary Frick. See Jacobs, Mary Frick (Garrett).
Garrett, Robert, 172
    Robert Garrett Fund for Surgical Treatment of Children, 172
Garrison, Fielding H., 36, 106, 129, 133, 212
Garrod, Sir Alfred Baring, 184
Garrod, Alfred Henry, 185
Garrod, Alfred Noel, 188
Garrod, Sir Archibald Edward, 101, 183–191
Garrod, Basil Raheer, 188
Garrod, Dorothy Annie Elizabeth, 184, 188–189
Garrod, Elizabeth Ann Colchester, 185
Garrod, Henry Baring, 188
Garrod, Laura Smith, 186
Garrod, Thomas Martin, 188
Gee, Samuel Jones, 185
George III of England, 124
Germ theory of disease, 8
Gerster, Arpad, 116
Gibbon, Edward, 123
Gibson, William C., 239